Clinical Genetics and Genomics at a Glance

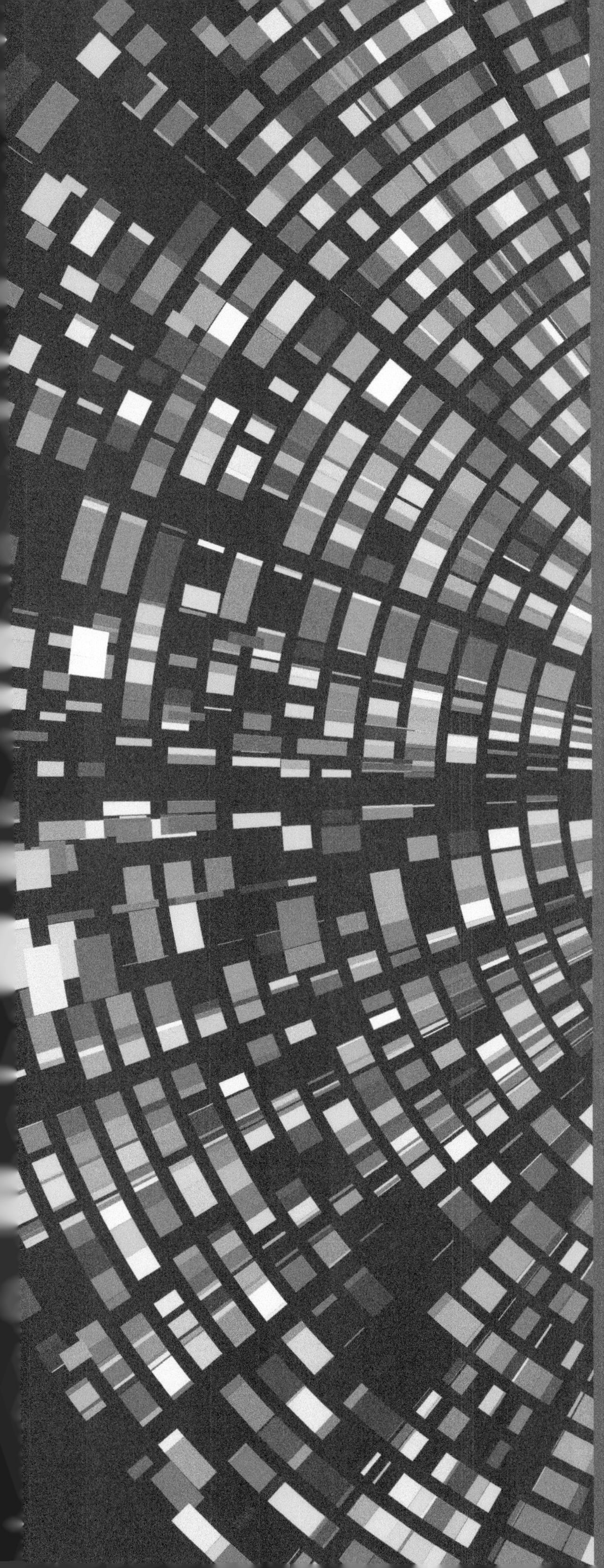

Clinical Genetics and Genomics at a Glance

Edited by

Neeta Lakhani

MBChB, BSc, MSc, MSt (Genomic Medicine), PG Cert, MRCPCH, Certificate in Medical Genetics
Specialty Registrar in Clinical Genetics
Department of Clinical Genetics, University Hospitals of Leicester NHS Trust, Leicester, UK

Kunal Kulkarni

BMBCh, MA (Oxon), MSc, FRCS (Tr&Orth), FEBHS, Dip Hand Surg (Br)
Consultant Trauma & Orthopaedic Surgeon
Department of Trauma & Orthopaedics, University Hospitals of Leicester NHS Trust, Leicester, UK

Julian Barwell

BSc, MBBS, PhD, FRCP (UK), AFHEA
Consultant in Clinical Genetics and Honorary Professor in Genomic Medicine
Department of Clinical Genetics, University Hospitals of Leicester NHS Trust, Leicester, UK

Pradeep Vasudevan

MBBS, FRCP, MRCPCH, DCH (London), MSc (Genomic Medicine)
Consultant in Clinical Genetics and Honorary Professor
Department of Clinical Genetics, University Hospitals of Leicester NHS Trust, Leicester, UK

Huw Dorkins

MA, MSc, MSt, FRCP, FRCPath, FHEA, FAcadMEd
Fellow and Senior Tutor in Medicine
St Peter's College, University of Oxford, Oxford, UK

WILEY Blackwell

This edition first published 2024

Registered Offices
John Wiley & Sons, Inc., 111 River Street, Hoboken, NJ 07030, USA
John Wiley & Sons Ltd, The Atrium, Southern Gate, Chichester, West Sussex, PO19 8SQ, UK

For details of our global editorial offices, customer services, and more information about Wiley products visit us at www.wiley.com.

Wiley also publishes its books in a variety of electronic formats and by print-on-demand. Some content that appears in standard print versions of this book may not be available in other formats.

Library of Congress Cataloging-in-Publication Data
Names: Lakhani, Neeta, editor. | Kulkarni, Kunal, editor. | Barwell, Julian, editor. | Vasudevan, Pradeep, editor. | Dorkins, Huw, editor.
Title: Clinical genetics and genomics at a glance / edited by Neeta Lakhani, Kunal Kulkarni, Julian Barwell, Pradeep Vasudevan, Huw Dorkins.
Other titles: At a glance series (Oxford, England)
Description: First edition. | Hoboken, NJ : Wiley-Blackwell, 2024. | Series: At a glance series | Includes bibliographical references and index.
Identifiers: LCCN 2023012124 (print) | LCCN 2023012125 (ebook) | ISBN 9781119240952 (paperback) | ISBN 9781119241034 (adobe pdf) | ISBN 9781119241027 (epub)
Subjects: MESH: Genetics, Medical–methods | Genomic Medicine–methods | Handbook
Classification: LCC RB155 (print) | LCC RB155 (ebook) | NLM QZ 39 | DDC 616/.042–dc23/eng/20230505
LC record available at https://lccn.loc.gov/2023012124
LC ebook record available at https://lccn.loc.gov/2023012125

Cover Design: Wiley
Cover Image: © Tartila/Shutterstock

Set in 9.5/11.5pt Minion by Straive, Pondicherry, India

SKY10052795_080923

Dedication

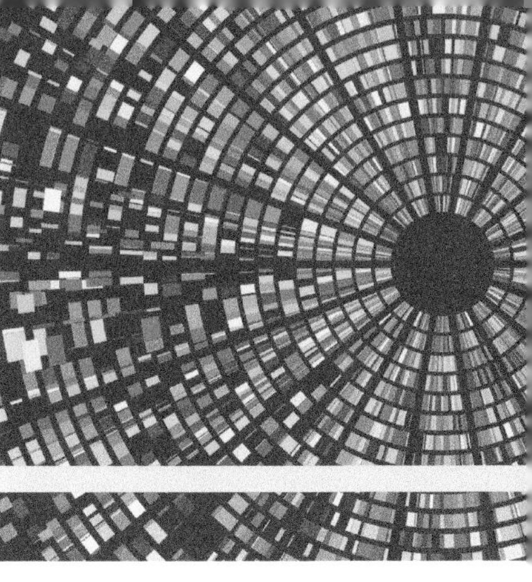

TTT TAG CGT TAA TCT GCT ATG ATT CGT TAA GCT AAT GAT TAA GCT AAT GCT ATT TAT GCT TAA GCT TCT TAA TTA ATT AAA GAA TAA ACT CAT GAA ATG TAA TGG GAA TAA ACT CAT TAG TGA GGT CAT ACT TAA ACT CAT ATT TCT TAA TGG GCT TCT TAA GCT TAA GGT TAG TAG GAT TAA ATT GAT GAA GCT TAA TAG GTT GAA CGT TAA GAT ATT AAT AAT GAA CGT TAA TAG AAT TGT GAA TAA CAT TAG TGG GAA GTT GAA CGT TAA ATT ACT TAA ACT TGA CGT AAT GAA GAT TAA ATT AAT ACT TAG TAA GCT TAA TTA TAG ACT TAA TAG TTT TAA CAT GCT CGT GAT TAA TGG TAG CGT AAA TAA TGG GAA TAA TGT TTA GAA GCT CGT TTA TAT TAA GAT ATT GAT TAA AAT TAG ACT TAA TTA GAA GCT CGT AAT TAA ATG TGA ATG TAA GCT AAT GAT TAA GAT GCT GAT TAA

Contents

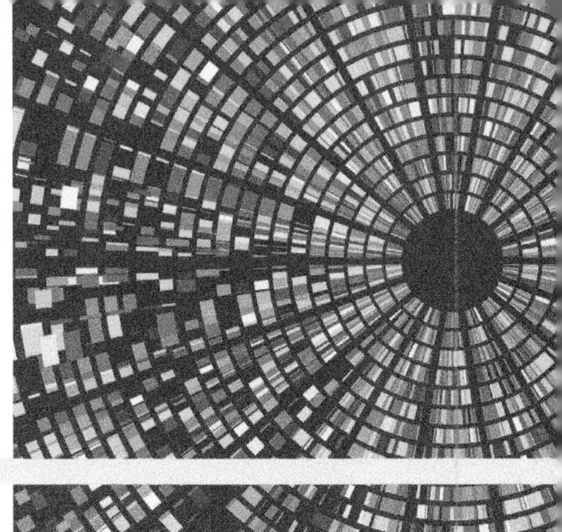

Part 5 Metabolic 71

Part 6 Gastroenterology 85

Part 7 Haematology 97

Part 8 Immunology 103

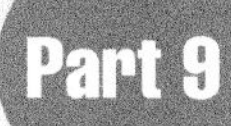

Part 9 Neurology 141

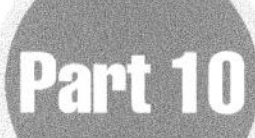

Part 10 Paediatrics and Obstetrics 157

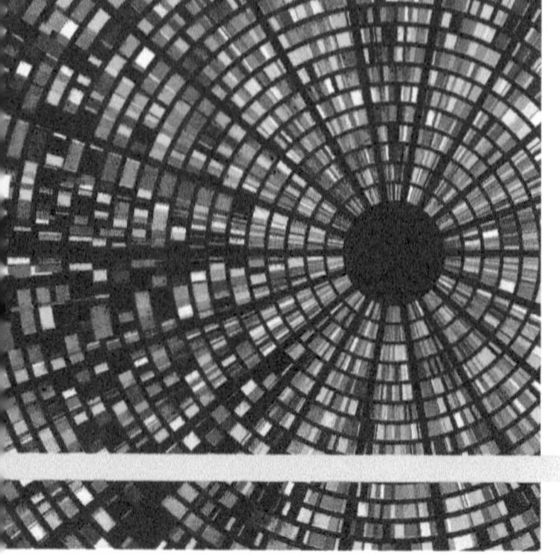

Contributors

Rebecca Allchin Department of Haematology, University Hospitals of Leicester NHS Trust, Leicester, UK

Aqua Asif Division of Surgery and Interventional Science, University College London, London, UK

Ashanti Sham Balakrishnan Department of Paediatrics & Neonatology, University Hospitals of Leicester NHS Trust, Leicester, UK

Micheal Browning Department of Immunology, University Hospitals of Leicester NHS Trust, Leicester, UK

Scott Castell Department of Emergency Medicine, Kettering General Hospital NHS Foundation Trust, Kettering, UK and Pre-hospital Emergency Medicine, The Air Ambulance Service, Northamptonshire, UK

Gemma Chandratillake East Genomic Laboratory Hub, Cambridge University Hospitals NHS Foundation Trust, Cambridge, UK

Emily Craft Department of Clinical Genetics, University Hospitals of Leicester NHS Trust, Leicester, UK

Maurice Dungey Department of Clinical Genetics, University Hospitals of Leicester NHS Trust, Leicester, UK College of Life Sciences, University of Leicester, Leicester, UK

Meghana Kulkarni Department of Urology, St George's University Hospitals NHS Foundation Trust, London, UK, Clinical Research Fellow - King's College London, London, UK

Gail Maconachie Division of Ophthalmology & Orthoptics, Health Sciences School, The University of Sheffield, Sheffield, UK

Karthick Manoharan Department of Cardiology, University Hospitals of Sussex NHS Trust, Brighton, UK

Titiksha Masand Department of Clinical Genetics, University Hospitals of Leicester NHS Trust, Leicester, UK

Jessica Myring Department of Clinical Genetics, University Hospitals of Leicester NHS Trust, Leicester, UK

Julian Omerod Oxford Heart Centre, John Radcliffe Hospital, Oxford University Hospitals NHS Foundation Trust, Oxford, UK

Manisha Panchal Department of Dermatology, University Hospitals of Leicester NHS Trust, Leicester, UK

Adithri Pradeep University of Sheffield Medical School, Sheffield, UK

Arthur Price Department of Immunology, University Hospitals of Leicester NHS Trust, Leicester, UK

Ataf Sabir Department of Clinical Genetics, Birmingham Women's and Children's NHS Foundation Trust and University of Birmingham, Birmingham, UK

Mervyn Thomas Ulverscroft Eye Unit, College of Life Sciences, University of Leicester, Leicester, UK

Zoe Venables Dermatology Department, Norfolk and Norwich University Hospital, Norwich, UK

Simon Wagner Department of Haematology, University Hospitals of Leicester NHS Trust, Leicester, UK

Foreword

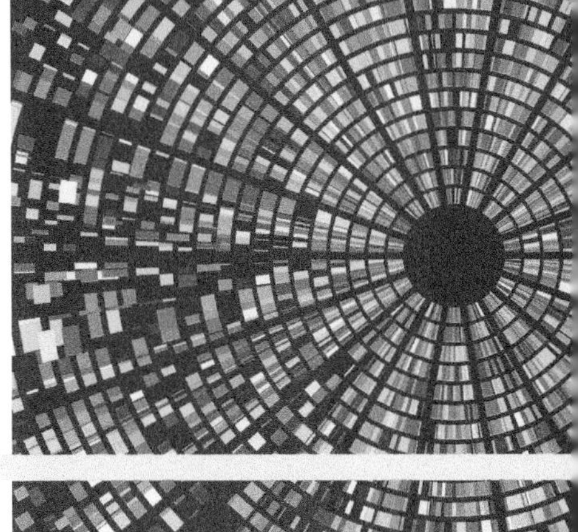

Genetics is coming in from the cold!

40 years ago, geneticists were specialists in a minority discipline, mainly involved in genetic diagnosis, testing, and counselling for relatively rare single gene or chromosomal disorders. Over recent years, we have become increasingly aware that there is a genetic component to all diseases, varying from a minor susceptibility to a very major component. Many diseases are multifactorial, with a variable genetic component. Genetic factors are involved in many aspects of disease susceptibility, including our ability to resist infections, and our susceptibility to certain cancers, so an understanding of genetics has become a necessary part of all aspects of medicine. This means that clinicians of all specialities need to know about inheritance and have a good working knowledge of the conditions in their specialty with a strong genetic component to their aetiology. A knowledge of the genetic aetiology of diseases can no longer be considered the sole domain of the geneticist but should be understood by all clinicians.

This novel book addresses this, by providing easily understood information about single gene disorders with the aim of empowering clinicians from all disciplines to understand and manage genetic disease and appreciate the impact of genomic medicine on clinical practice. The range of this book is wide, encompassing both, the more general specialities, and numerous subspecialties. Each topic is illustrated with key facts alongside informative and helpful diagrams for quick reference. It is an important and accessible reference for clinicians at all levels.

Professor Shirley Hodgson

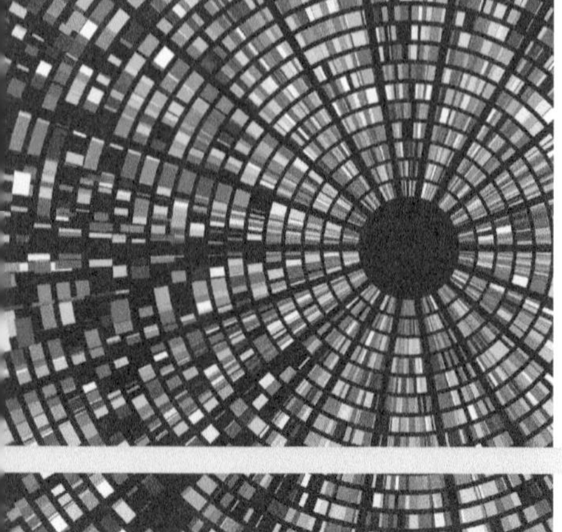

Preface

Welcome to Clinical Genetics and Genomics at a Glance!

This novel textbook provides concise and accessible information that will be useful to clinicians managing patients with potentially inherited disease with a Mendelian component, within a framework that incorporates the wider psychosocial experience of the individual and their concerns, and which may include reproductive advice or cascading of risk information to relatives.

This is particularly important as molecular testing through targeted tests, gene panels, or whole genome sequencing becomes more widely available through standardised care pathways. More extensive genetic testing increases the likelihood that gene variants of uncertain clinical significance or incidental genetic findings will be identified. For this reason, thorough pre-test consent and careful variant interpretation processes are key.

Within these pages we aim to summarise a range of common presentations and challenges patients face, arranged by different body systems, providing a succinct and digestible introduction to clinical management. We have consciously employed language that is used with patients in everyday practice, for example the term *gene* or *chromosome alteration*, rather than *mutation*, given the potentially negative connotations of the latter.

This book has been a labour of love of many different healthcare professionals from clinical genetics and beyond. We are indebted to numerous other specialists – including (but not limited to!) the orthopaedic surgeons, ophthalmologists, paediatricians, obstetricians, immunologists, dermatologists, cardiologists, neurologists, nephrologists, urologists, endocrinologists, gastroenterologists, and haematologists – who have all kindly contributed. This demonstrates the breadth of the coalition of clinicians establishing a genomic medicine-empowered service throughout the United Kingdom.

As genetics becomes increasingly embedded in the various clinical subspecialties, and as medical decision making becomes more dependent on integrated data science and computer-generated risk calculations, we hope that this book will provide a useful introduction to genetic aspects of individualised patient care. We trust that you find this book of value, and we would welcome your feedback to help shape future editions.

Neeta Lakhani, Kunal Kulkarni, Julian Barwell,
Pradeep Vasudevan, and Huw Dorkins

Introduction

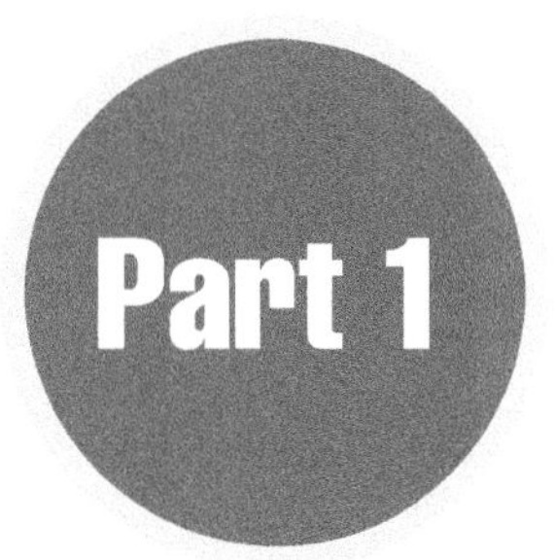

Part 1

Chapters

1 What is clinical genetics and genomic medicine?

What is clinical genetics?

Clinical Genetics involves the identification of individuals with, or at risk of, single gene inherited traits that could impact their health, alongside that of their relatives. Clinical geneticists are clinical doctors who diagnose and manage families with genetic disorders.

Their role encompasses coordinating the overall care of patients with rare disorders, diagnostics/genetic testing, and counselling regarding risk assessment (for example, with future pregnancies and for other potentially affected family members).

Geneticists work closely with their laboratory-based colleagues and genetic counsellors to perform and interpret the wealth of evolving molecular diagnostic tests in the clinical context.

Examples of conditions managed by clinical geneticists include:

- Chromosomal abnormalities
- Congenital (birth) defects with an underlying genetic basis
- Single gene disorders (for example, cystic fibrosis, muscular dystrophy, and Huntington's disease)
- Familial cancer and cancer-risk syndromes (for example, inherited breast or colorectal cancers; neurofibromatosis)
- Other inherited conditions that cause morbidity/mortality (for example, cardiac conditions at risk of causing sudden cardiac death)
- Developmental delay or learning difficulties in children (with other associated features suggestive of an underlying genetic aetiology)

How does clinical genetic testing help clinical care?

Clinical genetics is underpinned by making a correct clinical and molecular diagnosis. Rare diseases with Mendelian (single disease) traits affect 1 in 17 of the population, and 1/2 of the population are likely to develop cancer at some point in their lifetime caused by acquired pathogenic variants deregulating cell growth, differentiation, and cell death.

A highly suggestive medical diagnosis can be made by bringing together a series of symptoms and signs within either an individual patient, or by combining information from several relatives. For example, this could include linking bilateral vestibular schwannomas and a meningioma in a patient under 40 years of age with a diagnosis of neurofibromatosis type 2, or considering a pituitary adenoma with concurrent hyperparathyroidism in a proband with a story of her mother having had kidney stones and a pancreatic tumour being highly suggestive of Multiple Endocrine Neoplasia type 1. Genetic testing can then be used to either confirm this medical diagnosis or assist with family planning in the future. As testing costs fall and genetic and genomic testing becomes more readily accessible, molecular tests are increasingly being used to either make or further inform the suspected medical diagnosis. Improving the ability of clinicians to make a correct diagnosis leads to a better understanding of the natural history of the condition, thereby providing scope for potential interventions to reduce the burden of disease at an earlier stage.

Having the correct molecular diagnosis allows us to compare the patient to others in the medical literature to determine the inheritance pattern of the condition. When extensive case series have been studied, the penetrance of the condition can also be estimated. Note that this is not always assessed from probands (the first affected patient in the family that presents clinically), as sometimes these patients, by definition, tend to be more severely affected to be offered a test and hence may produce biased results when calculating future risk for relatives.

Pedigrees

Identifying familial risk is carried out by drawing a family tree (pedigree), which shows who is present in the family and their basic demographics in a pictorial form. Men are generally placed on the left and depicted as squares and women as circles. The consultant (the person seeking medical advice) has an arrow pointing towards the symbol and the symbol is shaded to represent if a patient is affected.

Apart from ascertaining who is at risk, the pedigree might indicate an inheritance pattern. As clinical geneticists work with family files, care must be taken in showing individuals the data collected from other relatives (such as including medical and molecular information on pedigrees) if consent has not been obtained to share.

Variant interpretation and the role of the clinical geneticist

Variant interpretation is an increasingly important component of a clinical geneticist's role, particularly as genetic testing and genomic sequencing becomes more widespread and it becomes clear that we all have multiple subtle variants that may impact on risk. This requires significant resource due to the sheer size of the human genome. Molecular biology expertise and framing within a clinical context is crucial in being able to explain risk effectively to patients, and this is an area where general physicians often struggle.

Classically, clinical geneticists have been highly effective in bringing together cohorts of patients for either research, governance, or shared experience. This has helped our understanding of the natural history of disorders and improved our ability to improve outcomes through large clinical research networks and patient support groups. Improved digital connectivity is making this more straightforward and effective.

Developing and championing a molecular culture within the wider NHS and public health is a key leadership role for geneticists. There are several competing acute medical and social care strains on our economy, and genetics has a potential role in improving some of this burden through targeted screening and prevention strategies, personalised medicine, and links to digital health. This involves education and training around molecular biology, innovation, and being early adopters of initiatives such as gene panels, genomic testing, and precision medicine. As artificial intelligence leads to improved integrated molecular, clinical, and social data sets, our ability to predict, prevent, and treat disease will improve. Clinical genetics therefore has a major role in Public Health, assisting with variant data collection and integrating this with health outcomes, as we generate an equation for life and well-being.

Clinical Genetics and Genomics at a Glance, First Edition. Edited by Neeta Lakhani, Kunal Kulkarni, Julian Barwell, Pradeep Vasudevan, and Huw Dorkins.

What is the impact of genetics on insurance and migration?

These are common areas of concern for patients undergoing diagnostic or predictive testing. Health insurance coverage can be a significant concern, particularly in countries with primarily private medical cover-based systems. Patients are therefore advised to investigate any specific policy exclusions, especially if planning to live or spend considerable periods of time overseas. Fortunately in the United Kingdom, this issue does not impact receipt of NHS care.

Unselected population-based genetic testing in the private sector for well individuals can create funding and capacity challenges, for example, when it comes to confirming any significant findings in a NHS accredited laboratory, which is required to act on any findings and arrange either screening or preventative measures.

Insurance companies in the United Kingdom are currently able to ask about family history or on-going investigations and screening. They can also currently ask about large amounts of cover for patients at risk of Huntington's (an autosomal dominant inherited condition with high penetrance), but not regarding other conditions. This is regularly reviewed with government oversight. The results from the 100 000-genome project are also exempt (but not any downstreamed medical investigations). It is currently unclear as to whether this advice is likely to change. Given the potential for genetics to target screening and healthcare to those most likely to benefit, it is hoped that policies would seek to maintain the current position with insurance companies to not impact the benefits of appropriate genetic screening on patient care.

What is genomic medicine?

There is no single agreed term that encompasses Genomic Medicine, but it can be broadly classified into three areas: personalised medicine, holistic and integrated care modelling, and integrated data science for the wider population. Each of these complement Clinical Genetics and whole genome sequencing to improve future health and disease modelling.

- In personalised medicine, additional nucleic acid-derived data from the closer analysis of a broader spectrum of genes, intronic coding regions, or single nucleotide polymorphisms are used in conjunction with tumour or microbial genetics and circulating biomarkers to try and personalise care. This includes tumour-specific therapies, pharmacokinetics, detection of potential antimicrobial resistance, and identification and monitoring of infectious agent outbreaks.
- In integrated and holistic care modelling, the aim is to work with patients and patient stakeholder groups to develop and design equitable access to patient-centred healthcare, building on patient involvement and empowerment to make informed decisions about their screening, management, and treatment in partnership with their doctors. This may involve the use of electronic care plans with access to additional support and red flag escalation alert systems for potential predictable complications and educational resources for clinicians and patients.
- The use of patient-centred and controlled electronic records provides opportunities to link health records to outcomes for artificial intelligence-based solutions. These models will be simple to start with, but in time, uploading data (such as our postcode, wearable technology-derived data, social media entries, supermarket store card and online purchase history, mental health questionnaires, alongside pathology, radiology, and genomic results) could provide a more accurate assessment of our health and well-being.

Genomic medicine involves integrating the results of nucleic acid-derived testing from blood and other biologically derived tissues with clinical and potentially social data. This aims to help predict future health outcomes more accurately via either the development of personalised treatments (intervention type and preferred dose of therapeutic agent if required) or through the design of more individualised and cost-effective screening programmes. These aim to treat disease for what it is rather than what it looks like, by planning screening based on calculated risk and not age, alongside smart prescribing to treat the right patient with the right drug at the right dose, first time, every time.

What does genomic medicine encompass?

Genomic medicine includes six areas beyond the analysis of the coding sequences of genes responsible for Mendelian traits (i.e. classical human genetics):

1 The role of single nucleotide polymorphisms (SNPs) in non-coding regions and epigenetic traits. Large genome wide association studies (GWAS) have identified many variants that are commonly found in the general population that are associated with risk. It is sometimes unclear if these have a cumulative effect when coupled with other variants or how they alter risk (through either altering gene expression from a distance), particularly when common in a population and inherited in close proximity (linked) to a true disease-causing variant that is yet to be identified (variant in linkage disequilibrium with the disease-causing variant).

2 Pharmacogenetics involves predicting the way that drugs are metabolised (and therefore the risk of side effects or lack of effectiveness) by identifying key variants in genes coding the relevant enzymes involved in their breakdown.

3 Testing other microorganisms can be helpful in identifying pathogens and predicting antibiotic or antiviral treatment resistance, as well as providing information about bacteria in the gut flora (microbiome) that is important for digestion. This could, for example, help possibly link food intake with the risk of obesity.

4 Testing other tissues for somatic mutations in either DNA or RNA can be particularly useful to identify circulating free DNA (cfDNA) released from tumours and predict either response to treatment or likelihood of relapse.

5 The use of other data sets, such as electronic patient records with linked radiology and pathology results, biometric data from smart handheld devices (e.g. fitbits) and background social data such as occupation, educational background, post code, supermarket store card/online purchases, and even social media interests, has the potential to be integrated with genomic results. Linking these large applied data sets to long-term health outcomes with machine learning algorithms will provide the opportunity to generate better predictors for disease and health and social well-being, thereby improving future health predictions.

6 Studying how gene expression can be altered by non-sequence variant changes, such as epigenetic changes in methylation patterns of promoters or DNA folding around modified histones, reducing planned transcription.

In a way, Clinical Genetics helps explain where – from an evolutionary perspective – we have come from and may possibly describe why we become unwell. Genomic Medicine tries to understand the more complex aspects of disease within an individual's broader genetic and environmental landscape, to make better future predictions about specific interventions.

2 Inheritance

Inheritance of characteristics and disorders may be chromosomal (due to aneuploidies, for example in Down syndrome), single-gene (also called Mendelian, named after Gregor Mendel), or multifactorial (multiple genes and environmental factors playing a role). In this chapter, we will consider the most common patterns of single-gene inheritances, with some examples of disorders more commonly encountered in clinical practice.

A gene located on chromosomes 1–22 is termed an *autosomal* gene; one on a sex chromosome (X or Y) is termed a *X- or Y-linked* gene, respectively. It is important to note that a particular condition is not dominant or recessive in itself, rather its inheritance is what may exhibit one of these Mendelian patterns.

Autosomal dominant (AD)

In autosomal dominant (AD) inheritance, only one copy of the pathogenic allele (alternate form of the same gene) needs to be inherited to cause the disorder (i.e. from a heterozygous parent).

The altered copy of the gene ('pathogenic' or 'mutant' allele) is dominant over the normal or 'wild-type' allele, causing the condition. When an affected individual has children (assuming the other parent is not affected), there is a 1 in 2 (i.e. 50%) chance that each child (son or daughter equally at risk in each pregnancy) will inherit the pathogenic gene alteration and therefore be affected with the condition (or unaffected if the child inherits the normal or wild-type allele) (Figure 2.1).

Examples of conditions with AD inheritance:

- Achondroplasia
- Autosomal dominant polycystic kidney disease
- Hereditary breast and bowel cancer
- Huntington's disease
- Hypertrophic cardiomyopathy
- Marfan syndrome
- Myotonic dystrophy
- Neurofibromatosis type 1 and 2
- Osteogenesis imperfecta
- Retinoblastoma

Figure 2.1 Autosomal dominant inheritance.

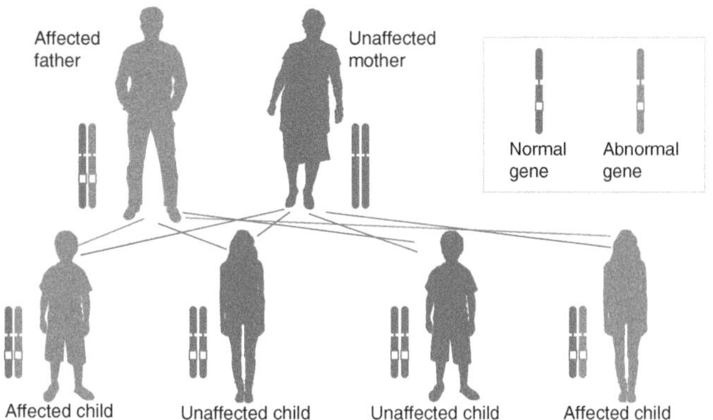

Variable expression and penetrance

These are features of this pattern of inheritance. *Expression* refers to the degree of severity of the disease, which may vary from individual to individual within the same family (e.g. in Neurofibromatosis type 1, there is variable expressivity between and within families).

Penetrance refers to the proportion of individuals expressing the condition to any degree (for e.g. Huntington disease, where there is age-dependent penetrance).

Anticipation

This refers to an increasing severity of the condition and earlier age of onset in successive generations. This occurs due to the expansion of tri-nucleotide repeat alterations (like 'CAG repeats' in Huntington disease or 'CTG repeats' in Myotonic dystrophy). Anticipation may also occur in conditions that follow X-linked inheritance, such as Fragile-X-syndrome ('CGG repeats').

Germline or gonadal mosaicism

This is when a new pathogenic gene alteration arises in some cells in the gonads (testis or ovary) and may not cause any phenotype in the parent, but can be passed on to their offspring.

Autosomal recessive (AR)

Autosomal recessive (AR) inheritance occurs when two copies of the defective gene are required for an individual to inherit a particular disease (i.e. the parent is homozygous or compound-heterozygous). Individuals that only have one copy of this allele are known as carriers. If both the parents are carriers of this 'abnormal' gene, the probability of the child being affected is 25% or a 1 in 4 chance.

Conditions following AR inheritance are more common in children of consanguineous relationships. Consanguinity is defined as a relationship between individuals who are previously related in the family by descent from a common ancestor, such as a cousin. This is because previously related parents (other than by marriage) are more likely to carry the same rare altered allele than unrelated individuals in the population (Figure 2.2).

Figure 2.2 Autosomal recessive inheritance.

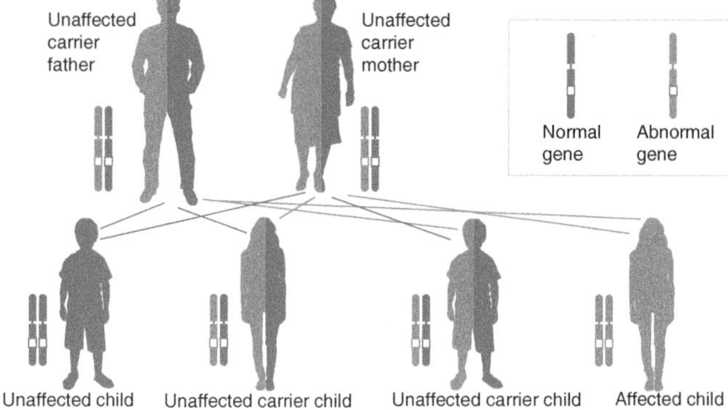

Clinical Genetics and Genomics at a Glance, First Edition. Edited by Neeta Lakhani, Kunal Kulkarni, Julian Barwell, Pradeep Vasudevan, and Huw Dorkins.

Examples of conditions with AR inheritance:

- Congenital adrenal hyperplasia (CAH)
- Cystic fibrosis (CF)
- Haemochromatosis
- Oculocutaneous albinism
- Phenylketonuria (PKU)
- Sickle cell anaemia/disease
- Spinal muscular atrophy (SMA)
- Thalassemia (alpha and beta)

X-linked recessive (XLR)

This inheritance pattern only concerns the genes on the X chromosome. These disorders are usually passed on from mother to son, and are more likely to affect males as opposed to females. This is because males only possess one copy of the X chromosome; therefore, if this contains a pathogenic gene alteration, a male individual would be affected by the condition (hemizygous). Females have two copies of the X chromosome and are generally unaffected (known as carriers); however, this is not always true. For example, in some disorders (such as like Duchenne Muscular dystrophy and Fragile-X-syndrome), some females who are carriers are also affected (albeit usually more mildly than males). Females tend to be carriers of the gene and have a 50% or 1 in 2 chance of passing the gene alteration to their sons (affected) or daughters (carrier). If an affected father goes onto have children, all of his daughters would be carriers, and all sons would be unaffected as male to male transmission cannot occur (as male parents do not pass on an X chromosome to their male offspring) (Figure 2.3).

Examples of conditions with XLR inheritance:

- Androgen insensitivity syndrome
- Becker and Duchenne muscular dystrophy
- Glucose-6-phosphate dehydrogenase deficiency
- Haemophilia (A and B)
- Hunter syndrome
- Fragile-X-syndrome
- Red-green colour blindness

Figure 2.3 X-linked recessive inheritance.

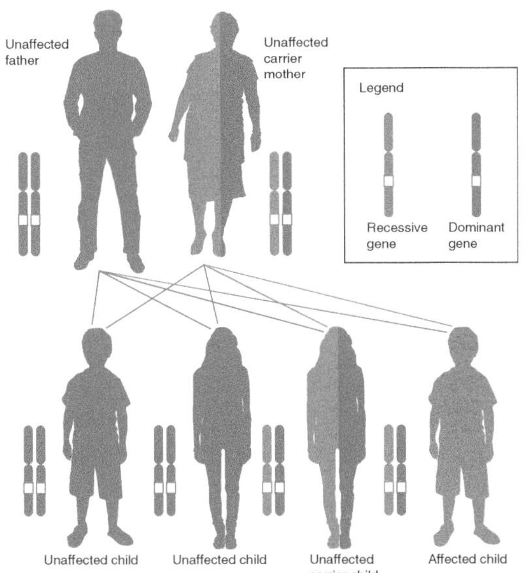

X-Chromosome inactivation

Also termed 'Lyonisation' (after Mary Lyon who first described it) is a process by which one X chromosome is inactivated (transcriptional silencing) in every cell in a developing female embryo 1–2 weeks after conception. This is to maintain dosage compensation of X-linked genes in females. Dosage compensation is required to achieve equilibrium in the expression of genes in females as they have two copies of the X chromosome. This is achieved by the *XIST* gene in the long arm of X-chromosome, which inactivates most of X chromosome except for a small part of its short arm (the pseudo-autosomal region). The process of X-inactivation is random, whereby approximately 50% of the maternal or paternal X chromosome is inactive in a female. Occasionally, the 50 : 50 ratio is skewed, a phenomenon known as skewed X-inactivation (80 : 20 or 90 : 10) and could lead on to manifesting carrier females.

Germline mosaicism (gonadal mosaicism)

As explained in the 'AD inheritance' section, this has been described in many X-linked recessive (XLR) disorders such as Becker and Duchenne muscular dystrophy.

X-linked dominant (XLD)

X-linked dominant (XLD) inheritance is caused by an alteration of a gene on the X chromosome, affecting heterozygous females. Both males and females are affected (very severe/lethal in males and less severe in females). There is a 1 in 2 or 50% chance that each son or daughter is affected when the source of transmission is an affected mother. The main difference from XLR inheritance is that the condition is expressed in heterozygous females (as opposed to being carriers), and some disorders in hemizygous males are lethal (Figure 2.4).

Examples of conditions with XLD inheritance:

- Incontinenta Pigmenti
- Oral-facial-digital syndrome type 1
- Rett syndrome
- Vitamin D-resistant rickets

Figure 2.4 X-linked dominant inheritance.

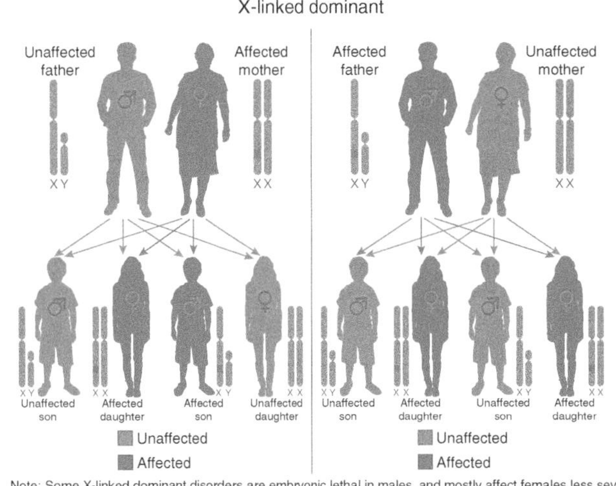

Y-chromosome inheritance

There are only a very small number of genes on the Y chromosome, and the function of these is mainly related to the maintenance of spermatogenesis. These include *SRY* and *DAZ* genes. The Y-chromosome abnormality is transmitted to all sons and no daughters through an affected father ('Holandric' inheritance).

Mitochondrial

Mitochondria are always inherited maternally, because during fertilisation only the sperm nucleus is used to form the zygote and almost all the mitochondria come from the egg cell. Mitochondrial DNA or mtDNA is quite different to nuclear DNA, being smaller, circular, and containing 37 genes. These genes are vital for the normal functioning and maintenance of the structure of mitochondria, and exhibit maternal inheritance in their transmission of disorders. *Heteroplasmy* is defined as a mixture of both normal (wild type) and altered mitochondrial genomes; therefore, the proportion of altered mtDNA must exceed a certain critical threshold level before an abnormality of the mitochondrial respiratory chain is expressed as a disorder in an affected individual. There is wide variability in clinical features depending on the percentage of altered mtDNA among individuals in a family, and also among organs and tissues in an individual.

Mitochondrial disorders could be caused by alterations in either the nuclear or mitochondrial genome. If nuclear, the inheritance could be AD, AR, or X-linked. If the alteration is in the mitochondrial genome, the inheritance is maternal and both sons and daughters could be affected with variable clinical features depending on the degree of heteroplasmy.

Examples of conditions with Mitochondrial inheritance:

- Kearns-Sayre syndrome
- Leber's hereditary optic neuropathy
- Leigh syndrome
- MELAS (mitochondrial encephalomyopathy with lactic acidosis and stroke-like episodes)
- MERRF (myoclonic epilepsy with ragged-red fibres)
- NARP (neurogenic weakness with ataxia and retinitis pigmentosa)

Imprinting and uniparental disomy

Genomic imprinting is a process by which a small number of genes are selectively expressed according to the parent of origin. Therefore, inheritance of both maternal and paternal copies ('imprinted genes') is required for normal growth and development. It is possible that disorders occur due to alterations in imprinted genes.

This can also result from *uniparental disomy* when both copies of the genes (chromosomes) are inherited from one parent and no copy from the other parent. Well-known examples of this phenomenon are Angelman syndrome (AS) and Prader–Willi syndrome (PWS), involving imprinted genes in the PWS/AS critical region on chromosome 15q11-13. AS and PWS are caused by loss of maternally and paternally inherited genes, respectively.

3 Cytogenetics and molecular genetic techniques

Cytogenetics and molecular genetics are two branches of genetics that focus on different characteristics of chromosomes. Cytogenetics studies diseases caused by either an abnormal number or structure of chromosomes. Molecular genetics studies hereditary, genetic variation, and alterations through chromosomes and gene expression.

Cytogenetics

Cytogenetics is a branch of pathology and genetics concerned with the study of normal chromosomes and chromosome aberrations. There are two broad subtypes of cytogenetics:

- **Classical cytogenetics** allows microscopic visualisation of whole chromosomes to assess their number and structure.
- **Molecular cytogenetics** uses specialised techniques such as fluorescence in situ hybridisation (FISH) and array comparative genomic hybridisation (aCGH) to evaluate submicroscopic chromosomal regions.

Both classical and molecular cytogenetic techniques are used to investigate congenital (i.e. present from birth) or acquired (e.g. cancer) changes in our genetic information. Cytogenetic study of chromosomes uses multiple techniques:

- **Banding:** The chromosome is stained with a dye, which gives a pattern of light and dark regions across the chromosome. These patterns can be read and identified. There are many forms of banding, but G-banding or Giemsa banding is the most used technique for the routine analysis of human chromosomes. The molecular mechanism and reason for these patterns remain unknown (Figure 3.1).
- **Karyotyping:** Analysis of the chromosome structure in the metaphase stage of cell division. For karyotying, the chromosomes are banded by using Giemsa and analysed under a microscope. Generally, 30 cells are reviewed to establish a sample representative of cell count (Figure 3.2).

Figure 3.1 G-banding (taken from https://onlinelibrary.wiley.com/doi/full/10.1038/npg.els.0001444).

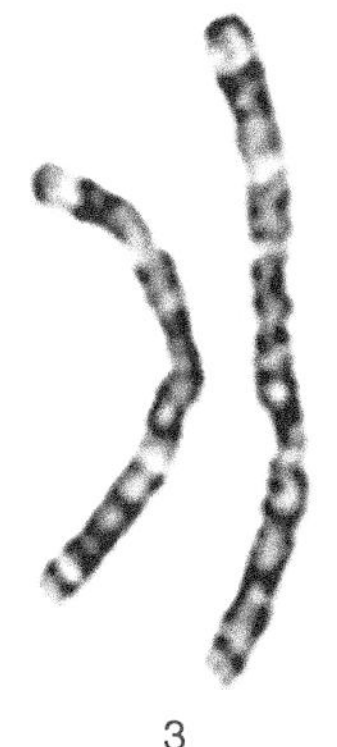

Figure 3.2 Karyotyping (taken from https://onlinelibrary.wiley.com/doi/full/10.1038/npg.els.0001444).

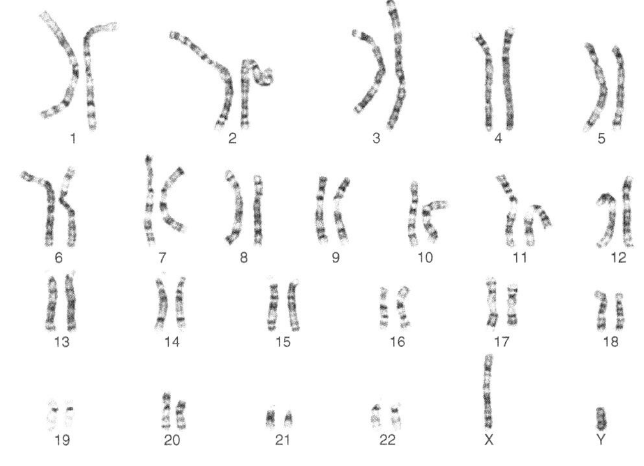

Figure 3.3 FISH - demonstrating the use of fluorescent probes to highlight specific nucleic acid sequences.

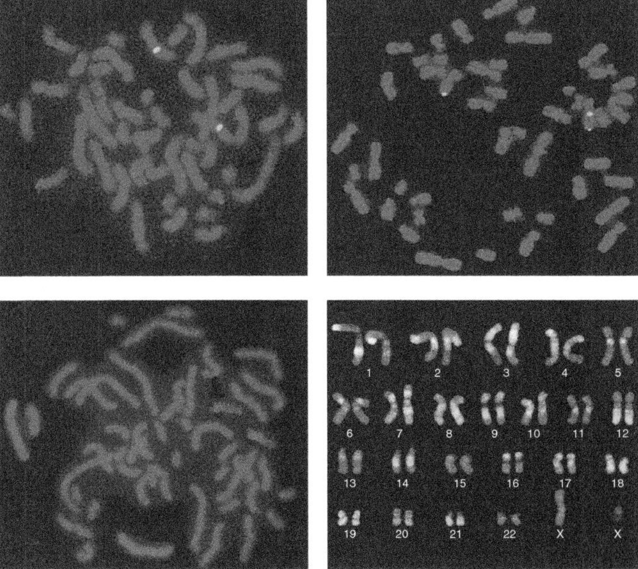

- **Fluorescent in situ hybridisation (FISH):** Allows chromosomes to be visualised using a fluorescent-labelled probe. The use of a probe that is labelled to a specific nucleic acid sequence allows that probe to be identified with the use of fluorescence. This technique allows for rapid identification of specific regions or volume (Figure 3.3).
- **Comparative genomic hybridisation:** Detects chromosomal copy number changes (chromosomal gains and losses) throughout the whole genome. If applied to the whole genome simultaneously in a method akin to multiple FISH analysis, a genomic overview on genetic volume can be conducted – 'array-CGH' (Figure 3.4).

Clinical Genetics and Genomics at a Glance, First Edition. Edited by Neeta Lakhani, Kunal Kulkarni, Julian Barwell, Pradeep Vasudevan, and Huw Dorkins.

Figure 3.4 Comparative genomic hybridisation (taken from https://onlinelibrary.wiley.com/doi/10.1111/j.1399-0004.2004.00322.x).

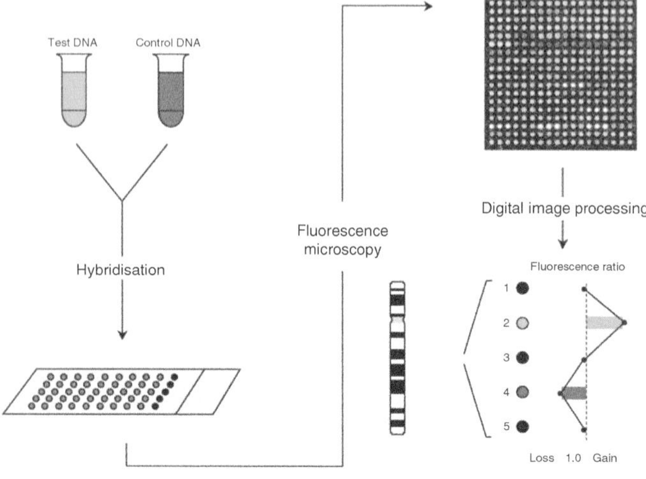

Molecular genetics

Molecular genetics is an area of genetics that studies the structure and function of genes at the molecular (DNA) level. It is a collaboration between genetic and molecular biology, which focuses on gene expression and their effect on heredity, genetic variation, and alterations. It is therefore apt for studying developmental biology and to aid the diagnosis and management of genetic disorders.

Several techniques used are to amplify DNA, and separate and identify nucleic acids:

- **Polymerase chain reaction (PCR):** An extremely versatile technique for copying DNA. PCR allows a single DNA sequence to be either copied millions of times or altered in predetermined ways. PCR has many variations, including reverse transcription PCR (RT-PCR) for amplification of RNA, and (more recently) real-time PCR, which allows for quantitative measurement DNA or RNA molecules (Figure 3.5).
- **Southern blots:** A method for probing for the presence of a specific DNA sequence within a DNA sample. Widely used in forensic laboratories to identify individuals who have left blood or other DNA-containing material at crime scenes. The number of bands that hybridise to a short probe provides an estimate of the number of closely related genes in an organism (Figure 3.6).
- **Northern blots:** Used to study the relative expression of patterns of a specific type of RNA molecule among a set of different samples of RNA. The RNAs on the blot can be detected by hybridising them to a labelled probe. The intensities of the band reveal the relative amounts of specific RNA in each sample (Figure 3.7).

DNA sequencing

This is the process of determining the nucleic acid sequence – i.e. the order of nucleotides in DNA. It includes any technique used to determine the order of the four bases: adenine, guanine, cytosine,

Figure 3.5 PCR (taken from https://www.britannica.com/science/polymerase-chain-reaction).

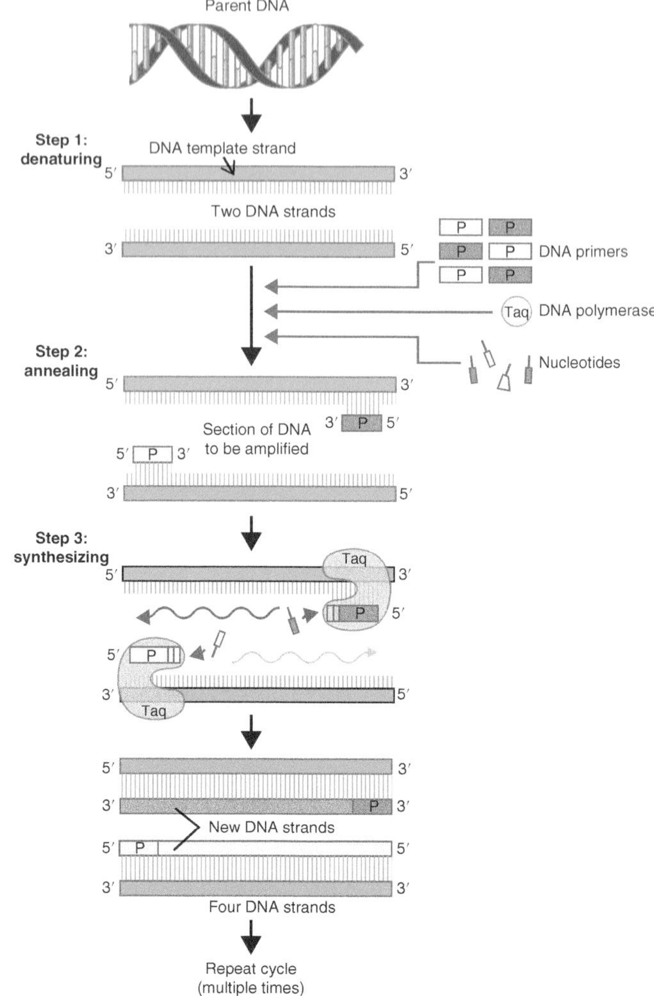

Figure 3.6 Southern blot.

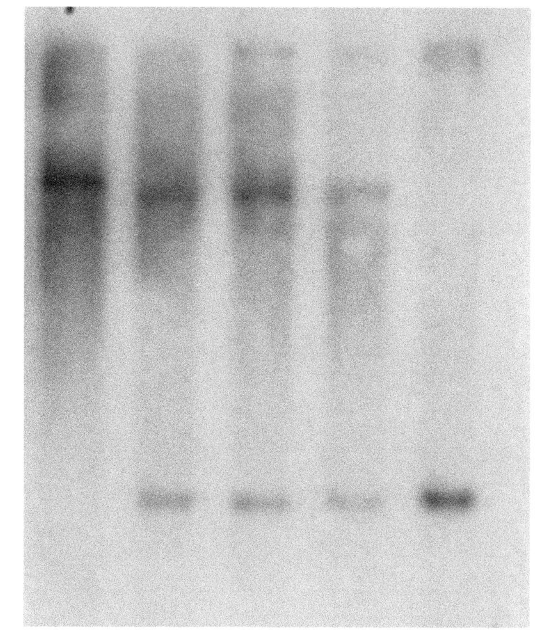

Figure 3.7 Northern blot.

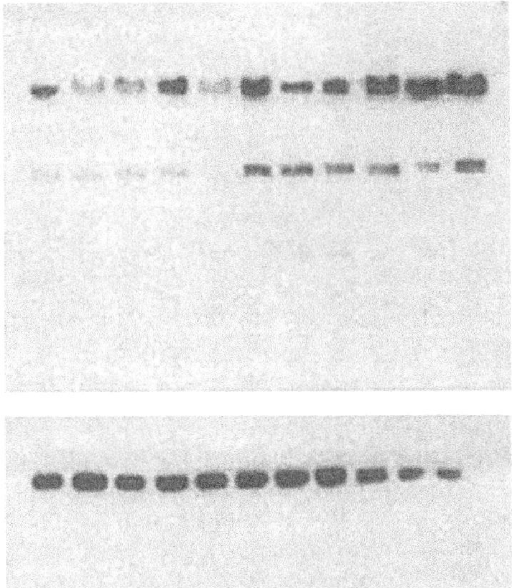

and thymine. The advent of rapid DNA sequencing methods has greatly accelerated genetic advances.

Sequencing an entire genome remains a complex task, requiring the DNA to be broken down into many smaller pieces, sequencing the pieces, and then re-assembling the sequences again.

There are many ways of sequencing DNA, with the list of techniques continually increasing. The first and most well-established method, Sanger sequencing, demonstrated the 'gold standard' art of sequencing that the newer techniques have since refined.

Sanger sequencing

Sanger sequencing was developed by the British biochemist Fred Sanger and his colleagues in 1977. In the Human Genome Project, Sanger sequencing was used to determine the sequences of many relatively small fragments of human DNA. The fragments were aligned based on overlapping portions to aid assembly of sequences of larger regions of DNA and, eventually, entire chromosomes.

The principle behind Sanger sequencing is to amplify the DNA needed to form sequences, denature the template (i.e. separate the strands), and then reassemble the DNA with the use of dye-labelled, chain-terminating dideoxynucleotides. The mixture is first heated to denature the template DNA and separate the strands, and then cooled so that the primer can bind to the single-stranded template. Once the primer has bound, the temperature is raised again, allowing DNA polymerase to synthesize new DNA starting from the primer. DNA polymerase will continue adding nucleotides to the chain until it happens to add a dideoxynucleotide instead of a normal nucleotide. At that point, no further nucleotides can be added, so the strand will end with the dideoxynucleotide.

This process is repeated in several cycles. By the time the cycling is complete, it is virtually guaranteed that a dideoxynucleotide will have been incorporated into every single position of the target DNA, in at least one reaction – i.e. the tube will contain fragments of different lengths, ending at each of the nucleotide positions in the original DNA, with the ends of the fragments labelled with dye that indicates their final nucleotide.

After the reaction is completed, the fragments are run through a long, thin tube containing a gel matrix in a process called capillary gel electrophoresis. Short fragments move quickly through the pores of the gel, while long fragments move more slowly. As each fragment crosses the 'finish line' at the end of the tube, it is illuminated by a laser, allowing the attached dye to be detected.

The smallest fragment (ending just one nucleotide after the primer) crosses the finish line first, followed by the next-smallest fragment (ending two nucleotides after the primer), and so forth. Thus, from the colours of dyes registered one after another on the detector, the sequence of the original piece of DNA can be built up, one nucleotide at a time. The data recorded by the detector consist of a series of peaks in fluorescence intensity. The DNA sequence is read from the peaks in the chromatogram.

The downsides of Sanger sequencing are that it is expensive and inefficient for larger-scale projects. However, it has remained the gold standard in the development of next-generation sequencing techniques.

Next-generation sequencing

Modern DNA sequencing technologies are collectively termed 'next-generation sequencing'. There are a variety of next-generation sequencing techniques, adopting different technologies. They are essentially highly parallel, fast, lower-cost versions of Sanger sequencing, implementable on a micro scale. This evolution in technology has enabled the routine sequencing of genomes and expanded the possibilities for molecular biology research, biomedical applications, and diagnostics, taking us one step closer to truly personalised medicine.

How to read a genetic test report

Introduction

Genetic disorders are caused by rare changes in the DNA sequence of a person's genome that cause particular genes not to function properly. To communicate specifically how a patient's DNA is different, and where that change is located in the genome, the international scientific community has agreed a system of co-ordinates for describing genetic changes. This system enables all biomedical professionals to refer to a particular change, or 'variant', in the same way, so that information about genetic variants can be shared. This chapter aims to explain the terminology used in genetic test reports as, at first glance, it can be confusing. Resources to find additional information about specific genes and variants are also included.

Explanation of report

Report summary

The summary tells you whether or not any potentially meaningful changes have been detected in the genes that were analysed. It will also state whether the change is present in one or both of the copies of the patient's gene. If no meaningful change was detected, i.e. the genetic test was 'negative', it does not necessarily mean that there is not a meaningful change present in the patient's DNA, just that the laboratory did not find one using the test that was performed (see 'caveats' box).

Gene

A genetic test can analyse from one to over a thousand genes, depending on the symptoms of the patient. The genes that were analysed will have been selected on the basis of their known link to the patient's symptoms. **It is important to clinically assess how well a gene in the report could explain the symptoms of each individual patient.** More information about the genetic disorders caused by particular genes can be found on the following websites:

Genetic Home Reference: https://ghr.nlm.nih.gov/
GeneReviews: https://www.ncbi.nlm.nih.gov/books/NBK1116/

Variant

The patient's DNA sequence is compared to a reference sequence for the gene(s) that is being analysed. Any differences between the patient's DNA sequence and the reference sequence are known as 'variants'. Everyone's DNA is different (with the exception of monozygotic twins), but most variants do not alter the function of genes. After detecting such variants, the laboratory must interpret them to decide whether each variant is likely to be meaningful, i.e. to affect the function of the gene(s) being analysed, or whether it is just normal genetic variation in the population.

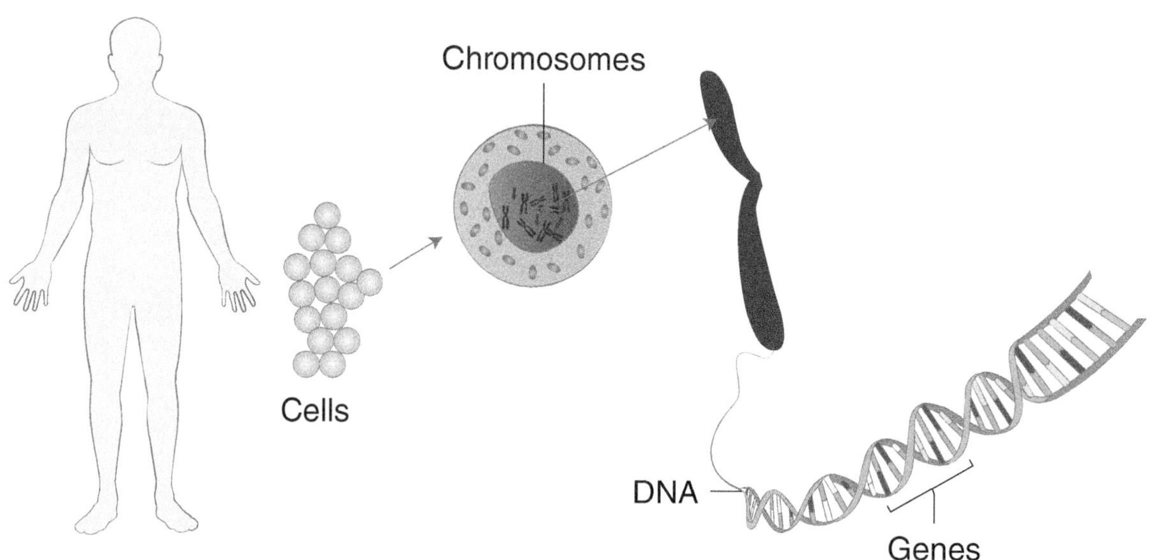

Clinical Genetics and Genomics at a Glance, First Edition. Edited by Neeta Lakhani, Kunal Kulkarni, Julian Barwell, Pradeep Vasudevan, and Huw Dorkins.

Genes are the instructions for building our bodies and making them work. Each person has ~20 000 genes. Genes are encoded in the DNA of the chromosomes in each cell. There are two copies of each gene, one inherited from each parent (except in males, who only have one copy of the genes that lie on the X and Y chromosomes).

How likely is it that a gene change is linked with a genetic condition?

Classification of variants: The laboratory interprets the variants that are found and classifies them into one of five categories. It is important to understand that this classification relies on the information that is currently available on the variant and that if new information becomes available in time, the classification of the variant may change. These five categories are:

Pathogenic: It is known that this variant affects the function of the gene and that it can cause a genetic disorder (Class 5).

Likely Pathogenic: It is probable that this variant affects the function of the gene and it is likely that it can cause a genetic disorder (Class 4).

Variant of Uncertain Significance (VUS): There is currently not enough information to know whether this variant can cause a genetic disorder or not (Class 3). Further information may become available in time. It may be helpful to test for this variant in other family members to help with the interpretation.

Unlikely Pathogenic/Likely Benign: It is probable that this variant is just part of normal genetic variation in the population and is unlikely to cause a genetic disorder (Class 2). Such variants are generally not included in genetic test reports.

Not Pathogenic/Benign: It is known that this variant is just part of normal genetic variation in the population and does not cause a genetic disorder (Class 1). Such variants are generally not included in genetic test reports.

More information on how variants are classified: https://www.acmg.net/docs/Standards_Guidelines_for_the_Interpretation_of_Sequence_Variants.pdf

Genetic terminology

Co-ordinates of a Variant: The exact location, or 'address', of a variant in the DNA sequence of the human genome is given by co-ordinates on the genetic test report. The location of a variant can be described in several ways:

A co-ordinate beginning with 'g.' or 'ChrN:' or 'N:' (where N is the chromosome number) describes the location of the variant in the whole genome sequence.

A co-ordinate beginning with 'c.' describes the location of the variant in the coding DNA sequence of the particular gene in which it was detected.

A co-ordinate beginning with 'p.' describes the change that results from the variant in the protein coded for by that gene.

A number that starts with 'LRG', 'ENST', 'NM_', or 'GRCh' refers to the sequence that is being used as a reference to derive the co-ordinates.

Using the co-ordinates of the variant, it is possible to look up whether any information is known about that particular genetic variant in various databases. Good places to start are:

Decipher: https://decipher.sanger.ac.uk/
ClinVar: https://www.ncbi.nlm.nih.gov/clinvar/

Homozygous/heterozygous/hemizygous: These words indicate whether a variant is present in one or both of the copies of the patient's gene.

Homozygous: The same variant was detected in both copies of the patient's gene.

Heterozygous: The variant is only present in one copy of the patient's gene.

Hemizygous: The patient only has one copy of the gene and that copy contains the variant.

Dominant genetic disorders: These are caused by a pathogenic variant in one copy of the gene.

Recessive genetic disorders: These require a pathogenic variant to be present in both copies of the gene. This can be due to a homozygous variant or due to two different heterozygous variants if each is present in a different copy of the gene. Sometimes the laboratory will request samples from the patient's parents in order to clarify whether the two changes are in the same or different copies of the patient's gene. A person can be a 'carrier' for a recessive genetic disorder if they have a pathogenic variant in only one copy of their gene.

X-linked genetic disorders: These are caused by a pathogenic variant in a gene on the X chromosome. These conditions generally affect males rather than females since males only have one X chromosome. Females may have a milder version of the condition or be unaffected 'carriers' of the disorder.

Caveats

Reasons that a genetic test can be 'negative':

- **The patient DOES NOT have a meaningful variant in the gene(s) that were tested**
  However, there may be **other genes** that can cause the patient's disorder that have not been examined because:
  - they were not included in the test, or
  - they are not yet known to cause a genetic disorder.
- **The patient DOES have a meaningful variant(s) in the gene(s) that were tested**
  But it **could not be detected** by the test method that was used (please refer to guidelines for testing particular genes/disorders and the reported analytical sensitivity of the test).

Further reading

NHS: http://www.nhs.uk/Conditions/Genetics/Pages/Introduction.aspx
EuroGentest: http://www.eurogentest.org/index.php?id=622
ACMG Guidelines: Richards, S., Aziz, N., Bale, S. et al. Standards and guidelines for the interpretation of sequence variants: a joint consensus recommendation of the American College of Medical Genetics and Genomics and the Association for Molecular Pathology. Genet Med 17, 405–423 (2015). https://doi.org/10.1038/gim.2015.30

5 Genetic and genomic counselling

Genetic counselling is the process of advising individuals and families affected by or at risk of genetic disorders to help them understand and adapt to the medical, psychological, and familial implications of genetic contributions to disease. Sheldon Clark Reed coined the term genetic counselling in 1947 and published the book *Counseling in Medical Genetics* in 1955. With the growth in knowledge of genetic disorders, genetic counselling has progressively become a key component of clinical genetics. In 1979, the National Society of Genetic Counselors (NSGC) was founded and the core principle and process was affirmed.

The genetic counselling process integrates:

- Interpretation of family and medical histories to assess the chance of disease occurrence or recurrence.
- Education about inheritance, testing, management, prevention, and resources.
- Counselling to promote informed choices, adaptation to the risk or condition, and support in reaching out to relatives that are also at risk.

The goals of genetic counselling are to increase the understanding of genetic disease, discuss disease management options, explain the risks and benefits of testing, and help the family to adjust to, and to communicate effectively about, the meaning of the genetic condition. Counselling sessions focus on providing genetic information in a way that can be understood by the patient to facilitate their decision-making process.

There are different approaches to genetic counselling. The reciprocal-engagement model of genetic counselling practice includes tenets, goals, strategies, and behaviours for addressing patients' genetic concerns. Genetic counselling is psychoeducational, as patients 'learn how genetics contributes to their health risks and then process what this means and how it feels'. Genetic counselling occurs in a reflective and non-judgemental way, using basic tenets of counselling practice such as unconditional positive regard, remaining aware of their own personal feelings and the effect they might have on the consultation. The aim is not to suggest one course of action over another; rather, the goal of the counselling process is to fully inform and empower patients so they may choose their preferred option based on accurate information and their own personal value system. This approach is often referred to as *nondirective* or *value neutral*.

Genetic counsellors are a uniquely skilled group of healthcare professionals with training and expertise in genetics and genomic medicine, allied with counselling skills, to deliver genetic counselling supported by evidence-based genetic counselling theory.

Seymour Kessler, in 1979, first categorised sessions into five phases: an intake phase, an initial contact phase, the encounter phase, the summary phase, and a follow-up phase. The intake and follow-up phases occur outside of the actual counselling session. The initial contact phase is when the counsellor and families first meet and build rapport. The encounter phase includes dialogue between the counsellor and the client about the nature of screening and diagnostic tests. The summary phase provides all the options and decisions available for the next step. If patients wish to go ahead with testing, an appointment is organised, and the genetic counsellor communicates the results.

The genetic counsellor role has continued to evolve, with increasing involvement in calculating genetic risk, explaining inheritance patterns, ordering genomic testing, interpreting variants, arranging medical and/or diagnostic testing (as well as testing of relatives), predicting risks of genetic disease, referring patients for appropriate disease screening, and supporting the psychosocial and ethical issues raised for individuals and their families.

In addition, genetic counsellors serve as patient advocates to signpost and refer individuals and families to community and charitable services. Many engage in research activities related to their field within genetics. Outcomes of their need include measures of improved patient knowledge, empowerment, lowering of anxiety or distress, satisfaction, knowledge of perceived risk, genetic testing, changed health behaviours, and lowered decisional conflict. Much of their role is conducted under the AGNC Code of Ethics, which advocates that genetic counsellors are encouraged to act under awareness of (see Table 5.1):

A Their own self-awareness and development.
B Relationships with service users including patients, families, and carers.
C Relationships with colleagues.
D Responsibilities to the wider society.

Table 5.1 AGNC Code of Ethics.

Self-awareness and development

1. Be aware of their own physical and emotional health and take appropriate action to prevent an adverse impact on their professional performance.
2. Report to an appropriate person or authority any conscientious objection that may be relevant to their professional practice.
3. Maintain and improve their own professional education and competence.
4. Acknowledge and disclose circumstances that may result in a real or perceived conflict of interest.
5. Inform the appropriate regulatory body without delay if, at any time, you have accepted a caution, been charged with or found guilty of a criminal offence, or if any finding has been made against you as a result of fitness to practice procedures, or if you are suspended from a scientific post, or if you have any restrictions placed on your scientific, clinical, or technical practice.

Clinical Genetics and Genomics at a Glance, First Edition. Edited by Neeta Lakhani, Kunal Kulkarni, Julian Barwell, Pradeep Vasudevan, and Huw Dorkins.

Table 5.1 Continued

Relationships with service users including patients, families, and carers

1. Never discriminate unfairly against patients, carers, or colleagues and the public.
2. Understand the need to respond and uphold the rights, dignity, values, and autonomy of service users including their role in the diagnostic and therapeutic process and in maintaining health and well-being.
3. Avoid any abuse of their professional relationship with service users.
4. Recognise that relationships with service users should be based on mutual respect and trust, and be able to maintain high standards of care even in situations of personal incompatibility.
5. Enable service users and their families to make informed independent decisions, free from coercion, through the use of a range of counselling theories and styles.
6. Protect all confidential information concerning service users obtained in the course of professional practice: disclosures of such information should only be made with the service user's consent, unless disclosure can be justified because of a significant risk to others.
7. Report to an appropriate person or authority any circumstance, action, or individual that may jeopardize patient care, or their health and safety.
8. Seek all relevant information required for any given patient situation.
9. Refer patients to other competent professionals if they have needs outside the professional expertise of the genetic counsellor.
10. Genetic Counsellors have a statutory duty to apply the principle of being open under the guidance of the Duty of Candour (Department of health 2014) to inform and apologise to patients if there have been mistakes in their care that have led to harm.

Relations with colleagues

1. Treat colleagues with dignity and respect.
2. Collaborate and cooperate with colleagues in order to provide the highest quality of service to the patients, carers, and families.
3. Foster relationships with colleagues across all area of service delivery as required to ensure that patients and families benefit from a multidisciplinary approach to care.
4. Assist colleagues to develop their knowledge of clinical genetics, genomics, and genetic counselling.
5. Maintain and apply quality standards, control, and assurance techniques.
6. Report to an appropriate person or authority any circumstance or action which may jeopardize the health and safety of a colleague.

Responsibilities within the wider society

1. Practice in accordance with the Genetic Counsellor Registration Board (GCRB) Code of Conduct or their designated regulatory body.
2. Provide reliable and expert information to the general public.
3. Adhere to the laws and regulations of society. However, when such laws are in conflict with the principles of practice, genetic counsellors should work towards change that will benefit the public interest.
4. Seek to influence policymakers on human genetic and genomic issues, both as an individual and/or through membership of professional bodies.

Further reading

https://www.agnc.org.uk/media/11805/agnc-code-of-ethics-january-2021.pdf

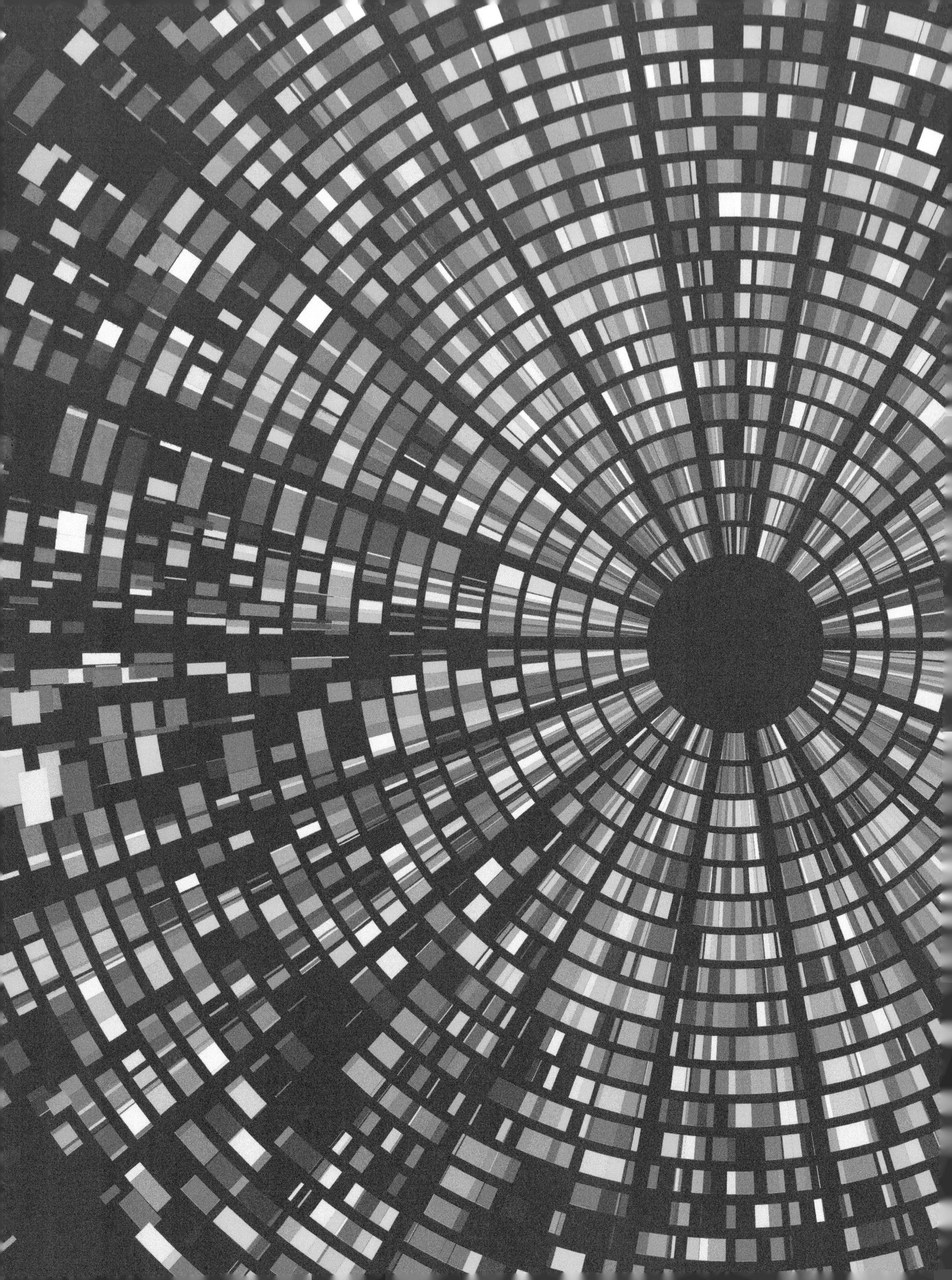

Cardiology

Chapters

6 Structural and congenital heart disease

Background

Congenital heart disease (CHD) is the commonest major congenital anomaly, occurring in 0.5–2% of neonates when including the most common lesion, bicuspid aortic valve. Improvements in both medical and surgical techniques have resulted in the growth of the adult CHD population and there are now more adults over the age of 18 than children with CHD.

Epidemiology

The aetiology of CHD is incompletely understood but is believed to be genetic with environmental contributions. CHD can occur as an isolated phenomenon or as part of a specific syndrome, with extra-cardiac and/or dysmorphic features.

Genetics

Several observations support the genetic basis of CHD. Concordance of CHD is more common in monozygotic than dizygotic twins; rates of CHD are substantially higher in families with consanguinity; CHD cases exhibit more cardiac candidate gene alterations than controls; finally sibling recurrence risk is substantial, though this varies between different types of CHD. Modifier genes and non-coding alterations likely affect both penetrance and type of CHD seen. Environmental factors are important: e.g. maternal diabetes mellitus increases the risk of CHD by ~4 times.

Most CHD is sporadic but there are important genetic causes (e.g. Noonan's syndrome, 22q11.2 deletion, and Holt-Oram syndrome). However, the phenotype in relatives may be subtle, and hence Mendelian disease may be misclassed as sporadic. Cardiac phenotype does not always correlate well with disease: different diseases may cause identical cardiac lesions and heterogenous phenotypes may be seen in the same disease. Alterations include:

- **Aneuploidy:** Variation in chromosome number is tested for by karyotyping and is seen in 10–20% of infants with CHD. Many different genes will be affected in each case. Aneuploidy syndromes are associated with a variety of cardiovascular phenotypes: most common are Down syndrome (trisomy 21; atrial septal defect, ASD; ventricular septal defect, VSD; atrioventricular septal defect, AVSD) and Turner syndrome (45,XO; bicuspid aortic valve, BAV; coarctation), less common are Edwards syndrome (trisomy 18; ASD, VSD, PDA) and Patau syndrome (trisomy 13; VSD, PDA).
- **Copy number variation:** Gains or losses of smaller regions of DNA can be detected by genome wide microarray or FISH. The most common disorders with cardiac involvement are del22q11 (DiGeorge syndrome; tetralogy of Fallot; interrupted aortic arch type B; PDA) and del7q11 (Williams syndrome; supravalvular aortic/pulmonary stenosis). Deletions or duplications may affect one or many genes, potentially affecting both function and expression through changes in coding and non-coding regions.
- **Point mutations:** These are found in coding regions and these may cause loss- or gain-of-function in a protein product. Most are dominantly inherited. Mendelian disorders causing CHD are uncommon but are important to recognise as they have a major effect on counselling patients and families. Table 6.1 illustrates several well-recognised conditions.

Pathophysiology

Three pathways are implicated:

- **Jag-Notch pathway:** The Jag-Notch pathway is involved in cell–cell communication and underlies a variety of vital processes in cardiac development including Left–Right organisation and the development of blood vessels and heart chambers. Unsurprisingly, dysregulation of this pathway (e.g. in Alagille syndrome) can present with a wide variety of cardiovascular phenotypes.
- **Ciliary disorders:** Cilia are hair-like motile structures on the surface of a variety of cell types. Vital in mucus clearance and sperm motility, in the heart their role is in Left–Right organisation. Disruption leads to ciliary dysfunction and heterotaxy disorders where the position of heart and other internal organs may be reversed or ambiguous. Loss of normal Left–Right organisation leads to *random* (not reversed) laterality; 50% of individuals with a mutation have normal organisation of their internal organs.
- **Ras/MAP kinase pathway:** RAS is a family of small GTPases that regulates cell growth, proliferation, and differentiation. This pathway was originally discovered in the context of somatic alterations in tumours. Dysregulation of the RAS/Mitogen-activated protein kinase (MAPK) pathway causes a group of diseases known as 'RASopathies'. These syndromes have many overlapping characteristics (see Table 6.1), including an increased risk of malignancy.

Symptoms and clinical features

See Table 6.1.

Diagnosis

Important Mendelian causes are recognised by relevant (family) history and distinctive clinical features. Many conditions are identifiable by earlier techniques but the advent of new sequencing technologies and an increased uptake of genetic testing in at risk groups has shed more light on the genetic basis and common biological pathways affected in CHD.

CHD is classified by the cardiac phenotype (see Table 6.1). Atrioventricular canal defects affect the mitral and tricuspid valves and atrioventricular septum (archetypal lesion in Down's syndrome); conotruncal disorders affect the ventricular septum, the right- and left-outflow tracts and the aorta (including Tetralogy of Fallot, coarctation, Patent Ductus Arteriosus [PDA] and Transposition of the Great Arteries); failure of development (hypoplasia) of the left or right ventricles leads to a univentricular heart; and heterotaxy disorders affect the left–right relationship of the heart and other structures. Also seen are isolated lesions of the LV outflow tract, individual valves (e.g. bicuspid aortic valve, BAV), or isolated defects of the atrial or ventricular septum (ASD, VSD).

Clinical Genetics and Genomics at a Glance, First Edition. Edited by Neeta Lakhani, Kunal Kulkarni, Julian Barwell, Pradeep Vasudevan, and Huw Dorkins.

Table 6.1 Overview of certain Mendelian disorders associated with congenital heart disease.

Disorder	Inheritance	Relevant genes	Clinical features	Cardiac phenotype
Holt-Oram syndrome	AD	*TBX5*, rarely *SALL4*	Upper limb abnormalities: wrist deformities; digital polydactyly; hypoplastic or triphalangeal thumb; partial/complete absence of forearm bones; abnormalities of humerus, clavicle, or scapula	ASD, VSD, conduction disease, hypoplastic left heart
Primary Ciliary dyskinesia	AR	Multiple *(~50)*, including *DNAI1, DNAH5, TXNDC3, KTU, RSPH4A, RSPH9, LRRC50*	Bronchiectasis, pneumonia, sinusitis, glue ear, infertility in males	Dextrocardia with situs inversus in up to 50% (Kartegener's syndrome), 6% have situs ambiguus (more commonly associated with intracardiac defects)
Oculofaciocardiodental (OFCD) syndrome	X-linked dominant	*BCOR*	Microphthalmia, distinctive facial features, dental abnormalities	ASD, VSD
CHARGE syndrome	AD	*CHD7*	**C**oloboma (hole/defect) of the eye, **H**eart defects, **A**tresia of posterior nasal apertures, **R**etarded growth and development, **G**enital abnormalities, **E**ar anomalies	CHD of almost any type is seen – conotruncal defects, ASD/VSD, AV canal defects, outflow tract obstruction
Alagille syndrome	AD	*JAG1, NOTCH2*	Characteristic facies, abnormalities of the liver (neonatal jaundice), eye, skeleton, and kidneys, mild-to-moderate learning delay	Stenoses of pulmonary tree, ASD, VSD, TOF, PDA, pulmonary atresia
Noonan syndrome (NS)	AD	*PTPN11, SOS1, RAF1, KRAS, NRAS, BRAF, SHOC2, CBL RIT1*	Distinctive facies and relative macrocephaly, short stature, mild developmental delay and cognitive impairment, cryptorchidism, webbed neck, pectus excavatum, myeloproliferative disorders	CHD in 80%: PS (50–62%), HCM (20%), ASD (6–10%), abnormal electrocardiogram (50%). HCM more frequent in RAF1 alterations (70%) and RIT1 alterations
NS with multiple lentigines (LEOPARD syndrome)	AD	*PTPN11, RAF1, BRAF*	Multiple lentigines, ocular hypertelorism, abnormal genitalia, retardation of growth and sensorineural deafness	HCM most common, ECG abnormalities (73%), PS (~23%), other VHD (50%), coronary abnormalities (15%)
Costello syndrome	AD	*HRAS*	Distinctive facies, short stature, failure to thrive and feeding difficulties, curly hair, palmar keratosis, increased risk of malignant tumours (~10 to 15%)	CHD in 44%: HCM (~60%), PS (~22%), and atrial tachycardia (48%)
Cardiofaciocutaneous (CFC) syndrome	AD. Usually caused by sporadic mutation	*BRAF MAP2K1 MAP2K2 KRAS*	Distinctive facies, short stature, failure to thrive, skin abnormalities including naevi, lentigines, and palmar-plantar keratosis, curly hair, severe intellectual disability, seizures	CHD in 75%: PS (~45%), HCM (~40%), ASD/VSD, VHD, arrhythmia, aortic dilatation
Neurofibromatosis type 1 (NF1)	AD	*NF1*	Multiple café-au-lait spots, skin-fold freckling, neurofibromas, short stature, macrocephaly, Lisch nodules	CHD in 2–3%: PS most common, other congenital heart defects and intracardiac neurofibromas

Management

Management depends on the specific defects and underlying cause. Most do not require intervention but may require investigation and monitoring. Medications (e.g. diuretics, digoxin) may be needed prior to intervention. Around 1/3 of patients with CHD are classified as severe and these will usually require either palliative or corrective surgery in childhood.

Extra-cardiac features and family history must be identified to estimate recurrence risk and to initiate family screening. Overall, recurrence risk in siblings/offspring is ~2–3% for children of affected males and ~5–6% for children of affected females. This difference in sex-specific transmission risk remains largely unexplored. Recurrence risk in certain types of CHD (e.g. heterotaxy disorders) or in Mendelian disease (i.e. 50% in AD disease) is much higher. Adult CHD patients were assessed in an era when genetic testing was limited, so may benefit from revisiting this option. Table 6.2 provides a guide to those for whom genetic counselling may be beneficial in adulthood.

Table 6.2 Factors suggesting adult CHD patients may benefit from counselling for clinical genetic testing.

Patients with a family history of CHD
Patients with CHD with high risk of 22q 11.2 deletion (TOF, TA, PA with VSD, AAA, IAA)
Patients who wish to have children (preconceptional counseling)
Patients with extracardiac abnormalities/disease:
Congenital Malformations
Dysmorphic features
Multisystem involvement
Psychiatric disorders
Intellectual disability

CHD, Congenital Heart Disease; IAA, Interrupted Aortic Arch, TA, Truncus Arteriosus; TOF, Tetralogy of Fallot; PA, Pulmonary Atresia, AAA, Aortic Arch Anomaly

Reprinted from van Engelen, K., Baars, M.J., Felix, J.P., et al., (2013). The value of the clinical geneticist caring for adults with congenital heart disease: diagnostic yield and patients' perspective. *American Journal of Medical Genetics Part A,* 161 (7): 1628–1637.

The future

Survival into adulthood was around 15% in the 1950s, now standing at around 90%. Early diagnosis and focused intervention is key to improving this further. The future of future research efforts will also involve management of any residual and associated pathology in those now living well into late adulthood, with the goal of improving life expectancy to near-normal.

7 Cardiomyopathies

Background

Cardiomyopathies are intrinsic disorders of heart muscle, excluding heart conditions caused by external factors such as ischaemic heart disease or infiltrative diseases such as amyloidosis or sarcoidosis. Cardiomyopathies may be limited to the heart or may be part of a multisystem disorder and are classified by clinical features into different subtypes, but there are also patients and families with overlapping conditions.

Epidemiology

Hypertrophic cardiomyopathy (HCM) affects approximately 1:500 of the general population. Dilated cardiomyopathy (DCM) is also relatively common, affecting between 1:250 and 1:2500 Arrhythmogenic cardiomyopathy is more uncommon, with prevalance estimates ranging from 1:1000 to 1:5000. The other subtypes are rarer. Aetiology is a combination of genetic and environmental factors, the latter including hypertension, ischaemic heart disease, cardiac valvular disease, drugs, inflammatory disorders, connective tissue disorders, pregnancy amongst others.

Genetics

HCM was the first cardiomyopathy to have the genetic causes identified. Table 7.1 provides an overview of the genetic alterations.

Pathophysiology

Heart muscle cells (*cardiomyocytes)* are rich in mitochondria to generate ATP, which fuels contraction of the sarcomere by powering the myosin heads to move along their actin scaffold. This process depends upon calcium release from the *sarcoplasmic reticulum,* triggered by inward calcium flow from outside the cell during the cardiac action potential. Cell–cell adhesion and transmission of the action potentials depend upon an agglomeration of cell wall proteins known as the *desmosome*. These different components of the cardiomyocyte may be disrupted in cardiomyopathy and are shown in Figure 7.1.

- **HCM:** The commonest pattern is asymmetric hypertrophy of the interventricular septum, though apical HCM is more common in the Far East. A combination of septal hypertrophy and mitral valve abnormalities leads to LV outflow tract obstruction (LVOTO). It is unclear how the identified alteration mutations

Table 7.1 Summary of some different cardiomyopathy subtypes and commonly involved genes (not exhaustive).

Condition	Inheritance	Genes commonly involved
Hypertrophic cardiomyopathy (HCM)	AD	50%–60% have an identified pathogenic alteration. Most affect proteins in the sarcomere β-myosin heavy chain (*MYH7*), myosin-binding protein C (*MYBPC3*), troponin T (*TNNT2*), troponin I (*TNNI3*), and tropomyosin (*TPM1*). Some are alterations in non-sarcomeric genes (e.g. *PRKAG2*) involved in energy metabolism.
Dilated cardiomyopathy (DCM)	Variable, 80–90% AD, rarely AR or XLR	Young age at onset or positive FH suggests a genetic cause. 40–50% of these have a pathogenic alteration identified. Four main genes: Titin (*TTN*), β-myosin heavy chain (*MYH7*), troponin T (*TNNT2*), and lamin A/C (*LMNA*). Lamin A/C aside. These encode proteins in the sarcomere (similarly to HCM); alterations usually loss-of-function and may relate to loss of calcium sensitivity.
Arrhythmogenic cardiomyopathy (AC)	Majority AD. Cardiocutaneous disorders (Naxos and Carvajal syndromes) AR	Desmosomal + non-desmosomal proteins. Plakophilin (*PKP2*), desmocollin (*DSC2*), desmoglein (*DSG2*), desmoplakin (*DSP*), and junction plakoglobin (*JUP*). Some present with a DCM-like phenotype but a more typically AC mutation; such individuals appear to have a worse prognosis than seen in typical DCM. Compound heterozygosity is quite common and can cause more severe disease.
Restrictive cardiomyopathy (RCM)	AD	Troponin I (*TNNI*), myosin light chain 3 (MYL3), desmin (*DES*).
LV non-compaction (LVNC)	Variable. Mostly AD, rarely AR or XLR	Sarcomere proteins; Myosin heavy chain (*MYH7*), myosin-binding protein C (*MYBPC3*), troponin (*TNNT2*), troponin I (*TNNI3*), and actin (*ACTC*).

Clinical Genetics and Genomics at a Glance, First Edition. Edited by Neeta Lakhani, Kunal Kulkarni, Julian Barwell, Pradeep Vasudevan, and Huw Dorkins.

Figure 7.1 The cardiomyocyte – the sarcomere, sarcoplasmic reticulum, nucleus, and desmosome.

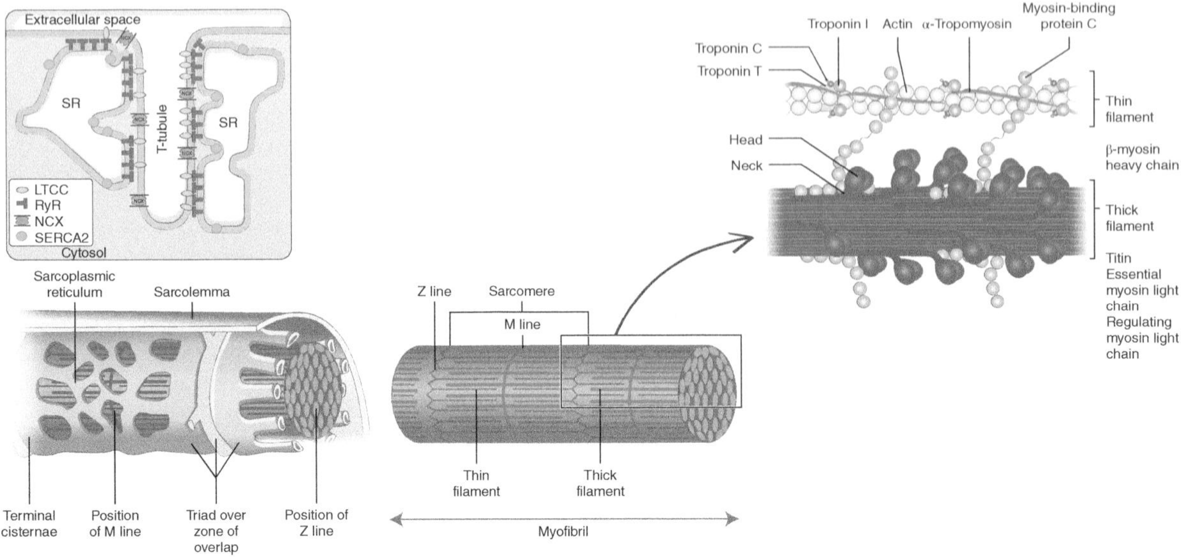

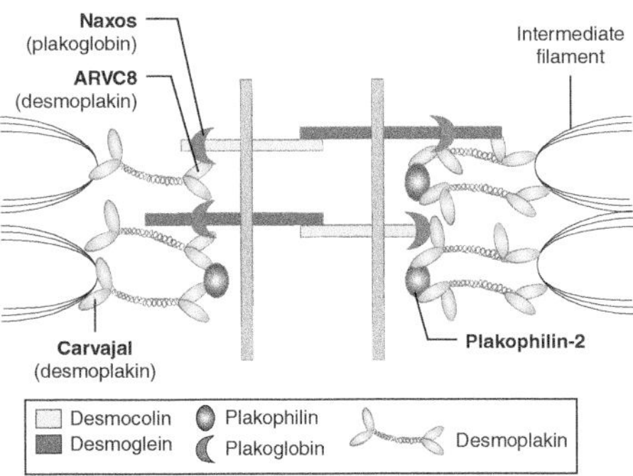

cause hypertrophy or the other clinical features of HCM, but one theory is that they lead to inefficiency in energy usage and a shortage of ATP. This causes hypertrophy and eventually dilatation of the ventricle and a declining ejection fraction ('burnt out' HCM).

- **DCM:** This may be caused by a number of factors (metabolic, toxic, and viral) but in some, it is clearly genetic. Four main proteins are implicated. One of these, Titin, is a very large structural protein. However, alterations in titin (even those causing large truncations) are often not enough to cause clinical disease, so additional environmental factors may be required. Another, Lamin A/C, encodes a nuclear envelope protein and causes a particularly malignant form of DCM associated with progressive conduction disease, ventricular arrhythmia, and sudden cardiac death. This is one of the rare examples of genotype–phenotype correlation in cardiomyopathy, another being DCM caused by mutations in the cytoskeletal protein desmin (DES).
- **AC:** This is characterised by progressive replacement of myocardium with fibrous and fatty tissue. This may affect either or both ventricles and around 10% of people will go on to develop heart failure. AC is often more malignant than HCM or DCM, and classically has a 'silent' phase where echocardiography is normal but a risk of fatal arrhythmia. There may be other clues, for example ECG abnormalities (frequent ventricular extra-systoles), and cardiac MRI may detect subtle early disease.

Symptoms

Patient may present with palpitations, shortness of breath (at rest or on exertion), peripheral oedema (e.g. pedal), orthopnoea, cough on lying down, chest discomfort, dizziness or light headedness, fatigue, or cardiac arrest.

Clinical features and diagnosis

Table 7.2 outlines the presentation and diagnosis of the commonly encountered cardiomyopathies.

Management

The principles of management are to identify and treat causative factors, prevent deterioration, manage symptoms and improve function, and to reduce risk of sudden cardiac arrest and other complications. Asymptomatic or minimally symptomatic individuals may require observation and/or lifestyle changes (e.g. diet change, exercise). Medications (antihypertensives, anticoagulants, diuretics, and antiarrhythmics) are commonly used. Invasive interventions (e.g. ablation, septal myectomy, and transplant) are uncommonly required. Implantable devices (e.g. left ventricular assist device (LVAD), implantable cardioverter defibrillator (ICD), and pacemaker) are more commonly utilised; for example, high risk groups (e.g. Lamin A/C and cytoskeletal protein DES alterations, associated with a particularly malignant DCM) should be considered for early therapy with a defibrillator.

The future

Novel pharmacological therapies, alongside developments in minimally invasive techniques and genetic techniques (e.g. editing) may play a role in reducing the morbidity and mortality of these conditions.

Table 7.2 Presentation and diagnosis.

Condition	Features
HCM	• Unexplained LV hypertrophy, LV outflow tract obstruction, arrhythmia. LVOTO manifests as exertional chest pain and shortness of breath. LVOTO occurs to some degree in 1/3 of HCM patients at rest (~2/3 on exercise). Energetic insufficiency may also cause arrhythmia (both atrial fibrillation and ventricular tachycardia/fibrillation are associated with HCM). Tend to have an above-normal ejection fraction. • Several uncommon multisystem conditions which mimic HCM ('phenocopies'), including Fabry disease, Friedreich's ataxia, and mitochondrial disorders. • Defined as hypertrophy (≥15mm) of any part of the left ventricle without an alternative explanation (in practice, usually hypertension or aortic stenosis), with decreased systolic (squeezing) function. Diagnosis in a first degree relative of a definite case with more modest hypertrophy (≥13mm).
DCM	• Dilatation of the LV ± RV with reduced systolic function, heart failure, and arrhythmia. • Can occur as part of a multisystem disorder, most commonly in muscular dystrophies. Cardiac involvement does not correlate with skeletal muscle disease, so patients with the less severe Becker muscular dystrophy or female Duchenne carriers may have severe cardiomyopathy. With the use non-invasive ventilation, heart disease is now the most common cause of death in Duchenne muscular dystrophy.
AC	• Frequent ventricular arrhythmia, may present similarly to DCM.
RCM	• Impaired ventricular relaxation and filling with preserved systolic function, poor prognosis without transplantation, and overlap with DCM/HCM.
LVNC	• Spongy layer of noncompacted myocardium, overlap with HCM/DCM but probably normal variant in some people. Risk of stroke/embolisation, arrhythmia.

8 Ischaemic heart disease

Background

Ischaemic heart disease (IHD), often referred to as coronary artery disease (CAD), is a leading global cause of morbidity and mortality. In the United Kingdom, one in five men and one in seven women overall die from this condition.

Epidemiology

Prevalence increases with age and it is known from *post-mortem* studies that almost all people in the United Kingdom will show some signs of atherosclerosis by the age of 40. Familial hypercholesterolaemia (FH) affects ~1 : 500. Homocystinuria is far rarer, affecting 1 : 200–400 000 (higher in certain countries). Risk factors for CAD include family history of premature CAD, hypercholesterolaemia, hypertension, diabetes mellitus, and smoking. It is clear from these associations that the development of CAD in an individual relies on a complex interplay between environmental and genetic factors.

Genetics

Twin and family studies suggest that CAD is highly heritable, accounting for 40–50% of susceptibility. Early attempts to find single gene drivers used traditional techniques such as linkage analysis and led to the discovery of the genetic basis of FH and homocystinuria. FH is usually AD, though AR forms are known. Homozygotes have more severe disease with up to a six-fold rise in plasma cholesterol and, untreated, up to 85% suffer a myocardial infarction (MI) by the age of 15. The first pathogenic mutation identified was in the gene encoding the LDL receptor (*LDLR*), and further pathogenic variants have been found in genes involved in lipid catabolism (*PCSK9*) and transport (*APOB*, encoding apolipoprotein B). However, these conditions are uncommon and do not explain the vast majority of CAD.

Some families have dominantly inherited early CAD without FH. Similar techniques have identified potentially pathogenic gene changes in cell signalling molecules, but such families are extremely rare so these findings remain largely unconfirmed. CAD is not a monogenic disorder in the vast majority of cases, but identification of these genes sheds light on the pathophysiological processes underlying more typical cases of CAD.

The first IHD GWAS was published in 2007, with more having followed. ~60 loci have been associated with risk of CAD (Figure 8.1). The variants involved are very common (usually >0.5% prevalence) but individual effect sizes are quite small (10–20%). Collectively, they are estimated to account for 30–40% of the total heritability of CAD. Many are found in non-coding regions and are presumed to affect the expression rather than the function of protein products.

A number of the risk alleles identified are biologically plausible, being associated with genes involved in production of LDL (*APOB, ABCG5, ABCG8, PCSK9, SORT1, ABO, LDLR, APOE,* and *LPA*) and HDL lipids (*ANKS1A*) and triglycerides (*TRIB1* and the *APOA5* cluster), with BMI and waist-hip ratio (*CYP17A1-CNNM2-NT5C2* and *RAI1-PEMT-RASD1*), and with blood pressure (*GUCY1A3* and *FES*). Others are implicated in signalling pathways that underlie inflammation and the development of atherosclerosis itself.

Pathophysiology

CAD is the clinical manifestation of atherosclerosis, which is characterised by the accumulation of oxidised LDL cholesterol in macrophages to form 'foam cells' which accumulate in lipid-rich plaques in arterial walls. These foam cells release pro-inflammatory cytokines (e.g. IL-1, IL-6, and matrix metalloproteinases) which stimulate muscle cell proliferation and initiate migration towards the lesion. This gradually narrows the calibre of the artery and impedes blood flow (Figure 8.2), leading to ischaemia of the heart muscle on exertion or emotional stress, known as angina pectoris. Pro-inflammatory cytokines reduce smooth muscle cell collagen secretion, which destabilises plaques and makes them prone to rupture. When this happens, plaque contents and inner parts of the artery wall are exposed to blood and this activated platelets and the clotting cascade. Layers of activated platelets and blood clot rapidly develop and can occlude the artery entirely.

Homocytinuria follows a different pathway, occurring secondary to enzyme deficiencies involved with methionine metabolism, particularly cystathionine beta synthase resulting in an accumulation of homocysteine. Up to 50% of those affected die of premature vascular disease. Aggregates of homocysteinylated lipoproteins can lead to ischaemia of arterial wall muscle cells, cell death, inflammation, and ultimately vulnerable atherosclerotic plaques.

Symptoms and clinical features

Atherosclerosis leads to necrosis of downstream heart muscle, known as a MI. Consequences include acute heart failure (pulmonary oedema or cardiogenic shock), arrhythmia, heart rupture, and sudden death. Survivors often suffer chronic heart failure which may be very disabling. FH is an uncommon subtype, presenting with raised plasma LDL, xanthomata (cholesterol skin eruptions), and early CAD.

Diagnosis

As adjuncts to history and clinical examination, useful investigations include bloods (anaemia, lipids), ECG, echo (transthoracic and transoesophageal), stress tests, catheterisation/angiography, and 3D imaging (e.g. CT/MRI). Risk calculators can help stratify individual risk and tailor preventative measures.

Management

This is complex and must address any underlying risk factors. Management involves both, preventative measures, alongside the acute management of complications such as MI. Lifestyle measures play an important role in all patients (exercise, weight

Clinical Genetics and Genomics at a Glance, First Edition. Edited by Neeta Lakhani, Kunal Kulkarni, Julian Barwell, Pradeep Vasudevan, and Huw Dorkins.

Figure 8.1 Circular Manhattan plot showing loci associated with CAD. Used with permission from: Nikpay N. et al. (2015). A comprehensive 1000 Genomes–based genome-wide association meta-analysis of coronary artery disease. *Nat Genet.* 47(10):1121–30.

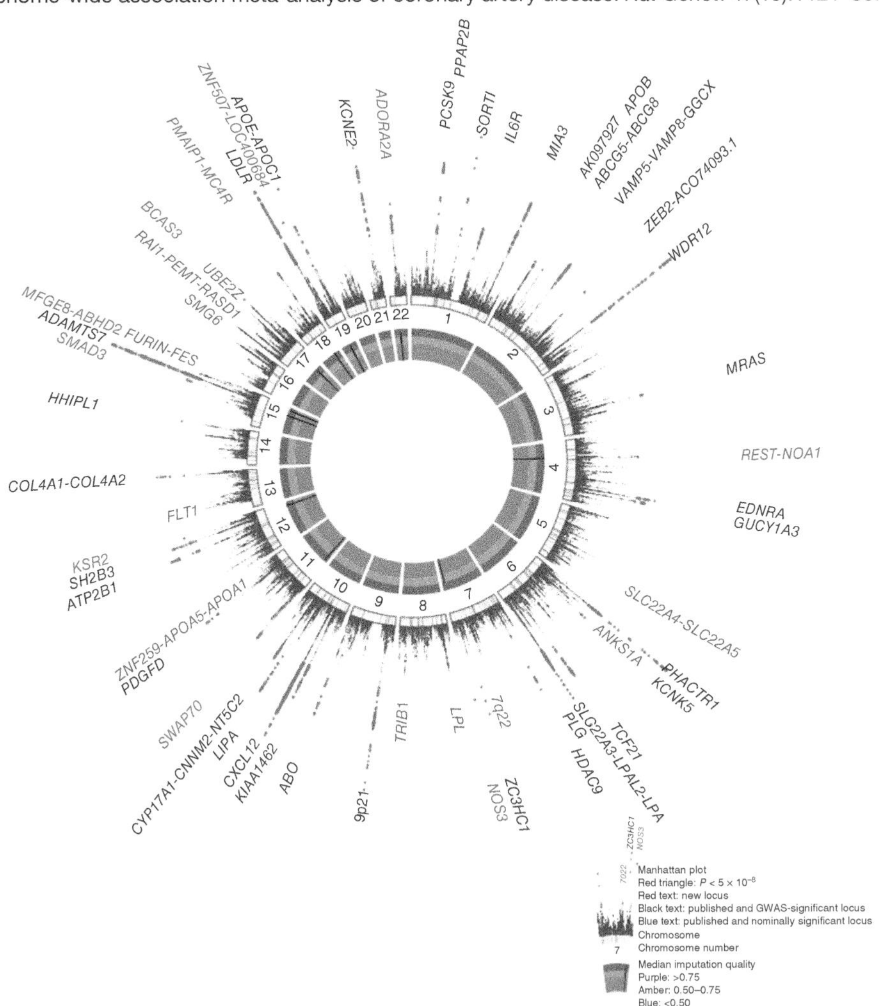

Figure 8.2 Development of atherosclerosis.

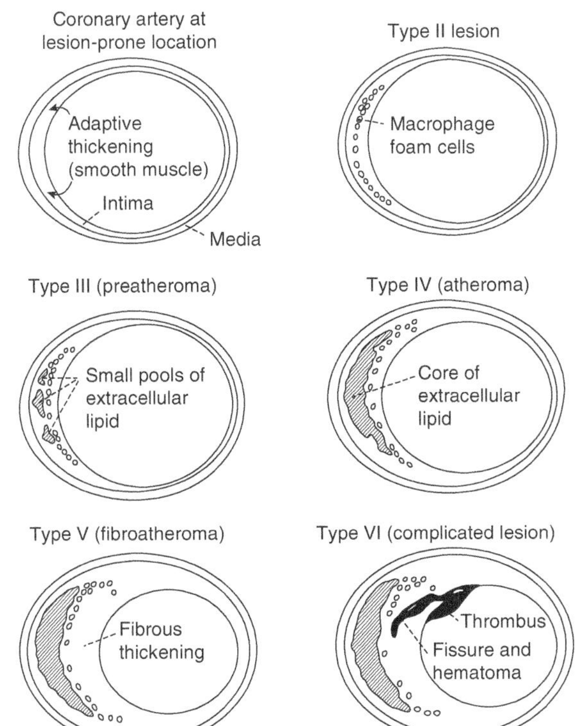

loss, dietary modifications, smoking cessation). Medications are the mainstay of long-term risk reduction, helping to improve glycaemic control in diabetic patients, blood pressure, and lipid levels, alongside controlling dysrhythmias and anticoagulants. Acute management of complications (e.g. MI) follows established pathways to restore and main cardiac perfusion. Percutaneous revascularisation (angioplasty/stenting) is commonly employed, whereas cardiac bypass grafting surgery plays a more selective role.

The future

New therapeutics may be developed through the identification of novel cellular targets, currently facilitated by the rapidly advancing area of functional genomics. The 9p21 locus has been linked with an increased risk of CAD. Its underlying mechanism is unclear, but it is thought that through its interference with cell cycle regulation and cellular proliferation, it contributes to plaque formation and progression. Rare genetic mutations have been shown to confer protection against CAD. Three variants (*PCSK9*, *NPC1L1*, and *ASGR1*) lower LDL cholesterol (risk reduction 88% with *PCSK9*), whilst *ASGR1*, *APOC3*, and *ANGPTL4* are associated with decreasing triglyceride-rich lipoproteins (risk reduction of 53% with *ANGPTL4*). Knowledge of these alleles can assist with drug design (e.g. the new PCSK9 inhibitors), and they could be targets for gene editing technology in future.

9 Arrhythmias and sudden cardiac death

Background

Arrhythmias are abnormalities of normal sinus rhythm. They can be divided into *bradyarrhythmias* (slow heart rhythms) and *tachyarrhythmias* (fast heart rhythms). Bradycardia (slow heart rate), heart block, and ventricular standstill can cause presyncope, syncope, or sudden death. Sudden cardiac death is defined as an unexpected death from cardiac causes ensuing within one hour of the onset of symptoms. The three main conditions considered in this chapter are Brugada syndrome (BrS), Long QT syndrome (LQTS), and Catecholaminergic polymorphic ventricular tachycardia (CPVT).

Epidemiology

The commonest cause of cardiac conduction disease is age-related fibrosis, but there are also rare infiltrative (e.g. sarcoid) and genetic (e.g. myotonic dystrophy) causes. Arrhythmias are more frequent in those with cardiomyopathy but also can occur in people with a seemingly normal heart. Where a cause is not found, it may be termed *idiopathic VF* and it maybe difficult to find affected family members; however, there are several heritable disorders of heart rhythm (*channelopathies*, see Table 9.1) which must be excluded. The three most common and best understood are discussed below.

- **BrS:** More common in men and most frequently causes arrhythmias and cardiac arrest in the fourth or fifth decade. It affects 1 : 1000–2000 of the UK population but is more common in South East Asia.
- **LQTS:** Certain situations are likely to provoke arrhythmia and genotype has an effect on this. Exercise (and particularly swimming) is most risky in LQT1. Emotional stress or loud noises, hormonal effects, and hypokalaemia commonly cause arrhythmia in LQT2. Events in LQT3 are most common at rest or whilst asleep.
- **CPVT:** Interestingly, this arrhythmia is also a feature of poisoning with digoxin, which affects the sodium–calcium ATPase leading to intracellular calcium overload. CPVT affects various proteins in the sarcoplasmic reticulum, which are thought to affect intracellular calcium handling.

Genetics

Victims of sudden cardiac death should have genetic material (e.g. from samples of spleen) stored to test for pathogenic gene variants (i.e. a 'molecular autopsy'). Unfortunately, all too often this is still not done. Panel testing for arrhythmia or cardiomyopathy may show a cause for the sudden death and this information can save lives in the wider family. If material is unavailable, then first-degree relatives should undergo clinical testing to look for these arrhythmia syndromes (as well as other forms of heart disease). Table 9.1 summarises some of the commonly involved genes.

Pathophysiology

Tachyarrhythmias can arise from either the atria or the ventricles. Atrial arrhythmias (atrial fibrillation/flutter or re-entry tachycardias) are rarely acutely dangerous though can be very symptomatically unpleasant, and are a major risk factor for cerebrovascular accidents (CVA). Ventricular arrhythmias include ventricular tachycardia (VT), torsades-de-pointes (TdP, a form of polymorphic VT), and ventricular fibrillation (VF). These are often less well tolerated by the patient and frequently lead to syncope or, untreated, sudden death.

Table 9.1 Genes commonly involved in inherited arrhythmia syndromes (not an exhaustive list).

Condition	Inheritance	Gene(s)
BrS	Usually AD, incomplete penetrance (can have single affected individual)	20% have an identified alteration commonly $Na_v1.5$ (*SCN5A*). Common variants in other genes have a strong influence on phenotype (careful clinical assessment mandatory). CACNA1C alterations account for <5% cases; other genes are much rarer.
LQTS	Romano-Ward syndrome: AD (without extra-cardiac features. Jervell and Lange Neilsen syndrome: AR with severe arrhythmia and congenital deafness. Rarer multisystem disorders incorporating LQTS (Andersen-Tawil and Timothy syndromes) also exist.	80–90% have identified mutation. Majority LQT1-3. LQT1: KVLQT1 (*KCNQ1*) LQT2: hERG (*KCNH2*) LQT3: $Na_v1.5$ (*SCN5A*)
CPVT	Usually AD, rare recessive forms	50–60% have identified alteration majority in the cardiac Ryanodine receptor 2 (*RYR2*) (or associated proteins such as calmodulin or calsequestrin) leading to cytosolic calcium overload and frequent ventricular extrasystoles in response to adrenaline, and sustained arrhythmia at higher stress levels.

Clinical Genetics and Genomics at a Glance, First Edition. Edited by Neeta Lakhani, Kunal Kulkarni, Julian Barwell, Pradeep Vasudevan, and Huw Dorkins.

Symptoms

Patients may report palpitations (noticeable heartbeat) due to an abnormally rapid, strong, or irregular rhythm. This may be triggered by an underlying illness or exertion (e.g. sport). Syncope (collapse) may also be manifestations of underlying arrhythmias.

Clinical features and diagnosis

Table 9.2 provides an overview of the common presentation and diagnosis of the common arrhythmias discussed. Figure 9.1 demonstrates common ECG patterns.

Management

- **BrS:** Affected patients should avoid certain drugs (www.brugadadrugs.org) or binge drinking alcohol and should treat fever promptly with paracetamol. High-risk patients or those who have suffered a cardiac arrest may require an implantable cardioverter-defibrillator (ICD). Asymptomatic patients with concealed (i.e. only seen with drug provocation) ECG changes may be at little greater risk than the background population, so clinicians should be cautious not to overtreat.
- **LQTS:** Affected patients should be treated with non-selective β-blocker drugs (e.g. nadolol, propranolol, and carvedilol) and avoid QT-prolonging drugs (as listed on www.crediblemeds.org). High-risk patients or those with symptoms despite maximal β-blocker therapy may require an ICD.
- **CPVT:** Affected patients should be treated aggressively with β-blockers at the maximal tolerated dose. Disconnection of the sympathetic nerve supply to the heart (an operation called left cervical sympathetic denervation) has been used to treat those who remain symptomatic despite β-blocker therapy, sometimes in an attempt to avoid an ICD. ICD therapy is generally a last resort as ICD shocks can cause more emotional stress and hence a vicious circle (leading to an 'electrical storm').

The future

Encouraging standardised mechanisms of diagnosis of underlying causes, particularly in cases of sudden cardiac death, will hopefully enable novel genetic variants to be identified. Ongoing research into disease-causing vs benign variants will help facilitate better risk stratification and monitoring of surviving family members.

Table 9.2 Clinical features and diagnosis.

Condition	Clinical features	Diagnosis
BrS	Syncope or sudden death at rest, while asleep, or provoked by drugs, typical ('type 1') ECG changes. Very fast, sometimes polymorphic, VT (>230–240bpm) or VF. Outward appearance of cardiac arrest in a sleeping patient is called 'nocturnal agonal breathing'.	Defined as a typical ECG appearance (a type 1 pattern, see Figure 9.1) either spontaneously or when provoked by sodium channel blocking drugs (e.g. ajmaline, flecainide).
LQTS	Syncope/Torsades-de-pointes/sudden death provoked by exercise (especially swimming, LQT1), emotion (LQT2), at rest/during sleep (LQT3) or by drugs (any); prolonged QT on ECG. Any age, either gender although some differences, e.g. higher risk in the post-partum period.	Congenital (as opposed to acquired - usually drug-induced - LQTS): Diagnosed by typical ECG appearances - especially, but not entirely, prolongation of the QT interval (measured between beginning of Q wave and end of T wave, see Figure 9.1) - and various supporting features such as syncope or documented arrhythmia and family history.
CPVT	Syncope/sudden death provoked by exercise/emotion/stress. Tends to present in childhood or young adulthood with syncope or sudden death in response to exercise or emotional stress.	It can be difficult to diagnose as the resting ECG is normal and, instead, arrhythmia is seen on exercise testing or adrenaline challenge. The hallmark feature of CPVT is bidirectional VT (with broad QRS complexes that alternate between positive and negative, see Figure 9.1).

Figure 9.1 Typical ECG appearances of inherited arrhythmia conditions. The black bar shows the QT interval.

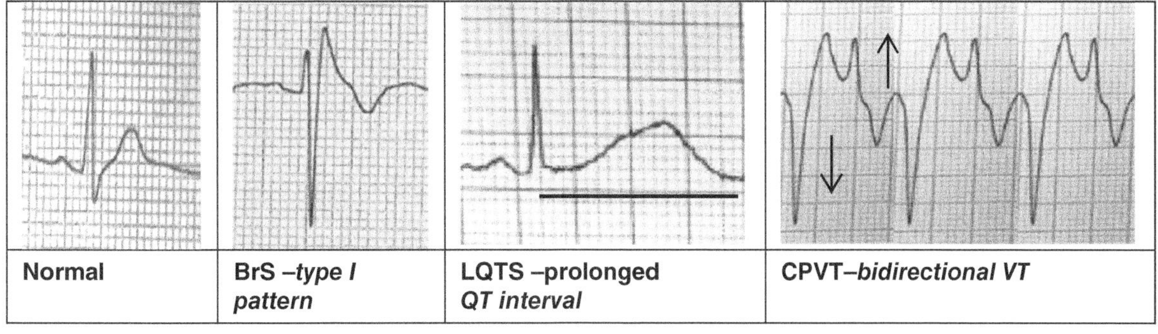

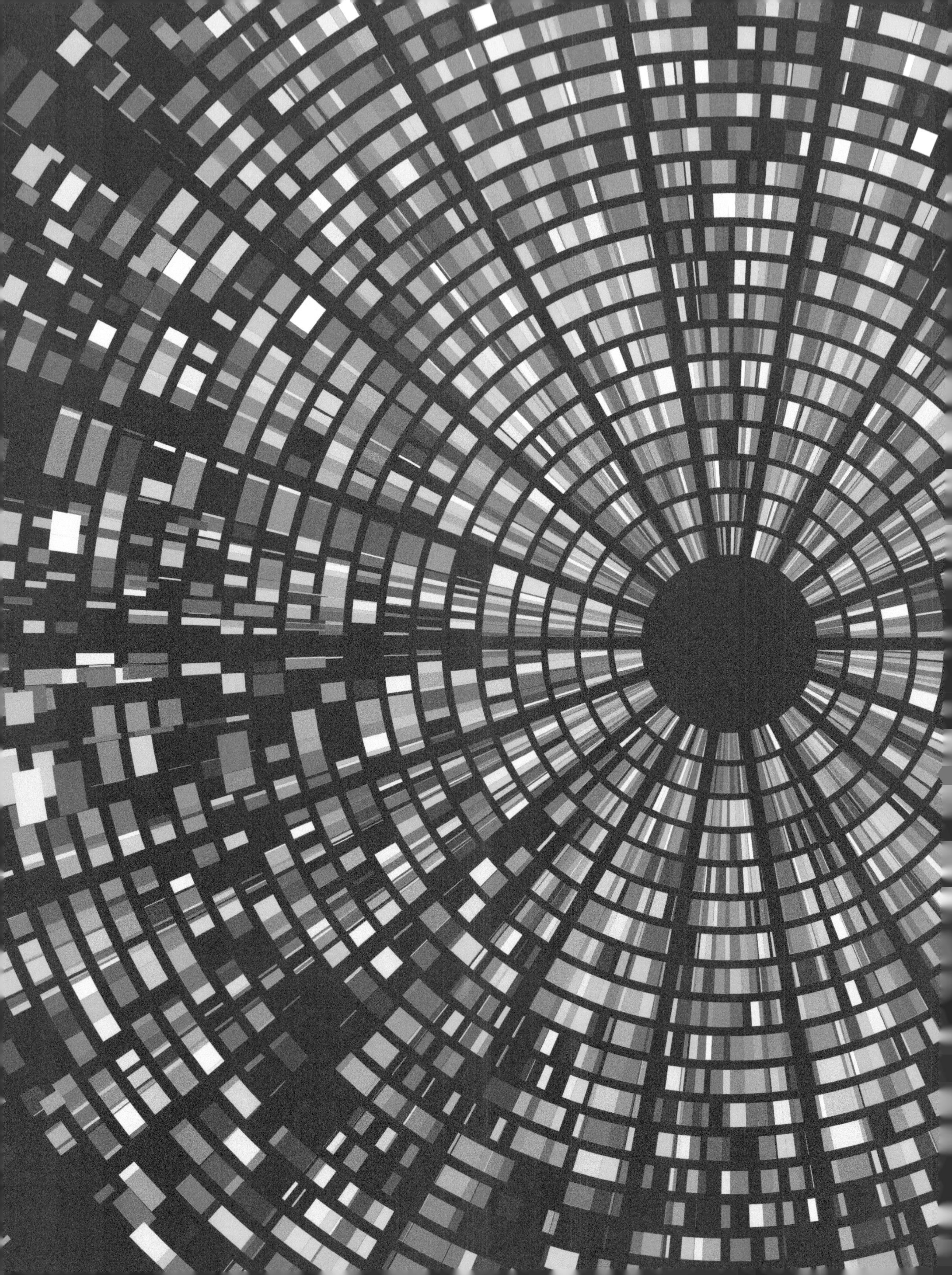

Dermatology

Chapters

Tuberous sclerosis complex

Background

Tuberous sclerosis complex (TSC) is a multisystem genetic condition that usually presents in infancy. It was previously known as tuberous sclerosis; however, the term 'complex' highlights the variability in disease phenotype and multiple organs often involved. It was first described over 150 years ago by Von Recklinghausen in 1862. It is characterised by the development of multiple benign tumours that commonly affect the skin, brain, eyes, kidneys, heart, and lungs. When tumours affect the brain, there may be associated epilepsy and learning difficulties.

Epidemiology

TSC is estimated to affect 1 in 6000–10,000 births.

Genetics

TSC is an AD-inherited condition, although two-thirds of alterations occur spontaneously. Penetrance is thought to be 100%; however, there is great variability of expression. It is most commonly (66% cases) caused by alteration in the *TSC2* gene, on chromosome 16p13. These are associated with a more severe phenotype.

In approximately 25% cases, it is caused by a heterozygous alteration in the *TSC1* gene on chromosome 9q34. In around 10% cases, no genetic cause is found; mosaicism may account for this. Some phenotype differences have been reported between families with *TSC1* or *TSC2* gene alterations.

Pathophysiology

TSC1 encodes the protein hamartin, whereas *TSC2* encodes a protein called tuberin. Although we do not fully understand the pathogenesis of TSC, it is thought to occur as a result of mammalian target of rapamycin (mTOR) pathway dysregulation and resultant disrupted embryogenesis. The defect in development can affect almost any organ resulting in benign tumours called hamartomas which are slow growing, do not metastasize, but through compression on local structures can cause significant morbidity including seizures and developmental delay.

Symptoms and clinical features

Common features of TSC listed by organ affected:

- **Skin:** The skin is affected in almost all patients with TSC. Changes include: hypomelanotic/ashleaf macules (pale patches that are usually present at birth or in infancy), facial angiofibromas (previously referred to as adenoma sebaceum - a misnomer - red or flesh coloured papules commonly affecting the medial cheeks and nose and usually develop between 3–10 years of age), Shagreen patches (connective tissue tumours which present as flesh coloured or orange plaques commonly affecting the lower back), (peri-)ungual fibromas (flesh coloured firm papules that develop around or under the nail), 'confetti' skin lesions (numerous 1–3 mm hypopogmented macules scattered across the body).
- **Brain:** Epilepsy affects 70% of those with TSC as a result of cortical tubers.
- Developmental delay and behavioural problems may also occur.
- Cortical tubers and nodules and giant cell astrocytoma affecting the subependymal zone (below the ependymal lining of the lateral ventricles of the brain) are major diagnostic criteria.
- **Eyes:** Can be affected by retinal hamartomas and achromic patches.
- **Renal:** Renal involvement can be caused by angiomyolipomas and hamartomas.
- **Other:** Dental enamel pits (randomly distributed pits in the dental enamel), lymphangioleiomyomatosis (LAM - interstitial smooth muscle infiltrates in the lungs), angiomyolipomas (benign tumours of vascular, smooth muscle, and adipose tissues which can affect kidneys and other organs), and cardiac tumours are other diagnostic features of TSC.

Diagnosis

Diagnosis is based upon history, identification of characteristic symptoms/signs, and molecular genetic testing. Clinical diagnostic criteria exist, with a clinical diagnosis made in individuals with ≥2 major features or 1 major feature and ≥2 minor features of the disorder (Table 10.1). A *possible clinical diagnosis* is suspected when 1 major feature or ≥2 minor features are present. Cardiac rhabdomyoma can be detected antenatally. Imaging (CT/MRI), cardiac echo, and ECG are also used to identify the various features of the condition.

Management

Although 60–70% alterations are thought to be spontaneous, unaffected parents of an affected child should both be fully investigated including a full skin examination using a Wood's lamp, ophthalmological examination, and consideration of renal imaging (CT, ultrasound, and intravenous pyelography). Facial angiofibromas can result in significant psychosocial upset and therefore curettage and electrodessication or laser surgery can be

Table 10.1 TSC clinical diagnostic criteria, International Tuberous Sclerosis Complex Consensus Group 2021.

Major criteria	Minor criteria
Facial angiofibromas ≥ 3	'Confetti' skin lesions
(Peri-)ungual fibroma ≥ 2	Dental enamel pits (>3)
Hypomelanotic macules ≥3, at least 5 mm diameter	Intraoral fibromas (≥2)
Shagreen patch	Retinal achromic patch
Multiple retinal hamartomas	Multiple renal cysts
Multiple cortical tubers	Non-renal hamartomas
Subependymal nodules > 2	Sclerotic bone lesions
Subependymal giant cell astrocytoma (SEGA)	
Cardiac rhabdomyoma	
Lymphangioleiomyomatosis (LAU)	
Angiomyolipomas (≥2)	

Clinical Genetics and Genomics at a Glance, First Edition. Edited by Neeta Lakhani, Kunal Kulkarni, Julian Barwell, Pradeep Vasudevan, and Huw Dorkins.

offered if disease is limited. mTOR inhibitors are now first-line therapies for enlarging SEGA and renal angiomyolipomas and LAM. Topical mTOR inhibitors are being developed for facial angiofibromas with promising initial results. Surgical debulking or removal of tumours is often unsatisfactory but neurosurgery can be considered where epilepsy is no longer controlled by medications or where there is a localised and stable electroencephalographic (EEG) focus. Most importantly screening of individuals is required. In 2021 The International Tuberous Sclerosis consortium updated the TSC guidelines for diagnosis, surveillance and management. Detailed recommendations have been published for screening and considerations that should be made in individuals at diagnosis and lifelong (Table 10.2). This includes routine interval imaging and investigations.

The future

Novel therapeutic agents are continually being investigated to help deal with the sequelae of TSC. For example, Epidiolex (cannabidiol) was licenced for seizures by the FDA in 2020. Building a better understanding of the molecular basis of the disease and management of the various sequelae will help develop better treatments.

Table 10.2 Surveillance and management recommendations for patients already diagnosed with definite or possible TSC (adapted from Updated International Tuberous Sclerosis Complex Diagnostic Criteria and Surveillance and Management Recommendations).

GENETICS:

- Offer genetic testing and family counselling if not performed previously.

BRAIN:

- MRI brain every 1-3 years in asymptomatic TSC patients younger than 25 years to monitor for new occurrence of SEGA. Frequent MRI in patients with large or growing SEGA, or with SEGA causing asymptomatic ventricular enlargement. Asymptomatic childhood SEGA should continue periodic imaging as adults to monitor growth.
- Surgical resection for symptomatic SEGA. Medical treatment with mechanistic target of rapamycin inhibitors (mTORi). For large tumours, neoadjuvant mTORi to facilitate surgery.
- Routine EEG in asymptomatic infants with TSC every 6 weeks up to age 12 months, then every 3 months up to age 24 months, as abnormal EEG frequently precedes onset of clinical seizures. Routine EEG in individuals with known or suspected seizure activity.
- Vigabatrin is the recommended first-line therapy for infantile spasms. Adrenocorticotropic hormone (ACTH), synthetic ACTH or prednisolone can be used if treatment with full-dose vigabatrin for 2 weeks has not correlated with clinical and EEG improvement.
- Antiseizure medications for other seizure types should follow that of other epilepsies. Everolimus and a specific cannabidiol formulation are approved by regulatory authorities.
- Epilepsy surgery should be considered for medically refractory TSC patients.
- TAND: Perform annual screening for TAND, using validated screening tools such as the TAND Checklist (tandconsortium.org/checklists/). Screening may be done more frequently.
- Comprehensive formal evaluation for TAND across all levels of TAND at key developmental time points: infancy (0–3 years), preschool (3–6 years), pre-middle school (6–9 years), adolescence (12–16 years), early adulthood (18–25 years), and as needed thereafter
- Many with TSC have learning difficulties requiring tailored education.

RENAL:

- MRI abdomen to monitor angiomyolipoma and renal cystic disease every 1-3 years.
- Assess renal function and blood pressure at least annually.
- Embolisation followed by corticosteroids is first-line therapy for angiomyolipoma presenting with acute haemorrhage. Avoid nephrectomy. For asymptomatic, growing angiomyolipoma measuring larger than 3 cm in diameter, treatment with an mTOR inhibitor is the recommended first-line therapy. Selective embolisation or kidney-sparing resection are acceptable second-line therapy for asymptomatic angiomyolipoma.

PULMONARY:

- Enquire about smoking, occupational exposures, connective tissue disease (CTD) symptoms, chyle leak, and pulmonary manifestations (e.g. dyspnoea, cough, and spontaneous pneumothorax) in all adult patients at each clinic visit.
- For females with negative CT, obtain HRCT to screen for LAM every 5 years through menopause. For patients with evidence of LAM on CT, follow-up HRCT after 1-3 years.
- Routine serial PFT monitoring at least annually in patients with evidence of LAM on HRCT and more frequently in patients with rapid growth/therapy response.
- mTOR inhibitors for treatment of LAM with abnormal lung function (FEV1 < 70% predicted), physiological evidence of substantial disease burden (abnormal DLCO (<80% or less than lower limit of normal, air trapping (RV > 120%), resting or exercise-induced oxygen desaturation, rapid decline (rate of decline in FEV1 > 90ml/year), and chylous effusions.
- Advice regarding risk of pregnancy and exogenous oestrogen use. Avoid routine hormonal therapy or doxycycline for LAM treatment. Advise against tobacco smoke exposure.
- Trial inhaled bronchodilators in patients with symptoms of wheezing, dyspnoea, chest tightness, or obstructive defect on spirometry. Consider measurement of annual VEGF-D levels in patients who are unable to perform lung function tests.

SKIN:

- Annual skin examinations for children. Adult dermatologic evaluation frequency depends on the cutaneous manifestations. Ongoing education on sun protection.
- For flat or minimally elevated lesions, topical mTOR inhibitor treatment is recommended.

TEETH:

- Detailed clinical dental inspection/exam at least every 6 months.

HEART:

- ECG every 1-3 years in asymptomatic children until regression of cardiac rhabdomyomas is documented. More frequent/advanced diagnostics if symptomatic.
- ECG every 3-5 years in asymptomatic patients of all ages to monitor for conduction defects. More frequent/advanced diagnostics (e.g. ambulatory/event monitoring if symptomatic).

EYE:

- Annual ophthalmic evaluation at baseline. Rare cases of aggressive lesions or those causing vision loss (affecting the fovea or optic nerve) may require intervention. mTOR inhibitors have been used with some success to treat problematic retinal astrocytic hamartomas.
- For patients receiving vigabatrin, there are specific concerns related to visual field loss, which appears to correlate with total cumulative dose.

OTHER:

- Unexpected functional and non-functional pancreatic neuroendrocrine tumours (PNETS) may be found on abdominal MRI, requiring endocrinology input.

11 Gorlin syndrome

Background

In 1960, Gorlin and Goltz first described this neurocutaneous condition characterised by a predisposition towards tumour formation (tumorigenesis). These are most commonly multiple cutaneous basal cell carcinomas (BCCs) that develop from adolescence or young adulthood, as well as jaw cysts (odontogenic keratocystic tumours) and developmental anomalies (bifid ribs and palmar pits). It is also referred to as Basal Cell Naevus syndrome (BCNS).

Epidemiology

It is estimated to affect 1 in 31 000 people, although <1% patients with BCC have Gorlin syndrome.

Genetics

This is an AD-inherited condition with variable penetrance, although approximately 40% are *de novo* alterations. It is caused by alterations in *PTCH1*, located on chromosome 9, and mapped to 9q22.32 or *SUFU*, located on chromosome 10. The most common alterations include insertions of deletions resulting in frameshift and premature termination of the *PTCH1* translation, although missense and nonsense alterations have also been identified.

Pathophysiology

PTCH1 is a tumour suppressor gene that encodes a protein called patched-1. Patched-1 functions as a receptor to the 'Sonic Hedgehog' ligand (named after its spiky appearance). Patched-1 blocks cell division until sonic hedgehog is attached; therefore, an abnormal patched-1 receptor results in uncontrolled cell proliferation.

The sonic hedgehog pathway is involved in the development of embryonic structures and tumours; therefore, dysregulation of this pathway results in developmental defects and tumorigenesis as seen in Gorlin syndrome.

Symptoms and clinical features

Gorlin syndrome can be diagnosed in the presence of either two major, or one major and two minor criteria (Table 11.1).

- Cutaneous BCCs are slow-growing skin cancers caused by a lifetime accumulation of ultraviolet radiation. They therefore tend to affect sun-exposed sites (face, neck, chest, and arms).
- BCCs are the most common type of skin cancer, with average age of onset is the seventh decade (it is unusual for them to develop <30 years of age). They present as slow-growing plaques or nodules with a characteristic appearance; a pearly, shiny surface, dilated blood vessels (telangiectasia), and central ulceration with a rolled raised edge. However, in Gorlin syndrome, BCCs can appear atypical, sometimes appearing more like a melanocytic naevus (mole), neurofibroma, or skin tag. Furthermore, they also tend develop from adolescence or early adulthood onwards. Although phenotype is variable, it is not unheard of for patients with Gorlin syndrome to develop hundreds of BCCs throughout their lifetime. A younger age of onset should always question an underlying genetic cause. Metastases from BCC are extremely rare; however, if left untreated, they can invade muscle and bone.
- Macrocephaly and rib anomalies are normally present from birth; palmo-plantar pits develop as the patient gets older.
- The highest risk of medulloblastoma is from age 1–3 years in around 1% patients with Gorlin syndrome.
- Jaw cysts (often the first symptom of Gorlin syndrome) tend to develop from the age of 10 years (Figures 11.1–11.4).

Table 11.1 Diagnostic criteria.

Major criteria	Minor criteria
>2 BCCs or one if < 20 years	Macrocephaly
Odontogenic keratocysts of the jaw	Congenital malformations; Cleft lip, prominent forehead, 'coarse' facies, hypertelorism
>2 palmar or plantar pits	Other skeletal and radiological abnormalities, e.g. pectus deformity, fusion or elongation of vertebral bodies
Calcification of falx cerebri	Ovarian fibroma
Bifid/splayed/extra ribs; bifid vertebrae	Medulloblastoma
First degree relative with Gorlin syndrome	

Figure 11.1 Palmar pits.

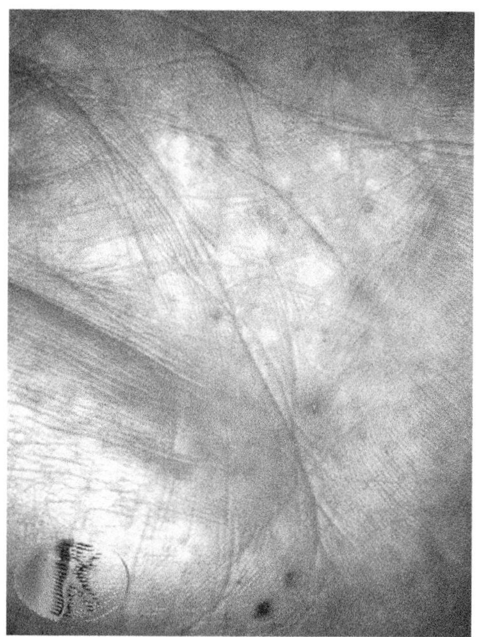

Source: DermNet New Zealand Trust.

Clinical Genetics and Genomics at a Glance, First Edition. Edited by Neeta Lakhani, Kunal Kulkarni, Julian Barwell, Pradeep Vasudevan, and Huw Dorkins.

Figure 11.2 Multiple BCC.

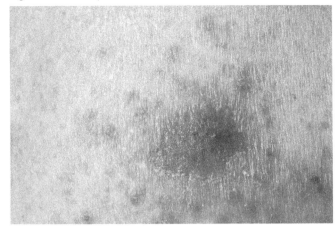

Source: Laura Ballard/Adobe Stock.

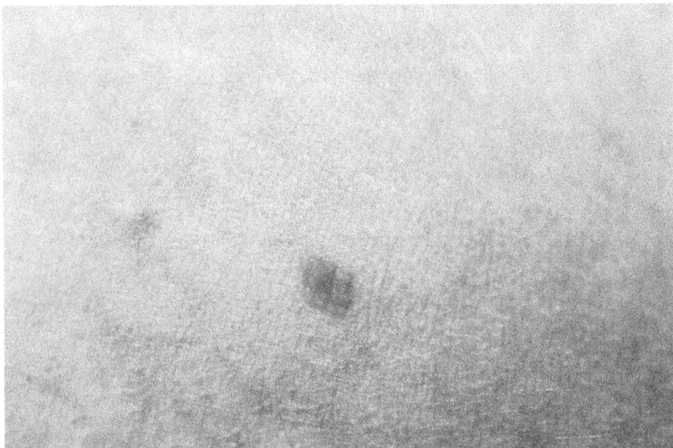

Source: ImagESine/Adobe Stock.

Figure 11.3 Odontogenic keratocysts.

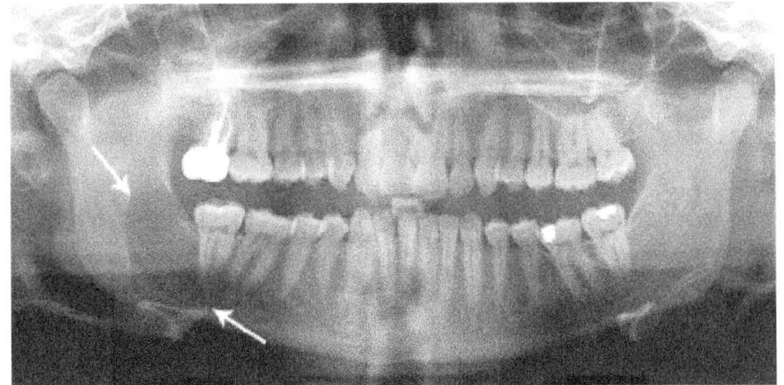

Source: Coronation Dental Specialty Group / Wikimedia / CC By 3.0.

Diagnosis

This is normally made clinically, although genetic testing can be performed. BCCs developing from a younger age are often the most striking clinical feature. Associated phenotypic features and a family history aid diagnosis. Although the appearance of BCCs can appear macroscopically slightly differently to BCCs in the normal population, histologically they are identical; therefore, a skin biopsy can confirm the presence of a BCC but clinical context is required to diagnose Gorlin syndrome.

Figure 11.4 Relative macrocephaly, hypertelorism, ectusexcavatum, kyphoscoliosis.

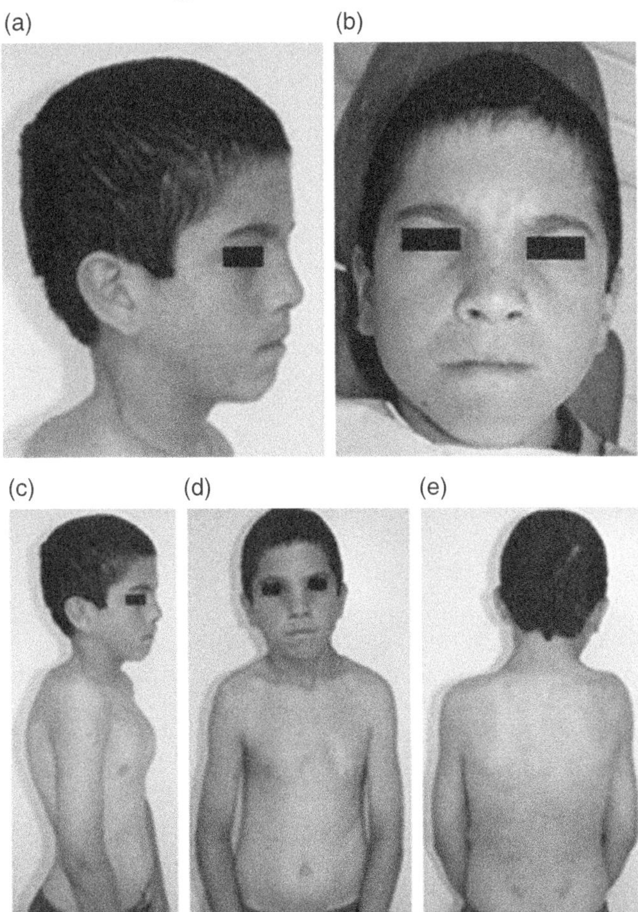

Management

- Preventing the development of BCCs through education and protection from UV exposure is important, alongside monitoring of vitamin D levels.
- Surgical excision is the gold standard treatment for BCC; consideration of the site, number of lesions, and patient preference are extremely important in managing multiple BCCs in Gorlin syndrome. Complete surgical excision is not always suitable; other options include curettage and cautery, cryotherapy, laser, photodynamic therapy, and topical treatments such as Imiquimod and Efudix (5-fluorouracil) cream. However, there is a higher risk of recurrence with these.
- Radiotherapy is often used as a treatment option for BCCs, but in patients with Gorlin syndrome, it must be avoided as it has been shown to result in an increased development of BCCs in the treated site that are often more aggressive.

The future

A recently developed small molecule biologic agent that inhibits smoothened (SMO), a component of the sonic hedgehog receptor, is FDA approved for the treatment of BCCs. It is the first of its kind and has shown promising results in treating BCCs and preventing their development although side effects such as nausea, muscle aches, and hair loss have limited its use.

Research into targeting different aspects of the sonic hedgehog pathway is likely to impact the management of BCCs and Gorlin syndrome in the future.

12 Darier's disease

Background

Also known as Darier-White disease and keratosis follicularis, Darier's disease was first described independently by White and Darier in 1889. It is characterised by a persistent eruption of hyperkeratotic papules that tend to present later than most genetic conditions, often in the second or third decade.

Epidemiology

Prevalence is estimated to be 1 in 30 000–50 000 in the United Kingdom. It affects males and females equally.

Genetics

Darier's disease is an AD-inherited condition that occurs as a result of alterations of the *ATP2A2* gene located on 12q24.11. Penetrance is 100%, although expressivity is variable. Sporadic cases are common, occurring in 40–50% cases.

Pathophysiology

The *ATP2A2* gene encodes the calcium pump Ca(2+)-ATPase-2 on the sarcoplasmic reticulum. This is considered to have a role in the Ca(2+)-signalling pathway that regulates cell-to-cell adhesion and differentiation of the epidermis. The late-onset of Darier's disease may be explained by an age-related critical dependence on the *ATP2A2*-encoded calcium pump in the epidermis.

Symptoms and clinical features

- Onset is usually in adolescence although this can vary.
- It is characterised by the onset of yellow-brown greasy firm rough or scaly papules in a classical distribution described as 'seborrhoiec,' i.e. trunk, flexures, scalp, and forehead. Papules may coalesce to form warty plaques. The papules may be itchy and become macerated and malodorous if secondarily infected.
- Other classical features include pits on the palms and soles, and distinctive nail changes including V-shaped nicks at the distal free margin of the nail, red and white longitudinal streaks. A cobblestone appearance of the oral mucosa may also be present (Figures 12.1–12.4).
- The severity of the phenotype can vary within families but also over time.
- It is a chronic condition with flares which can be triggered by sunlight, heat, stress, infection (bacterial, fungal, and viral), and some medications including lithium and trauma.
- When Darier's disease was first being described, it was said to be associated with neurological conditions such as mild learning disabilities, epilepsy, and depression. However, as we become more aware of the disease, more recent research suggests these associations may be coincidental.
- There are also linear and segmental variations of the disease.

Figure 12.1 Keratotic papules with pigmentation on (a) the neck and (b) armpit.

(a)

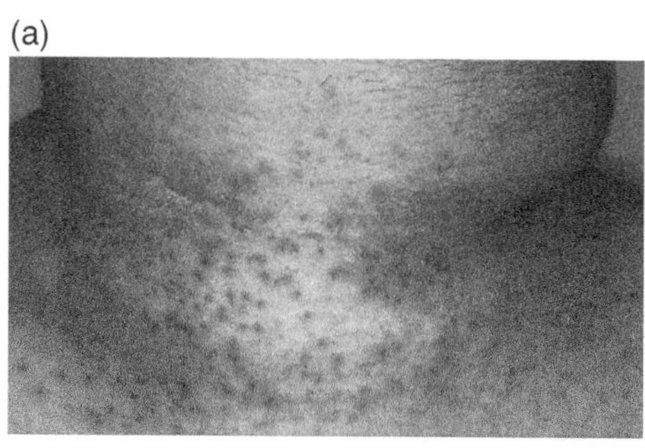

(b)

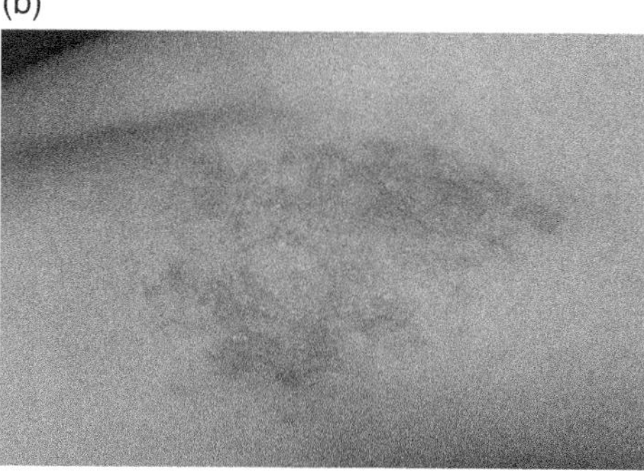

Source: Atsushi Takagi et al. (2016), John Wiley & Sons.

Figure 12.2 Verrucous lesions with keratotic crusts on the leg.

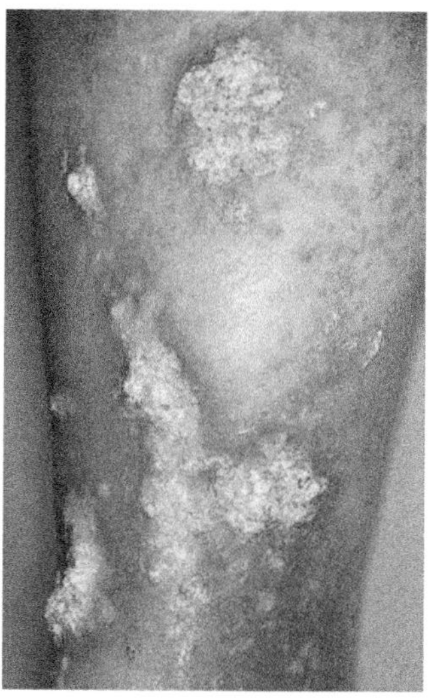

Source: Atsushi Takagi et al. (2016), John Wiley & Sons.

Clinical Genetics and Genomics at a Glance, First Edition. Edited by Neeta Lakhani, Kunal Kulkarni, Julian Barwell, Pradeep Vasudevan, and Huw Dorkins.

Figure 12.3 Papillomatous and macerated lesion in the groin.

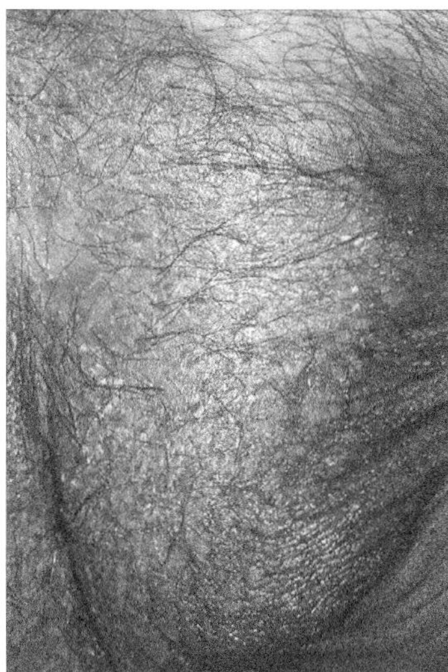

Source: Atsushi Takagi et al. (2016), John Wiley & Sons.

Figure 12.4 Pits and keratotic plugs on the sole.

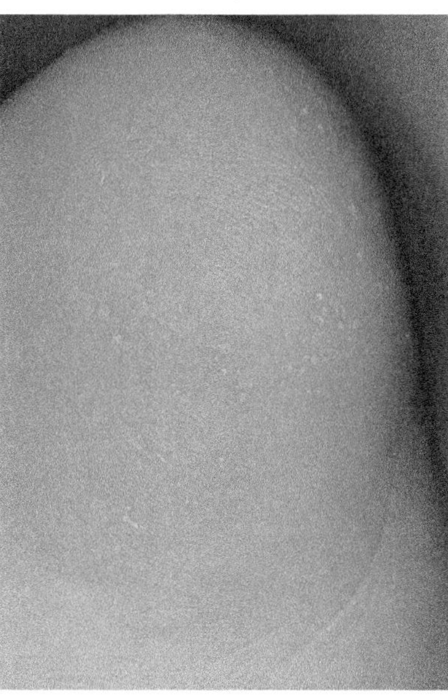

Source: Atsushi Takagi et al. (2016), John Wiley & Sons.

Diagnosis

- A diagnosis of Darier's disease can be made based upon clinical features alone; however, histological findings and gene testing can be supportive. Classical histological features include 'corps ronds and grains,' a term used to describe the suprabasal cleavage, acantholysis (loss of intracellular connections between keratinocytes), and abnormal keratinocytes (Figures 12.5 and 12.6).
- Differential diagnoses includes seborrhoiec dermatitis (greasy scaly erythematous plaques affecting face, scalp, and chest) and Hailey-Hailey disease (familial benign pemphigus resulting in erosions and plaques affecting the flexures).

Management

- A majority of patients manage their symptoms with regular emollients, simple hygiene, and avoidance of triggers. Antiseptic emollients may help prevent infection.

Figure 12.5 Example of suprabasal cleavage of the epidermis containing acantholytic cells (hematoxylin–eosin, original magnification x40).

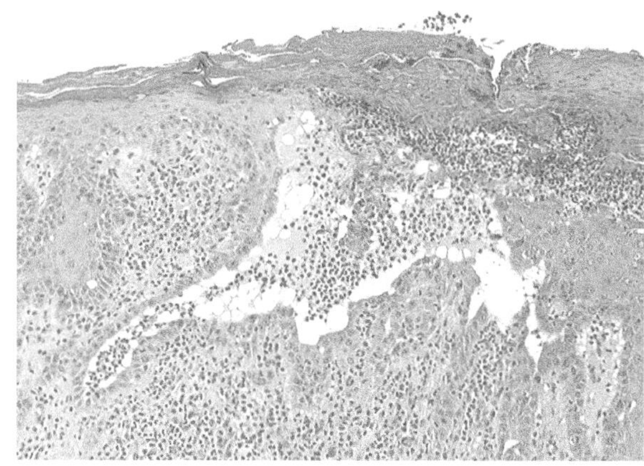

Source: Atsushi Takagi et al. (2016), John Wiley & Sons.

Figure 12.6 Keratotic plug and parakeratotic cells in the horny layer with abnormal keratinocytes comprising corps ronds in the granular layer (hematoxylin–eosin, original magnification x100).

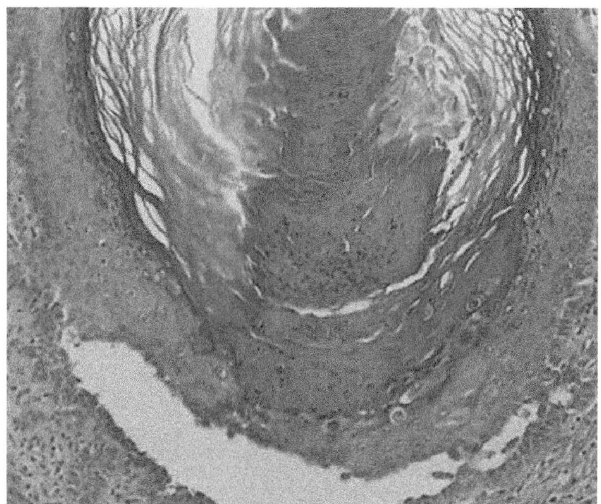

Source: Atsushi Takagi et al. (2016), John Wiley & Sons.

- Patients have an increased susceptibility to Herpes Simplex Virus and secondary bacterial and fungal infection; therefore, early treatment is essential to prevent severe flares. Bacterial and viral skin swabs and fungal scrapings are important, especially when flares do not respond to treatment.
- Topical retinoids or topical steroids can be used for flares and for those severely affected, oral retinoids can be effective; however, are highly teratogenic.

The future

It has been reported that UV exposure induces *COX2* which in turn suppresses *ATP2A2* expression; therefore, *COX2* inhibitors are being considered as a potential therapeutic option for Darier's disease awaiting clinical trials. Furthermore, Miglustat, a glucosylceramide synthase inhibitor, was reported to improve cell adhesion; therefore, it may be developed as a future treatment.

13 Lamellar ichthyosis

Background

Ichthyosis are a group of conditions that share a common feature of dry thick scaly skin. The word ichthyosis derives from the ancient Greek term for 'fish scales', so called due to the appearance of the thick brown scales that are associated with the condition. They occur mainly as a result of defects in the skin barrier function.

This section focuses on lamellar ichythyosis, also known as non-bullous congenital ichthyosiform erythroderma, which is a disorder of keratinisation, mostly limited to the skin (Table 13.1).

Epidemiology

Lamellar ichthyosis is estimated to affect 1 in 100 000 individuals. Two-thirds of patients are severely affected.

Genetics

This AR condition is caused by *TGM1* alterations in around 90% cases. *TGM1* encodes transglutaminase 1 (involved in the formation of the cornified envelope that forms a structural barrier in the upper epidermis). Its loci is 14q11. Individuals without a *TGM1* alteration may have an alteration affecting the *ABCA12* gene (ATP binding cassette A12), which encodes proteins responsible for the transport of molecules across cell membranes and is essential for skin barrier function.

Pathophysiology

The alterations associated with lamellar ichthyosis result in abnormal structure of the epidermis as well as altered epidermal fatty acids. This results in impaired thermoregulation, increased risk of infection, and water loss from the epidermis with an impaired skin barrier.

Symptoms and clinical features

- This condition classically presents at birth, where a neonate may have a 'collodion membrane', a tight translucent outer layer of skin that dries and sheds in the first few weeks of life. However, several other conditions can result in a collodion membrane at birth. An underlying erythroderma (where >90% of the skin is red) is evident.
- Most patients have palmoplantar keratoderma (PPK), which is abnormal keratin production of the palms and soles that results in thickened yellow rough skin which can be associated with painful fissuring and digital contractures.

Table 13.1 Main ichthyosis types and syndromes

Condition	Inheritance	Gene	Phenotype
Ichthyosis vulgaris	AD	*Profilaggrin*	Commonest type, presents after birth/early childhood with ichthyosis. Flexural sparing, hyperlinear palms and atopy.
X-linked ichthyosis	XLR	*Steroid sulfatase*	Presents in infancy with mild erythroderma and ichthyosis over extremities, trunk, and neck. Associated with corneal opacities and cryptorchidism.
Nethertons syndrome	AR	*SPINK5*	Presents at birth with erythroderma and scaling ± collodion membrane. Ichthyosis, bamboo-like hair, atopy.
Congenital ichthyosiform erythroderma	AR	*Transglutaminase 1*, *ALOXE3* or *ALOX12B*	Presents with collodion membrane at birth, erythroderma, scaling, flexural involvement, PPK, scarring alopecia, and heat intolerance.
Epidermolytic hyperkeratosis	AD	*KRT1, KRT10*	Presents at birth with erythroderma, bullae, erosions which develop into verrucous hyperkeratotic plaques, flexural involvement, PPK, and recurrent infections.
Harlequin ichthyosis	AR	*ABCA12*	Presents at birth with a hard, thickened restrictive stratum corneum. Death occurs within a few days due to respiratory difficulties and sepsis.
KIDS syndrome (Keratosis, ichthyosis, deafness)	AD	*GJB2* (connexion 26)	Presents at birth with hyperkeratotic plaques on extensor surfaces and face, PPK, sensorineural deafness, blindness, abnormal teeth/nails, and infections.
Conradi Hunermann syndrome	XLD	*EBP* (emopamil binding protein)	Presents at birth with ichthyosiform erythroderma developing into hyperkeratosis and then ice-pick-like scarring. Stippled appearances of bony epiphyses on X-ray, cataracts, deafness, and scarring alopecia.
Sjogren Larsson syndrome	AR	*FALDH* (fatty aldehyde dehydrogenase)	Presents at birth with erythema, generalised ichythosis, pruritis, PPK, and spastic tetraplegia.

Clinical Genetics and Genomics at a Glance, First Edition. Edited by Neeta Lakhani, Kunal Kulkarni, Julian Barwell, Pradeep Vasudevan, and Huw Dorkins.

- Other associations include nail dystrophy (ridging and thickening), scarring alopecia, ectropion *(eversion of eyelids)*, eclabium *(eversion of lips)*, loss of eyebrows and eye lashes, heat intolerance, and hypernatraemia.
- In later life, patients develop thickened brown scaling that is more prominent in the flexures but may cover the entire body surface area. Erythema is often minimal (Figure 13.1).

Figure 13.1 Thickened brown scaling.

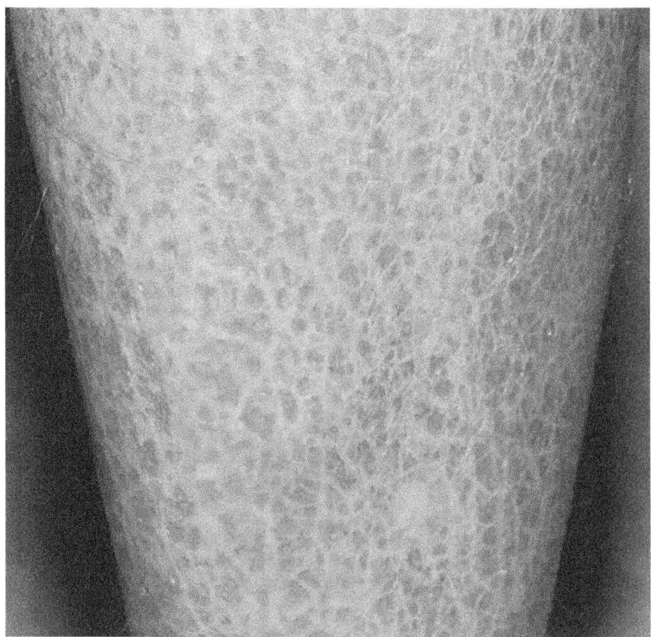

Diagnosis

Diagnosis can usually be made clinically, although a diagnostic skin biopsy and genetic testing can be supportive. Histology findings include massive orthokeratotic hyperkeratosis and acanthosis.

Management

- Regular application of urea-containing or bland emollients alleviates dry itchy skin. Urea-containing products are considered more effective for ichthyosis as urea has keratolytic properties and is therefore more effective in removing the thick scale found in ichthyosis. Prevention and treatment of secondary infection (including viral, bacterial, or fungal) is very important.
- Retinoids (vitamin A derivative), such as Acitretin, can be helpful where symptoms are not controlled with emollients alone. However, they are highly teratogenic for up to three years after withdrawing treatment.

The future

With greater availability of whole exome genome sequencing, further genes have been associated with lamellar icthyosis, including *ABCA12*, *ALOXE3*, *ALOX12B*, *CERS3*, *CYP4F22*, *NIPAL4/ICHTHYIN*, and *PNPLA1*. Improved understanding of the molecular and genetic basis of these conditions will help develop our understanding of the complex interactions of the skin barrier and identify more focused therapeutic targets.

14 Mal de Meleda

Background

Mal de Meleda is one of over 25 different types of inherited palmoplantar keratodermas (PPKs). PPKs all have one feature in common: hyperkeratosis resulting in yellowed thickened skin affecting the palms and soles. Inherited PPK can be divided into focal or diffuse forms. Mal de meleda results in a diffuse PPK that tends to present at or soon after birth. This condition is also known as keratoderma palmoplantaris transgrediens and acro-erythrokeratoderma. It is named after the Croatian Island of Meleda, where it was first described, and it remains more common in Mediterranean populations.

Epidemiology

Mal de Meleda is a rare condition, with estimated overall prevalence of 1 in 100 000.

Genetics

This AR-inherited condition is most commonly associated with alterations in the *SLURP-1* gene at 8q24.3. *SLURP-1* encodes the secreted LY6/urokinasetype plasminogen activator receptor (uPAR)-related protein-1. Sporadic cases are rare.

Pathophysiology

SLURP-1 is involved in inflammatory responses as well as regulation of keratinocyte apoptosis. Dysfunction therefore results in hyperkeratosis and abnormal inflammatory responses.

Symptoms and clinical features

- Presentation is usually at or soon after birth. Erythema of the palms and soles (with a well-defined boundary) often precedes the development of waxy thickened yellow plaques, extending across the surface of the palms and soles.
- Over time, transgrediens (hyperkeratosis progressing to the dorsal surface of hands and feet) and progrediens (worsening with age) develop. The PPK is sharply demarcated in a 'glove and stocking' distribution. Hyperhidrosis may also be present.
- If severe, the PPK can result in painful fissuring, loss of finger pulp volume, and restricted function.
- Nail abnormalities such as subungual hyperkeratosis, beau's lines, and onycholysis are commonly associated.
- Secondary bacterial or fungal infection is common.

Diagnosis

Diagnosis can be made clinically; however, a skin biopsy and genetic testing can support diagnosis. On skin histology, features observed include hyperkeratosis (thickening of the stratum corneum), acanthosis (thickening of the epidermis) without epidermolysis (splitting of the epidermis from dermis), and often an infiltration of lymphocytes within the dermis.

Differential diagnosis includes other forms of inherited PPK, ectodermal dysplasia, pachyonychia congenital, and epidermolysis bullosa simplex.

Management

- Regular application of emollients is important to protect the skin barrier and hydrate the skin. Keratolytic emollients, such as those containing urea, should be used to improve the hyperkeratosis.
- Prevention and treatment of secondary infection is important.
- Acitretin, a vitamin A-derived oral retinoid, can prove effective for some affected individuals, although it is highly teratogenic for up to three years after stopping treatment.
- Genetic counselling is warranted for families with a history of PPK (Table 14.1).

The future

TNF alpha may be involved in the inflammatory pathways associated with Mal de Meleda and may be a potential focus for future clinical trials.

Clinical Genetics and Genomics at a Glance, First Edition. Edited by Neeta Lakhani, Kunal Kulkarni, Julian Barwell, Pradeep Vasudevan, and Huw Dorkins.

Table 14.1 Summary of Palmoplantar keratodermas.

Disease	Key characteristics	Inheritance	Gene affected
Diffuse PPKs			
Non-epidermolytic PPK	Non-epidermolytic PPK, non-transgrediens, hyperhidrosis	AD	*KRT1*
Epidermolytic PPK	Epidermolytic hyperkeratosis, non-trangredient, hyperhidrosis	AD	*KRT9*
Vohwinkle syndrome, Classic	Mutilating keratoderma and deafness, scarring alopecia	AD	*GJB-2 (connexin 26)*
Olmsted syndrome	Mutilating keratoderma with periorificial plaques and autoamputation	AD	*TRPV3*
Papillon Lefevre syndrome	Transgredient PPK with periodontitis, early loss of teeth, hyperhidrosis	AR	*Cathepsin C*
Naxos disease	PPK, wooly hair, and right ventricular cardiomyopathy	AR	*Plakoglobin*
Carvajal syndrome	PPK, wooly hair, and dilated cardiomyopathy	AR	*Desmoplakin*
Focal PPKs			
Striate PPK	Linear hyperkeratotic plaques, onset in teens/early adulthood	AD	*Desmoglein 1 and desmoplakin 1*
Punctate PPK	Punctate keratoses on palms and soles presenting in adolescence. More common in those of Afro-Caribbean descent	AD	?
Acrokeratoelastoidosis	Crateriform papules over lateral and medial aspect of soles and palms. More common in those of Afro-Caribbean descent.	AD	?
Howel-Evans syndrome	Focal PPK over pressure areas, oral leucokeratoses, and associated with oesophageal cancer	AD	*TOC*
Tyrosinaemia type II	Painful focal PPK, corneal ulcers, hyperhidrosis, treat with diet restriction of tyrosine and phenylalanine	AR	*TAT (hepatic tyrosine amino transferase)*
Other causes of PPK			
Epidermolysis bullosa simplex, localised	PPK in areas of trauma plus blistering	AD	*KRT5, KRT14*
Pachyonychia congenita	Painful focal PPK, dystrophic nails, oral leukokeratosis	AD	*KRT6, KRT16, KRT17*
Ectodermal dysplasia	Many different types, features may include diffuse PPK, conical teeth, dystrophic nails, abnormal hair growth and abnormal sweating,	AD	*GJB6, EDA, p63, plakophilin-1*

15 Cutaneous porphyria

Background

Porphyria are a rare group of conditions that are caused by enzyme deficiencies in the biosynthesis of haem. Porphyrias can be divided into acute and cutaneous reflecting their primary presenting feature as shown below and conditions within these groups can have overlapping features (Table 15.1).

Table 15.1 Acute vs cutaneous porphyrias.

Acute	Cutaneous
• ALA dehydratase porphyria (ADP) • Acute intermittent porphyria (AIP) • Hereditary coproporphyria (HCP) • Variegate porphyria (VP)	• Congenital erythropoeitic porphyria (CEP) • Porphyria cutanea tarda (PCT) • Hepatoerythropoietic porphyria (HEP) • Hereditary coproporhyria (HC) • Variegate porphyria (VP)

Epidemiology

Overall prevalence of the acute porphyrias is around 5 per 100 000. The most common acute porphyria, AIP, has a prevalence of around 1 in 20 000. PCT, the commonest overall, has a prevalence of 1 in 10 000. Others, such as CEP, are extremely rare, with an estimated prevalence of <1 in 1 000 000.

Genetics

The majority are inherited in an AD manner with the exception of congenital erythropoeitic porphyria (CEP) and hepatoerthryopoietic porphyria (HEP), which are inherited as AR. *See descriptions of each condition for further details.*

Pathophysiology

Porphyrin is a compound made up of four pyrrole rings that are linked by methane bridges into a large ring structure. Haem is formed when ferrous iron inserts into the centre of the porphyrin molecule allowing it to carry out its function of oxygen delivery. In skin disease, singlet oxygen produced as a result of photons of

Figure 15.1 A simplified illustration of enzyme defects and associated porphyrias.

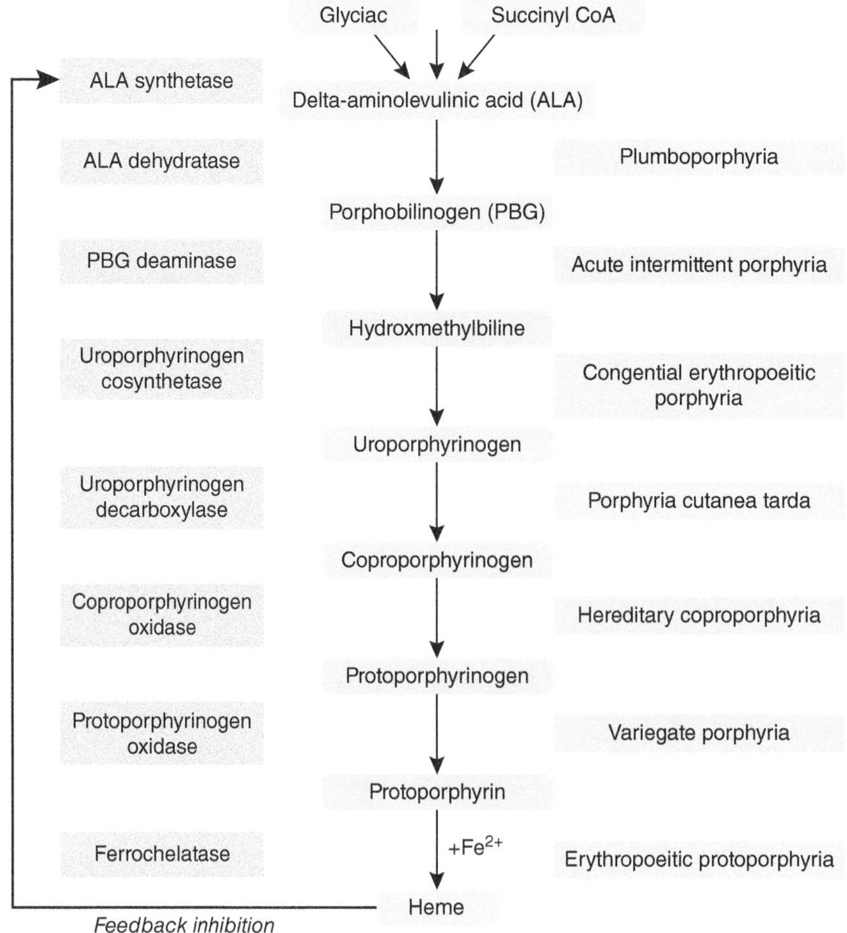

Clinical Genetics and Genomics at a Glance, First Edition. Edited by Neeta Lakhani, Kunal Kulkarni, Julian Barwell, Pradeep Vasudevan, and Huw Dorkins.

violet light altering the porphyrin molecule leads to direct tissue damage, mast cell degranulation, matrix melanoproteinase activity, and complement activation. Enzyme deficiencies along the pathway involved in the synthesis of haem results in porphyria. Figure 15.1 demonstrates the enzyme deficiencies involved in the particular conditions.

Symptoms and clinical features

Acute porphyrias tend to present with a range of non-specific neuro-visceral symptoms including abdominal pain, psychiatric complaints, and neurological symptoms. Cutaneous porphyrias tend to present with skin fragility and blistering usually on sun-exposed sites.

Cutaneous porphyrias can be further subdivided into ones that cause cutaneous disease only and others that cause cutaneous disease and acute attacks as shown below (Table 15.2).

Table 15.2 Different types of cutaneous porphyrias.

Cutaneous disease and acute attacks	Cutaneous disease only
• Porphyria cutanea tarda (PCT) • Congenital erythropoietic porphyria (CEP) • Erythropoietic protoporphyria (EPP) • Hepatoerythropoietic porphyria (HEP)	• Hereditary coproporphyria (HC) • Variegate porphyria (VP)

- **PCT:** There are two types. Type I (sporadic – 75% of patients) is acquired and Type II (familial – 25% of patients associated with *UROD* gene alterations) is inherited in an AD manner. Type II PCT usually presents at a younger age. Patients present with fragility and bullae on areas of sun-exposed skin in particular dorsal aspects of hands and forearms. These heal leaving scars, milia, and mottled hyper/hypopigmentation. Scarring alopecia following bullae on scalp hypertrichosis on upper face and forehead, ears, or arms are also seen. Melasma-like hyperpigmentation in the periorbital region. Morphea like plaques on the trunk and morpheic changes on the scalp have been reported.
- **CEP:** This is a rare AR condition leading to deficiency of uroporphyrinogen III cosynthatase enzyme. Presentation can vary from mild disease to severe disease starting in infancy. There is extreme photosensitivity in infancy with bullae formation and subsequent mutilated scarring. Patients often have hypertrichosis of the face and upper arms. CEP can affect the teeth causing brown staining that fluoresce red under Wood's light. Eyes and bone marrow involvement can occur. Patients are at a high risk of skin cancer and avoidance of sunlight may lead to impaired vitamin D metabolism. Urine is often pink or brown which fluoresces red under Wood's light.
- **EPP:** This is an AD-inherited condition caused by deficiency in ferrochelatase enzyme. Patients present with immediate pain on sun exposure, severe photosensitivity, and burning. There is subsequent waxy scarring. This condition can rarely cause hepatic disease.
- **HEP:** HEP is caused by a deficiency in uroporphyrinogen decarboxylase enzyme same as PCT. It is inherited in an AR manner and has clinical features that are between PCT and CEP.
- **HC:** This condition is inherited in an AD manner and results in a deficiency of coproporphyrinogen oxidase enzyme. Skin features are found in approximately 10-20% of patients suffering from this disease. Clinical features include bullae and skin fragility in sun-exposed areas which mimic PCT or VP. HC may reflect liver disease and may be worsened with liver involvement.
- **VP:** This is a rare AD condition. Protoporphyrinogen oxidase is the deficient enzyme. Patients usually present during adolescence with 70% of patients having skin manifestations. Clinical features are indistinguishable from PCT. Patients tend to develop intercurrent biliary obstruction which worsens skin disease.

Diagnosis

This is based on clinical biochemical correlation together with genetic testing. Measurement of porphyrins and porphyrin precursors in urine, stool, blood, and plasma will help confirm the diagnosis (Table 15.3). Knowing the haem synthesis pathway is key to interpreting and understanding the biochemical abnormalities. Uroporphyrin and Coproporphyrin are excreted into the urine. Coproporphyrin and Protoporphyrin into faeces (Table 15.1).

Table 15.3 Biochemical measurements of porphyrias and porphyrin precursors in urine, stool, and blood.

Condition	Urine	Stool	RBC	Plasma
PCT	↑↑Uroporphyrin III > Hepatocarboxyporphyrin Pink - Wood's lamp	↑Isocoproporphyrin Heptacarboxy-porphyrin	Normal levels	Peak at 615–620 nm
CEP	↑↑Uroporphyrin I/ Coproporphyrin I	↑↑Coproporhyrin I	Zinc and free protoporphyrin; ↑Uroporphyrin I; Coproporphyrin I	Peak at 615–620 nm
EPP	Normal	↑↑Protoporhyrin	↑↑Free protoporphyrin	Peak at 626–634 nm
HEP	↑Uroporphyrin	↑Uroporphyrin, Coproporphyrin	↑Protoporhyrin	Peak at 615–620 nm
HC	Corporphyrin III	Corporphyrin III	Normal levels	Peak at 615–620 nm
VP	Coproporphyrin III	Protoporphyrin, Coproporphyrin III, X-porphyrin	Normal levels	Peak at 624–627 nm

Management

Photoprotection is vital for all forms of cutaneous and mixed porphyrias. Information on adequate clothing, eye protection, and use of sun block on exposed and covered skin needs to be provided (Table 15.4).

The future

The variable clinical expression of the porphyrias depends on the nature and severity of the underlying enzymatic abnormality and the activity of the first/rate-limiting enzymes, alongside the ALA-synthase in the liver and bone marrow. While current therapies mostly address symptoms, advances in understanding of the pathophysiology of porphyrias are driving development of novel therapeutic strategies.

Table 15.4 Management of porphyrias.

Condition	Treatment
PCT	Phlebotomy, Chloroquine, Interferon, Desferoxamine, and Erythropoietin (Haemodialysis)
CEP	Vitamin D supplementation Ophthalmic and dental care Red cell transfusions Allogenic haematopoietic transplant
VP	Phlebotomy
HCP	Phlebotomy
HEP	Same as CEP
EPP	Subcutaneous afamelanotide to improve sunlight tolerance Betacarotene Vitamin D supplementation Patients with cirrhosis or severe protoporphyric hepatopathy should be referred for liver transplant

16 Cowden syndrome and Cowden-like syndrome

Background

Cowden syndrome is a cancer predisposition syndrome characterised by multiple benign growths called hamartomas. This condition has been seen to overlap with other cancer predisposition syndromes that produce hamartomas called Bannayan-Riley-Ruvalcaba syndrome and Proteus-like syndrome. Alongside segmental overgrowth lipomatosis arteriovenous malformation epidermal nevus (SOLAMEN) syndrome, these conditions are thought of as a spectrum of overlapping conditions known as '*PTEN* hamartoma tumour syndrome', due to their aetiology.

Epidemiology

Some studies have shown a female predominance in Cowden syndrome. Most patients reported in the literature are Caucasian. Some estimates show the incidence to be approximately 1 in 200 000.

Cowden syndrome is also associated with a increased risk of endometrial cancer. Inherited alterations in fumarate hydrates can cause severe fibroids and retroperitoneal sarcomas and alterations in the *SMARCA4* gene can cause small cell hypercalcaemic type ovarian cancer. Squamous cell cervical cancer is usually partially due to the human papilloma viruses but adenocarcinoma can be seen in *BRCA* affected families.

Genetics

- Cowden syndrome is inherited in an AD manner.
- These syndromes can be caused by alterations in one of four genes: *PTEN* (phosphatase and tensin homolog), *SDHB* (succinate dehydrogenase complex iron sulphur subunit B), *SDHD* (succinate dehydrogenase complex subunit D), and *KLLN* (killin), inherited in an AD fashion. Most cases (80%) are secondary to an alteration in *PTEN*, located at 10q23.
- A small proportion have variations in *SDHB* or *SDHD*, which produce succinate dehydrogenase (SDH), although this is controversial.
- When Cowden syndrome and Cowden-like syndrome are not related to changes in the *PTEN*, *SDHB*, *SDHD*, or *KLLN* genes, their cause is unknown.

Pathophysiology

- *PTEN* produces a protein product that is a tumour suppressor gene. An alteration within this gene is deemed as highly penetrant. Specifically, the phosphatidylinositol 3-kinase (PI3K)/AKT/mammalian target of rapamycin (mTOR) pathway is downregulated by the *PTEN* gene product, resulting in decreased cellular proliferation and survival, leading to uncontrolled cell division and the formation of hamartomas and cancerous tumours. The *PTEN* gene likely has other important functions within cells; however, it is unclear how alterations cause the other features of Cowden syndrome, such as macrocephaly and intellectual disability.
- Other cases are otherwise secondary to *KLLN* alterations. This gene provides instructions for making a protein called killin, which also likely acts as a tumour suppressor (p53-regulated DNA replication inhibitor). The genetic change that causes Cowden and Cowden-like syndrome is known as promoter hypermethylation. The promoter is a region of DNA that controls gene activity (expression). Hypermethylation occurs when too many small molecules called methyl groups are attached to the promoter region. The extra methyl groups reduce the expression of *KLLN*, resulting in less killin produced, which may allow abnormal cells to survive and proliferate inappropriately, leading to the formation of tumours.
- SDH is an important enzyme for energy production in cells, as well as playing a role in signalling pathways that regulate cell survival and proliferation. Defective SDH may allow cells to grow and divide unchecked, leading to the formation of hamartomas and cancerous tumours. However, it is unclear whether the identified variants are directly associated with Cowden and Cowden-like syndrome, as some of the variants described above have also been identified in people without the features of these conditions.

Symptoms and clinical features

- Individuals with Cowden syndrome almost inevitably develop hamartomas involving mucocutaneous and extracutaneous sites with an increased risk of malignancy. These growths are found all over the body, although most are found on the skin and mucous membranes. The skins manifestations usually occur in the 20s–30s (Figure 16.1).
- As a cancer predisposition syndrome, there is an increased risk of multiple types of cancers, including breast, thyroid, and endometrium. Cancers such as colorectal, kidney, and melanomas can also occur. These cancers present at a younger age, and can occur in an affected individual's 30s.
- Other associated signs and symptoms are a relative macrocephaly, and a rare and benign brain tumour called Lhermitte-Duclos disease, delayed development, and learning difficulties (Table 16.1).

Table 16.1 Clinical features.

Mucocutaneous lesions	• Skin-coloured lichenoid papules in perioral and periocular areas • Acral keratoses on palms and soles on palmar and plantar aspects • Papillomatous lesions on labial and buccal mucosa, fauces, and oro-pharynx and may extend to larynx • Lipomas • Fibromas
Extracutaneous lesions	• Intestinal polyps • Fibrocystic disease of the breast • Uterine fibroids • Thyroid adenoma • Multinodular goitre
Malignancies	• Thyroid carcinoma • Breast carcinoma • Renal carcinoma • Endometrial carcinoma

Clinical Genetics and Genomics at a Glance, First Edition. Edited by Neeta Lakhani, Kunal Kulkarni, Julian Barwell, Pradeep Vasudevan, and Huw Dorkins.

Table 16.2 Major and minor criteria.

Major	Minor
Breast cancer Endometrial cancer (epithelial) Thyroid cancer (follicular) GI hamartomas (including ganglioneuromas, but excluding hyperplastic polyps; ≥3) Lhermitte-Duclos disease (adult) Macrocephaly (≥97 percentile: 58 cm for females, 60 cm for males) Macular pigmentation of the glans penis Multiple mucocutaneous lesions (any of the following): Multiple trichilemmomas (≥3, at least one biopsy proven) Acral keratoses (≥3 palmoplantar keratotic pits and/or acral hyperkeratotic papules) Mucocutaneous neuromas (≥3) Oral papillomas (particularly on tongue and gingiva), multiple (≥3) OR biopsy proven OR dermatologist diagnosed	Autism spectrum disorder Colon cancer Esophageal glycogenic acanthoses (≥3) Lipomas (≥3) Intellectual disability (i.e. IQ ≤75) Renal cell carcinoma Testicular lipomatosis Thyroid cancer (papillary or follicular variant of papillary) Thyroid structural lesions (e.g. adenoma, multinodular goiter) Vascular anomalies (including multiple intracranial developmental venous anomalies)

Diagnosis

The National Comprehensive Cancer Network (NCCN) diagnostic criteria are most widely used in suspected cases of Cowden syndrome. Diagnostic criteria (NCCN 2016) are divided up into two categories (Table 16.2).

An operational diagnosis of Cowden is made if an patient meets either of the following:

- ≥3 major criteria, but one must include macrocephaly, Lhermitte-Duclos disease, or GI hamartomas; or
- Two major and three minor criteria.

Patients who meet the diagnostic criteria for Cowden syndrome should have their risk assessment and counselling undertaken by the clinical genetics team. Family status of suspected individuals needs to be assessed and in patients with no known familial *PTEN alteration,* comprehensive genetic testing of the individual and a family member needs to be conducted.

Some individuals have some of the characteristic features of Cowden syndrome, particularly the cancers associated with this condition, but do not meet the strict criteria for a diagnosis of Cowden syndrome and are described as having Cowden-like syndrome.

Management

Management is multidisciplinary and is largely based upon the clinical features. Patients who meet the diagnostic criteria for Cowden syndrome should have their risk assessment and counselling undertaken by the clinical genetics team. Family status of suspected individuals needs to be assessed and in patients with no known familial *PTEN alteration,* comprehensive genetic testing of the individual and a family member needs to be conducted (may have varying facets of the condition).

Cutaneous lesions are often troublesome and can be managed by surgical excision, 5-fluorouracil, mTOR inhibitors, laser, or isotretinoin.

Management largely involves a lifelong screening programme (Table 16.3):

- Children should have neurodevelopmental assessments
- Adults require baseline thyroid ultrasound examination

Table 16.3 NCCN surveillance guidelines.

Men and Women

- Annual comprehensive physical exam starting at age 18 yr or 5 yr before the youngest age of diagnosis of a component cancer in the family (whichever comes first), with particular attention to thyroid exam.
- Annual thyroid ultrasound starting at time of PHTS diagnosis.
- Colonoscopy, starting at age 35 yr unless symptomatic or if close relative with colon cancer before age 40 yr then start 5–10 yr before the earliest known colon cancer in the family. Colonoscopy should be done every 5 yr or more frequently if patient is symptomatic or polyps found.
- Consider renal ultrasound starting at age 40 yr, then every 1–2 yr.
- Dermatologic management may be indicated for some patients.
- Consider psychomotor assessment in children at diagnosis and brain MRI if there are symptoms.
- Education regarding the signs and symptoms of cancer.

Women

- Breast awareness starting at age 18 yr.
- Clinical breast exam, every 6–12 mo, starting at age 25 yr or 5–10 yr before the earliest known breast cancer in the family (whichever comes first).
- Breast screening.
- Annual mammography and breast MRI screening starting at age 30–35 yr or 5–10 yr before the earliest known breast cancer in the family (whichever comes first).
- Age >75 yr, management should be considered on an individual basis.
- For women with a *PTEN* alteration who are treated for breast cancer, screening of remaining breast tissue with annual mammography and breast MRI should continue.
- For endometrial cancer screening, encourage patient education and prompt response to symptoms (e.g. abnormal bleeding). Consider annual random endometrial biopsies and/or ultrasound beginning at age 30–35 yr.
- Discuss option of hysterectomy upon completion of childbearing and counsel regarding degree of protection, extent of cancer risk, and reproductive desires.
- Discuss option of risk-reducing mastectomy and counsel regarding degree of protection, extent of cancer risk, and reconstruction options.
- Address psychosocial, social, and quality-of-life aspects of undergoing risk-reducing mastectomy and/or hysterectomy.

Relatives

- Advise about possible inherited cancer risk to relatives, options for risk assessment, and management.
- Recommend genetic counselling and consideration of genetic testing for at-risk relatives.

Reproductive options

- For women of reproductive age, advise about options for prenatal diagnosis and assisted reproduction including pre-implantation genetic diagnosis. Discussion should include known risks, limitations, and benefits of these technologies.

- Women aged >30 years require regular breast screening
- Men and women aged >35 years require colonoscopy

Long term follow-up and surveillance guidelines have been recommended by NCCN. These are shown in the table below.

The future

Clinical trials often focus on the improved management of the respective cancers that arise, including on the use of sirolimus and other novel therapeutic agents.

Figure 16.1 Clinical features.

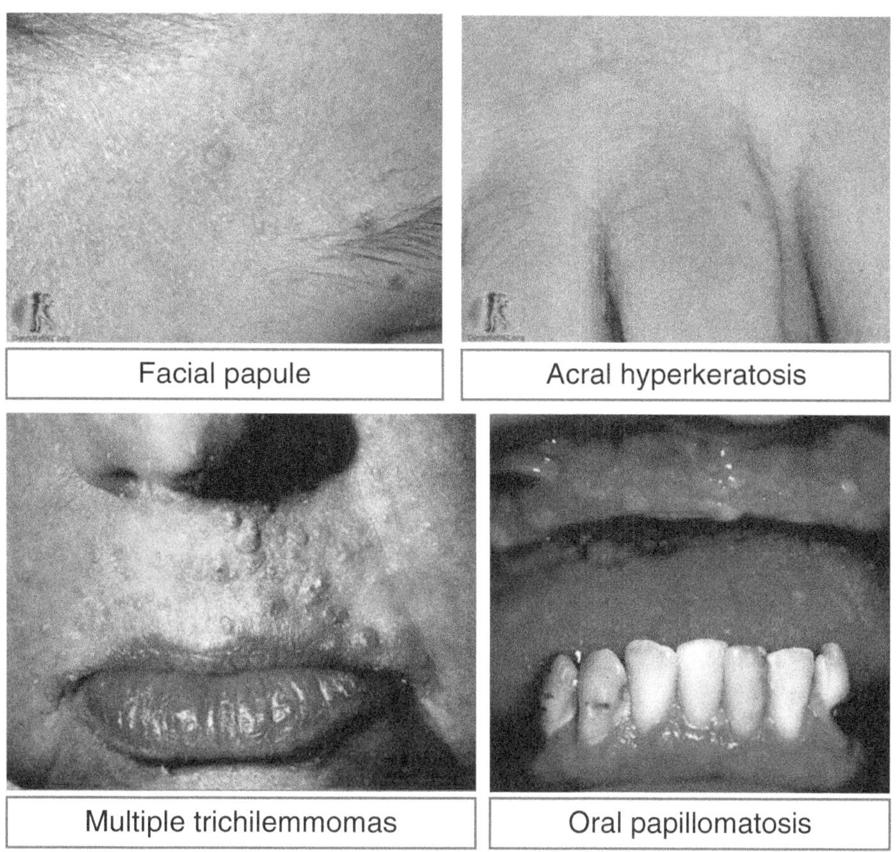

Source: DermNet New Zealand Trust.

17 Epidermolysis bullosa

Background

Epidermolysis bullosa (EB) encompasses a group of inherited disorders that are characterised by the common feature of skin and mucous membrane blistering lesions. Internal membranes are also susceptible, including in the respiratory tract and gut. Lesions are often, although not always secondary to minor trauma or friction.

Epidemiology

1 in 17 000 live births are affected. Males and females are equally affected, with no specific ethnic preponderance.

Genetics

Both AD-inherited and AR-inherited forms exist. There are four main variants of EB, each causing blister formation at different skin layers (Figure 17.1). These include:

- Epidermolysis bullosa simplex (EBS) – epidermis (keratinocytes). Around 12 subtypes. AD or AR. Genes affected include *Keratins 5, 14; Plectin.*
- Junctional epidermolysis bullosa (JEB) – lamina lucida (within basement membrane). Around 6 subtypes. AR. Genes affected include *Collagen XVII, Integrin,* and *Laminin.*
- Dystrophic epidermolysis bullosa (DEB) – lamina densa and upper dermis. Around 13 subtypes. AD or AR. Genes affected include *Collagen VII.*
- Kindler syndrome – a mixed pattern affecting multiple levels within and below the basement membrane. AR. Genes affected include *FERMT1.*

Pathophysiology

EB results from defects in skin adhesion molecules. Around 30 subtypes (variants) exist within these four categories (Table 17.1).

Figure 17.1 Alterations affecting different skin layers.

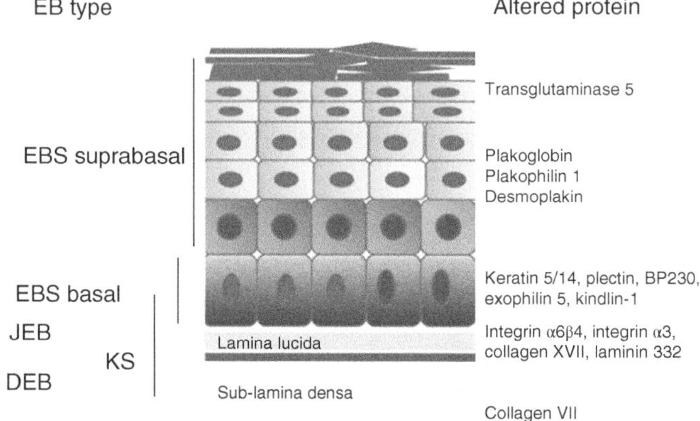

Symptoms and clinical features

Presentation is usually at birth or in early childhood, although can rarely be early adulthood. Presentation depends on the particular variant (Figure 17.2).

Table 17.1 Features of different types of epidermolysis bullosa.

Major EB type	Major subtype	Minor subtype	Affected gene (protein)	Typical inheritance	Clinical features
Simplex	Suprabasal	Lethal acantholytic EB	*DSP* (desmoplakin)	AR	Rare, rapidly progressive erosions, fatal in neonatal period
		Plakophilin deficiency (ectodermal dysplasia with skin fragility)	*PKP1* (plakophilin)	AR	Spontaneous erosions and fissures – perioral area, fissured keratoderma, wooly hair, nail dystrophy, growth failure
		EBS superficialis	*COL7A1* (type VII collagen)	AD	Superficial erosions
	Basal	Localised (Weber-Cockayne)	*KRT5, KRT14*	AD	Blisters of hands and feet, mild oral disease
		Generalised severe (Dowling – Meara)	*KRT5, KRT14*	AD (30% cases sporadic)	Blisters occur in groups. Mucocutaneous blistering severe in infancy with shedding of nails and formation of milia Spontaneous annular blistering on trunk limbs and neck Irregular hyperkeratosis of palms and soles confluent keratoderma – tends to improve with age
		Other generalised (Koebner)	*KRT5, KRT14*	AD	Blisters appear within first year and may be present at birth. Infancy – occiput, back, legs. Childhood – hands and feet. Hair nails and teeth normal
		With mottled pigmentation	*KRT5*	AD	Associated pigmentary changes present at birth or appear during infancy. Small tan coloured macules spread from acral sites to trunk and fade with age
		With muscular dystrophy	*PLEC1* (plectin)	AR	Blisters present skin and mucosa present at birth. Muscle weakness and waisting severe and evident in early childhood. Supraglottic hoarsness and scarring

Clinical Genetics and Genomics at a Glance, First Edition. Edited by Neeta Lakhani, Kunal Kulkarni, Julian Barwell, Pradeep Vasudevan, and Huw Dorkins.

Table 17.1 Continued

Major EB type	Major subtype	Minor subtype	Affected gene (protein)	Typical inheritance	Clinical features
		With pyloric atresia	*PLEC1, ITGA6, ITGB4* (intergrin)	AR	Poor prognosis. Widespread blisters and erosions that increase infection risk
		Autosomal recessive	*KRT14*	AR	Blisters are scattered usually minor palmoplantar keratoderma, varying degrees of nail dystrophy, atrophic scarring, hyperpigmentation, oral and genital blistering
		Ogna	*PLEC1*	AD	Seasonal blistering, generalised bruising, haemorrhagic bullae, and onychogryphotic toenails
		Migratory circinate	*KRT5*	AD	Present at birth, generalised in distribution, migratory circinate erythema, and postinflammatory hyperpigmentation
Junctional	Generalised	Severe	*Laminin-332*	AR	Blistering erosions soon after birth and rapidly becomes generalised, oropharyngeal involvement, hoarseness, stridor (laryngeal involvement). Lesions occur symmetrically around nose and mouth, neck trunk, buttocks, upper respiratory tract, teeth nail, eye, and GU involvement
		Intermediate	*Laminin-332, type XV11 collagen*	AR	Early clinical course similar to generalised severe JEB but patients usually survive to adulthood. Mucocutaneous disorder. Nail involvement. Lesions heal with atrophic scarring. Alopecia, pigmented naevi or acquired macular hyperpigmented lesions with irregular border. Oesophageal stricture, laryngeal involvement, corneal involvement, urethral stricture
		Late onset	*Type XVII collagen*	AR	Aged 5–8 initially trauma-induced blisters on hands and feet – may precede nail dystrophy. Later knees and elbows are involved
		With pyloric atresia	*A6, B4* (intergrin)		Teeth hypoplastic lacking normal enamel. Nails are dystrophic. Feeding results in vomiting. Haematuria dysuria and recurrent UTI
		With respiratory and renal involvement	*A3 intergrin*		Congenital nephrotic syndrome, ILD, and skin fragility
	Localised	Localised	*Laminin-332, type XVII collagen a6, and b4 intergrein*	AR	Nail dystrophy, dental enamel changes, and blistering involving lower legs and feet. In some, blistering can happen as a neonate but in others late onset disease
		Inversa	*Laminin-332*		Neonatal period whole skin may be fragile with generalised blistering. Later predilection for groins, perineum, and axillae. Dysplastic teeth, erosions of cornea feet, and nail dystrophy
		Laryngo-onycho-cutaneous syndrome	*Laminin a3a*	AR	Starts in infancy. Chronic erosions affecting the face (around nose and mouth). Erosions are also seen on limbs, trunk, and genitalia. Periungual and subungual inflammation on nails. Hoarseness
Dystrophic	Dominant	Generalised Acral Pretibial Pruriginosa Nails only Bullous dermolysis of newborn	*COL7A1*	AD	Skin fragility Blistering Scarring Nail dystrophy Milia formation Mucosal involvement is common Erosions and scarring can affect the mouth oesophagus genitalia and anus
	Recessive	Severe generalised Generalised other Inversa Pretibial Pruriginosa Centripetalis Bullous dermolysis of newborn	*COL7A1*	AR	
Kindler syndrome			*FERMT1* (kindlin-1)	AR	Skin blistering lessens during childhood. Signs of progressive poikiloderma develop. Gingivitis, Ectropion, Corneal erosions, periodontal disease, scarring of external urethral meatus. Increased risk of SCC

Diagnosis

It is important to exclude other differentials of blistering, including infection (bacterial, viral, and fungal), trauma (common friction blisters), metabolic (acrodermatitis enteropathica, Aminoacidureas), and autoimmune (bullous pemphigoid, pemphigus; non-inherited epidermolysis bullosa acquisita, EBA, which often develops in later adult life) (Figure 17.3).

Figure 17.2 Clinical features of different subtypes.

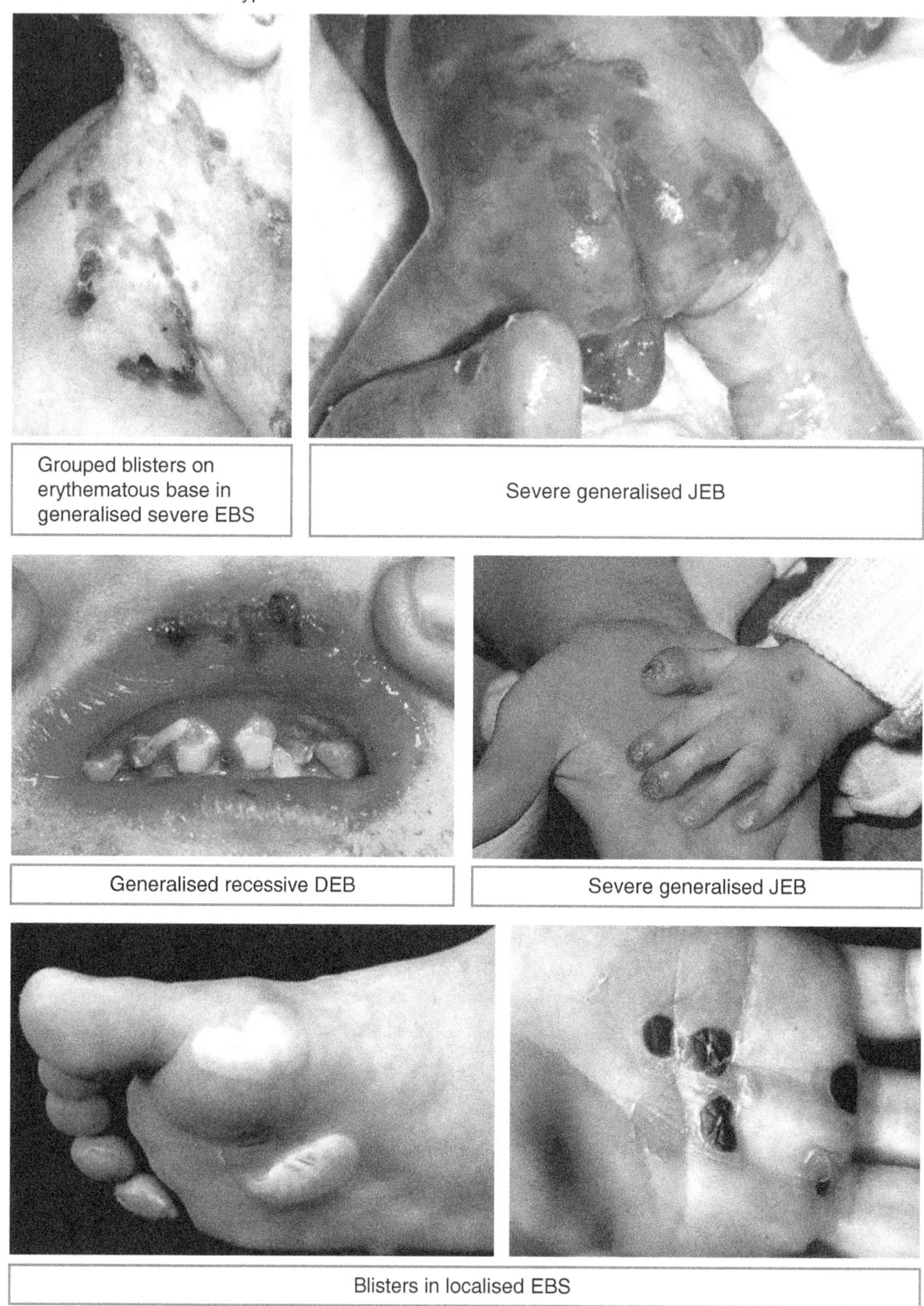

Management

There is no cure, so management focuses on skin protection and avoidance of provoking factors.

- **Neonates and infants:** Expert nursing care is required (paediatric nurse specialists in EB care), with nursing on thick foam pads covered by a silk sheet. Erosions are cleaned with sterile normal saline and covered in comfortable non-adherent dressing.
- **EBS:** Heat and humidity lower the threshold for blistering, so steps should be taken to reduce both of these factors. Individuals with localised or generalised EB should wear well fitted and ventilated shoes with a soft inner lining. Use of aluminium hydroxide or Botox can be used to reduce sweating.
- **JEB (generalised severe):** This is a severe form of JEB, usually with poor prognosis and so most affected individuals do not survive. There is mucocutaneous fragility, so extreme care must be taken in handling. Extracutaneous abnormalities include muscular dystrophy and pyloric atresia. Tracheostomy may be required for vocal hoarseness and airway obstruction.

Figure 17.3 Diagnostic algorithm.

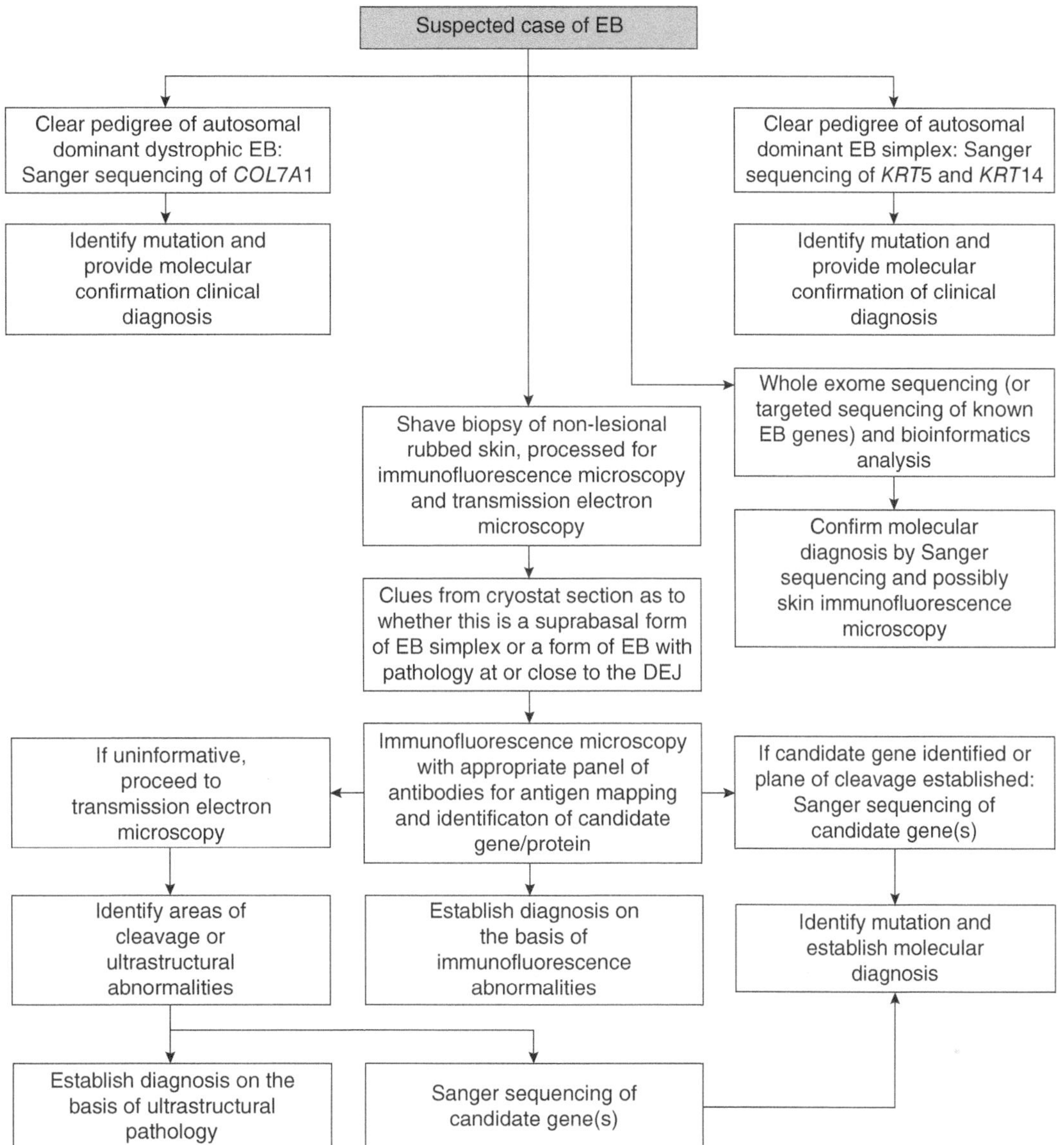

- **AR (generalised severe):** A MDT approach is needed, with six monthly visits. Areas of focus include: oral and dental care, GI tract and nutrition, ophthalmology, orthopaedic team input, management of anaemia of chronic disease, genito-urinary abnormalities, squamous cell carcinoma (SCC) surveillance, pain management, and skin grafting for chronic ulcers or erosion.

Grouped blisters on erythematous base in generalised severe EBS.

The future

There remains no cure, but ongoing research into the underlying mechanisms may yield more focal targets. Currently the aim is to develop improved wound care and pain management strategies for affected individuals.

18 Muir-Torre syndrome

Background

Muir-Torre syndrome (MTS) is characterised by the association of one sebaceous skin tumour and one visceral malignancy (colorectal, endometrial, ovarian, or urothelial cancers). Caused by germline alterations in the DNA mismatch repair (MMR) genes, it is considered a phenotypic variant of Lynch syndrome.

Epidemiology

MTS is a rare disorder, with approximately only 200 patients reported. However, it is felt that the condition is probably more common than reported. It occurs in both sexes, with a male-to-female ratio of 3 : 2.

Genetics

MTS is inherited in an AD manner, with high penetrance, caused by germline alterations in one allele of the DNA MMR genes *MLH1*, *MSH2*, or *MSH6*. The MMR system consists of human mutS homolog 2 (hMSH2), human mutS homolog 3 (hMSH3), human mutS homolog 6 (hMSH6), human mutL homolog 1 (hMLH1), and human postmeiotic segregation increased 2 (hPMS2) proteins. These are responsible for maintaining genomic integrity by correcting base substitution mismatches and small insertion–deletion mismatches generated by errors in base pairing during DNA replication.

Pathophysiology

Microsatellite instability (MSI) is the hallmark of MMR gene deficiency. Microsatellites are short repetitive DNA sequences, typically mononucleotide or dinucleotide tandem repeats, that are susceptible to mutations during DNA replication. The loss of DNA MMR function due to germline and/or somatic inactivating mutations of MMR genes leads to the accumulation of alterations across the genome and mainly in the microsatellite repetitive sequences, creating a molecular phenotype known as MSI.

Alterations in *MLH1* and *MSH2* have the most severe effect, producing a high-frequency MSI phenotype (MSI-H). A MSI-H phenotype can be demonstrated in nearly all cutaneous and visceral tumours from patients with MTS. In contrast with Lynch syndrome, in which germline alterations are almost equally distributed across all MMR genes, most patients with MTS have alterations in *MSH2*.

Symptoms and clinical features

MTS is characterised by the association of one sebaceous skin tumour and/or keratoacanthoma and one visceral malignancy. Sebaceous adenomas and carcinomas are the most commonly seen tumours noted in these patients (Figure 18.1). Although common, they do not indicate a timeline and can occur before, during, and after a visceral malignancy.

Age of onset ranges with a median age of 53 years. Unlike sporadic cases of sebaceous adenoma and sebaceous carcinoma (which are commonly on the head and neck), MTS patients present with these on their trunk. Other skin manifestations such as Fordyce spots (ectopic sebaceous glands) are deemed additional identified features.

Colorectal cancer is the most commonly associated visceral malignancy. Unlike their sporadic colorectal cancer counterparts, these malignancies are more proximal and can occur 20 years earlier. Associated tumours are urogenital tract (endometrium, ovary, bladder, ureter, and kidney), breast, pancreatic, gastric, lung, and hematologic cancers.

Diagnosis

The following diagnostic criteria are used:

- ≥3 relatives with a Lynch-associated cancer (i.e. colorectal, endometrial cancer, small bowel, ureter, or renal pelvis).
- Cancer affecting at least two successive generations.
- One person with cancer is a first-degree relative of the other 2, at least 1 case of colorectal cancer age <50 years, a diagnosis of familial adenomatous polyposis has been excluded, tumours are verified by histologic examination.

It is now recommended that all patients with breast cancer and ovarian or endometreial cancer diagnosed <70 years are tested for *MSI*.

Management

Patients diagnosed with MTS and at-risk family members (first-degree relatives) should undergo a preventive cancer screening program similar to that indicated for patients with HNPCC syndrome which involves:

- Annual skin examination for lesion suspicious of sebaceous carcinoma or keratoacanthoma.
- Colonoscopy every two years, beginning at age 25–35 years, depending on the gene involved, or 2–5 years before the youngest age of diagnosis of colorectal cancer in the family, if diagnosed before age 25 years.
- A gynaecological review at the age of 40 years with consideraton of preventative surgery.

The future

As a rare condition, it is likely that better diagnosis and treatment of the respective tumours will serve most effective in improving outcomes.

Clinical Genetics and Genomics at a Glance, First Edition. Edited by Neeta Lakhani, Kunal Kulkarni, Julian Barwell, Pradeep Vasudevan, and Huw Dorkins.

Figure 18.1 Clinical features.

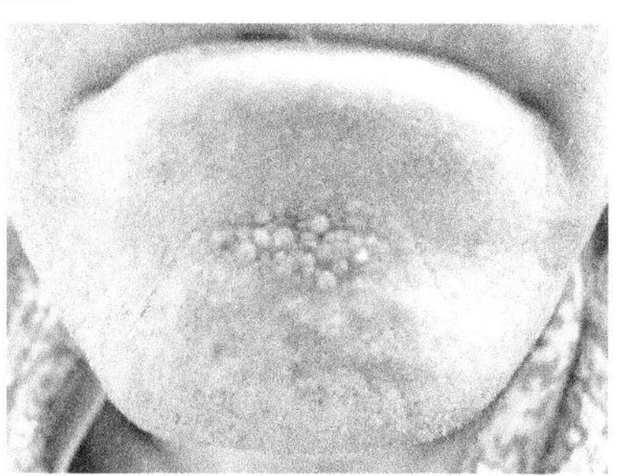

Sebaceous adenoma
Source: WebMD LLC.

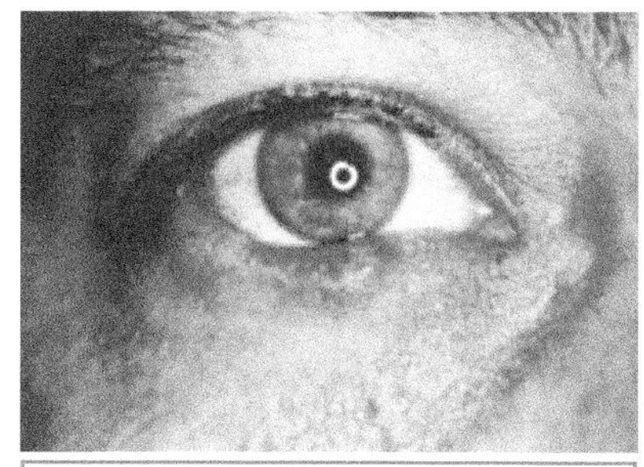

Sebaceous carcinoma

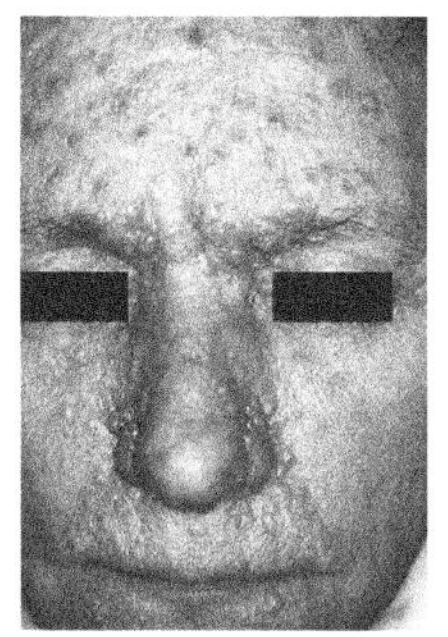

Multiple sebaceous adenomas
Source: WebMD LLC.

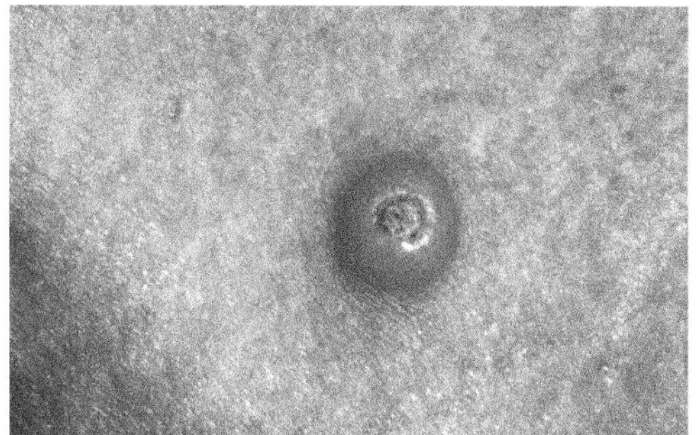

Keratoacanthoma
Source: The Primary Care Dermatology Society.

19 X-linked ichthyosis

Background

X-linked ichthyosis (XLI) is a rare genetic disorder affecting males, with a largely dermatological manifestation. It is caused by a deficiency of the enzyme steroid sulfatase, which normally breaks down cholesterol to maintain the integrity of the skin. As a result, there is an abnormally excessive accumulation of dead squames (skin cells) in the epidermis.

Epidemiology

XLI is a rare disorder that affects around 1 in 2000–6000 males.

Genetics

This condition is caused by an alteration in the *STS* gene located at Xp22.3. It is therefore X-linked and affects females and males differently. This gene is seen to escape X inactivation and therefore its expression is higher in females than males. *STS* encodes for the enzyme arylsulfatase C; a hemizygous deletion/alteration results in an absence in enzyme activity and the hence the observed phenotype. The majority of individuals inherited the alteration, whereas a small proportion are *de novo*. Affected females are observed on occasion, for example when an affected male and carrier female have offspring. The vast proportion of XLI is caused by a complete deletion of the *STS* gene. The remaining are secondary to a point alteration or partial deletion. Continuous gene deletions are also commonly seen and contribute to a wider phenotype which includes learning difficulties.

Pathophysiology

The enzyme steroid sulfatase is expressed in skin cells throughout the body. It is also expressed in liver, lymph nodes, placenta, breast tissue, and the brain. Steroid sulfatase catalyses the sulphated steroid to a non-sulphated steroid. This enzyme is required for normal skin maintenance; a deficiency results in breakdown of the skin barrier and retention of corneocyte due to the accumulation of cholesterol sulphate in the outer epidermis (Figure 19.1).

Figure 19.1 Functional consequences of the Epidermal cholesterol sulphate cycle.

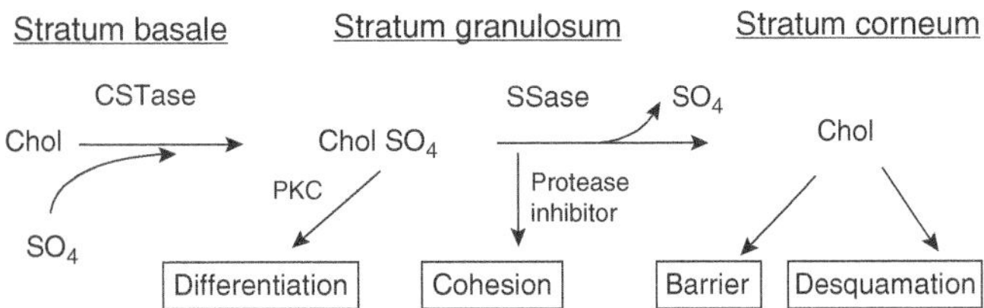

Symptoms and clinical features

Clinical features are not normally present at birth, but can rapidly develop within the first year of life. The dermatological manifestation is darker scales over the skin. The location of the scales varies but most frequently affects the back and legs. The scaling is troublesome to resolve and is often unresponsive to first-line medications. It can be described as symmetrical, palm, and sole sparing, with minimal hair and nail involvement. There is a typical improvement in signs and symptoms over the warmer months.

In addition to the dermatological manifestations, 'comma shaped' corneal opacities are observed that do not normally affect vision. An association with undescended testicles has been reported. As the enzyme is also expressed in the placenta, lower estriol levels in the placenta can cause a failure to initiate or progress labour. *STS* is also expressed in the human brain, predominantly in the subcortical structures. It is therefore felt to be related to the higher than expected rates of neurological features, including epilepsy, learning difficulty, and reduced ability to smell (hyposmia).

Diagnosis

As with many dermatological presentations of genetic conditions, the diagnosis is often suspected clinically. However, due to the varying range of symptoms, it is often not picked up until later on in infancy once all routine treatments for drying skin have failed. Molecular testing may be performed for confirmation of diagnosis, and also to aid cascading to unaffected carrier females. XLI can be diagnosed antenatally by amniocentesis or chorionic villus sampling. Low maternal estriol levels may suggest a diagnosis.

Ichthyoses are disorders of cornification, which present as large accumulations of dead skin in the top layer of the skin matrix. Other ichthyosis to exclude include ichthyosis collodion, which also has a genetic basis (AR). This is usually seen in babies and presents as large areas of red, dry, and coarse skin with fine white scales. Other forms of ichthyosis include Sjogren-Larsson syndrome, Netherton syndrome, ichthyosis hystrix, lamellar ichthyosis, Darier disease, and epidermolytic hyperkeratosis (Refer to chapter 13 - Lamellar ichthyosis).

Management

By the time the diagnosis is made, patients have often tried many of the routine skin treatments with minimal success. The ultimate aim is to reduce the scaling and build-up of flakes, in addition to keeping the skin hydrated. Skin softening is key, with emollient applied when the skin is soft after baths.

The acceleration of the shedding of dead skins cells can be aided by topical keratolytic containing lactic acid, glycolic acid, salicylic acid, and urea. Ammonium lactate (Lac-hydrin) can be used to remove retained corneocytes. Topical isotretinoin/topical receptor selective retinoid tazarotene can also be used.

Genetic counselling and cascade testing should be offered to the family of affected individuals. Males should be advised to perform regular testicular self-examinations for features of malignancy.

The future

XLI is potentially a recessive enzyme deficiency gene disorder that may be a target for cutaneous gene transfer. In 1997, Freiberg et al. demonstrated a highly efficacious retroviral gene transfer followed by grafting of genetically engineered cells to improve the skin's tissue architecture, gene expression, clinical appearance, and function. Improvements have not yet been sustained, but this area of research does offer an opportunity for possible future treatments.

Clinical Genetics and Genomics at a Glance, First Edition. Edited by Neeta Lakhani, Kunal Kulkarni, Julian Barwell, Pradeep Vasudevan, and Huw Dorkins.

20 Birt-Hogg-Dubé

Background

Birt-Hogg-Dubé (BHD) syndrome is a complex genetic disorder characterised by the development of skin papules, most commonly on the head, face, and torso. A proportion of patients may also develop renal tumours and pulmonary cysts. It was first described in 1977 by three Canadian physicians, after whom the disease was named.

Epidemiology

BHD is rare; approximately 600 affected families have been identified to date.

Genetics

Most commonly inherited in an AD fashion. BHD is caused by germline alterations in the *FLCN* gene, which encodes folliculin. The gene is located on the short arm of chromosome 17. The most common alteration in this region is the insertion or deletion of a cytosine residue, found in 50% of BHD families. The function of this protein is largely unknown, although *FLCN* has been linked to the mammalian target of rapamycin (mTOR) pathway and as a tumour suppressor.

Pathophysiology

FLCN is expressed strongly in the skin, nephrons, and pneumocytes. It can also be found in other organs including the brain, breast, and pancreas. Alterations in the *FLCN* gene may interfere with the ability of folliculin to control cell growth and division, leading to the formation of benign and malignant tumours. Folliculin's participation in the mTOR pathway may explain the similarity in phenotype between this condition and others such as Cowden syndrome and tuberous sclerosis complex (TSC).

Symptoms and clinical features

- BHD syndrome is characterised by the development of multiple benign skin tumours, named fibrofolliculomas, on the face, neck, and chest. They are generally 2–3 mm in size, dome shaped, skin-coloured, and do not cause pain or discomfort.
- Affected individuals also have an increased chance of developing cysts in the lungs and the development of pneumothoraces. Lung function is typically unaffected.
- Approximately 15–30% of patients develop multiple renal neoplasms. These are typically oncocytomas and chromophobe histologic cell types.

Diagnosis

- Diagnosis is based upon clinical evaluation, with the identification of characteristic manifestations, including ≥2 fibrofolliculomas, history of a spontaneous pneumothorax, or bilateral and multiple chromophobe or hybrid oncocytic renal tumours. Excision and histological evaluation of these skin lesions is diagnostic.
- Identification of the *FLCN* alteration by DNA-based genetic testing also aids definitive diagnosis. Due to the significant risk of developing renal tumours at a young age, genetic testing is recommended for at-risk family members.
- Lung CT is recommended to detect pulmonary cysts and pneumothoraces.
- Surveillance for renal tumours maybe undertaken with ultrasound, CT, or MRI.

Management

Management is based on the development of the specific clinical features:

- Skin lesions may be treated with laser ablation, although recurrence is not uncommon.
- Prompt aspiration of a pneumothorax is required. If recurrent, pleurodesis or surgical treatment may be required.
- Partial or radical nephrectomy may be required for any malignant renal tumours. A nephron-sparing approach is generally preferred as patients are likely to develop multiple tumours over the course of their lifetime. Patients should undergo regular surveillance to actively screen for tumour development.

The future

The antibiotic mithramycin can inhibit the growth of cells lacking the *FLCN* and may be an effective treatment for BHD-associated renal cell carcinoma (RCC). Additionally, the activation of certain apoptosis genes and decreased cell viability in FLCN-null cells suggests that therapies targeting SSH2 activity may also prove an effective treatment for these cancers. mTOR inhibitors (e.g. everolimus) are approved for sporadic metastatic RCC, but have not been specifically trialled in BHD-associated and sporadic chromophobe RCC.

Clinical Genetics and Genomics at a Glance, First Edition. Edited by Neeta Lakhani, Kunal Kulkarni, Julian Barwell, Pradeep Vasudevan, and Huw Dorkins.

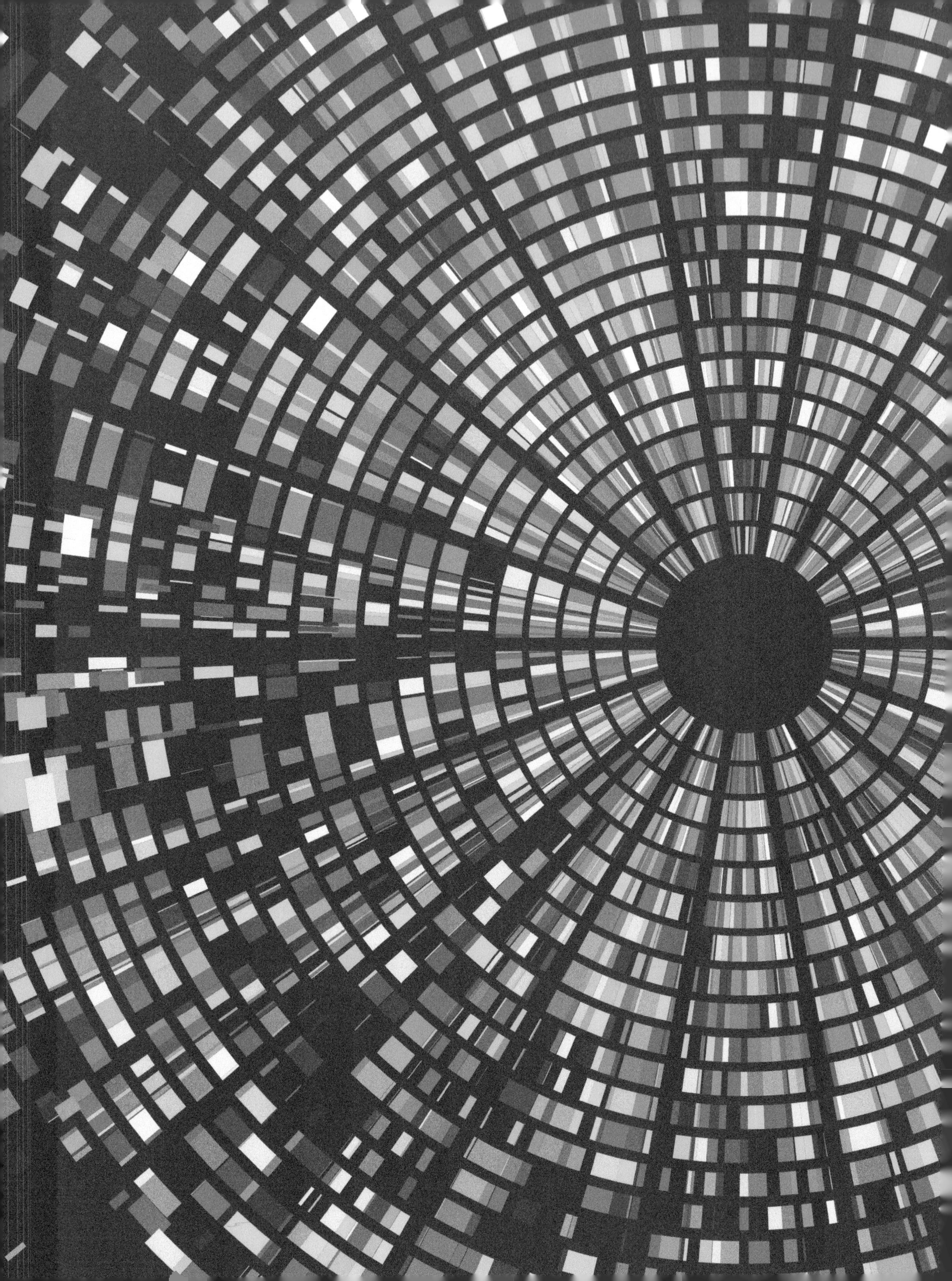

Endocrinology

Chapters

21 Disorders of sexual development and differentiation

Background

Disorders of sex development (DSD) encompasses a wide range of conditions. In general, these are conditions where chromosomal, gonadal, or anatomical sex development is atypical. Children born with ambiguous genitalia present challenges to clinicians and parents alike. Education of the parents and patient is essential, with discussion of the child's *sex* (bimodally categorised and tied to biology, i.e. the physical structure of the reproductive system internally and externally) and *gender* (individualised expression of identity). 'Intersex' has conventionally been used to refer to ambiguous external genitalia. The Chicago Consensus in 2005 led to the establishment of revised nomenclature with newly defined 'disorders of sex development' and removal of terms such as intersex, pseudohermaphroditism' and hermaphroditism.

Aetiology

The estimated incidence of DSDs is approximately 1 in 4500 to 5500 globally. Accounting for all congenital genital abnormalities, the incidence increases to roughly 1 in 200 to 300. XY females present at a rate of 6.4 per 100 000, while males with androgen insensitivity present at a rate of 4.1 per 100 000.

Genetics

This wide range of disorders have different underlying basis. Examples of inheritance patterns include:

- **AD or AR: Ovotesticular DSD:** 10% have a SRY translocation from Y to X. Less commonly, alterations of other genes (*SOX9, RSPO1, NR5A1, DMRT1,* and *MAP3K1*).
- **AR:** 5 alpha reductase deficiency (*SRD5A2* alteration), 21 and 11-OH-deficiency, and aromatase deficiency.
- **Not inherited:** Most cases of Turners, Kleinfelters, and Swyer syndrome (complete gonadal dysgenesis).

The larger categories of DSDs are represented in Table 21.1. There are broadly three groups: sex chromosome DSDs, 46, XY DSD, and 46,XX DSD. Sex chromosome DSDs are primarily categorised by an atypical arrangement of sex chromosomes often due to missing chromosomes. 46,XY DSDs are found in individuals who typically develop male sex characteristics, but there is an impediment to sex development that can lead to more feminine appearances. 46,XX DSDs present in individuals who develop female sex characteristics, but individuals with 46,XX DSDs are often exposed to increased levels of male sex hormones *in utero*. Although the downstream effects of any specific type of DSD will vary depending on the exact condition and patient, understanding DSDs categorically provides causal insight and leads to more effective treatment and management of the condition.

Pathophysiology

The urogenital ridges develop by 4–6 weeks of gestation as outgrowths of coelomic epithelium (Figure 21.1). These ridges then develop into the adrenal cortex, kidneys, gonads, and reproductive tracts. Bipotential embryonic tissues develop into gonads, internal genital ducts, and external genitalia. Gonadal differentiation is the first step in the sex development process. The sex-determining region on the Y chromosome (*SRY* gene) leads to the male/testicular development (Figure 21.2). In 46 XY embryos, factors both activate the determination of male gonads and repress female sex differentiation. Testosterone and anti-Müllerian hormone, both produced by the testes, induce normal male development (scrotum and penis) and cause Müllerian structures to regress. Without these hormones and the *SRY* gene, ovaries are typically developed in females (46,XX). Absence of these hormones leads to Wolffian duct structure regression and Müllerian duct structures persisting - the uterus and Fallopian tubes develop. External genitalia develop into the labia, clitoris, and vagina through the absence of androgens. Therefore, through a specific sequence of synergistic activation and repression of factors, sex determination and development are established. Divergence from this sequence can lead to DSDs.

Table 21.1 Classification of DSDs, based on the 2005 Chicago Consensus.

Loss or gain of sex chromosome DSD	46,XY DSD		46,XX DSD		
	Disorders of testicular development	**Disorders of androgen synthesis / action**	**Disorders of ovarian development**	**Fetal androgen excess**	
				CAH	**Non CAH**
- 45,X Turner and variants - 47,XXY Klinefelter and variants - 45,X/46,XY MGD - Chromosomal ovotesticular DSD	- Complete gonadal dysgenesis - Partial gonadal dysgenesis - Gonadal regression - Ovotesticular DSD	- Androgen synthesis defect - LH-receptor defect - Androgen insensitivity - 5α–reductase deficiency - Disorders AMH - Timing defect - Endocrine disrupters - Cloacal extrophy	- Ovotesticular DSD - Testicular DSD - Gonadal dysgenesis	- 21-OH-deficiency - 11-OH deficiency	- Aromatase deficiency - *POR* gene defect - Maternal luteoma - Iatrogenic

DSD: Disorders of sex development, MGD: Mixed Gonadal Dysgenesis, AMH: anti-Müllerian hormone, CAH: Congenital adrenal hyperplasia

Clinical Genetics and Genomics at a Glance, First Edition. Edited by Neeta Lakhani, Kunal Kulkarni, Julian Barwell, Pradeep Vasudevan, and Huw Dorkins.

Figure 21.1 Embryology of gonadal development.

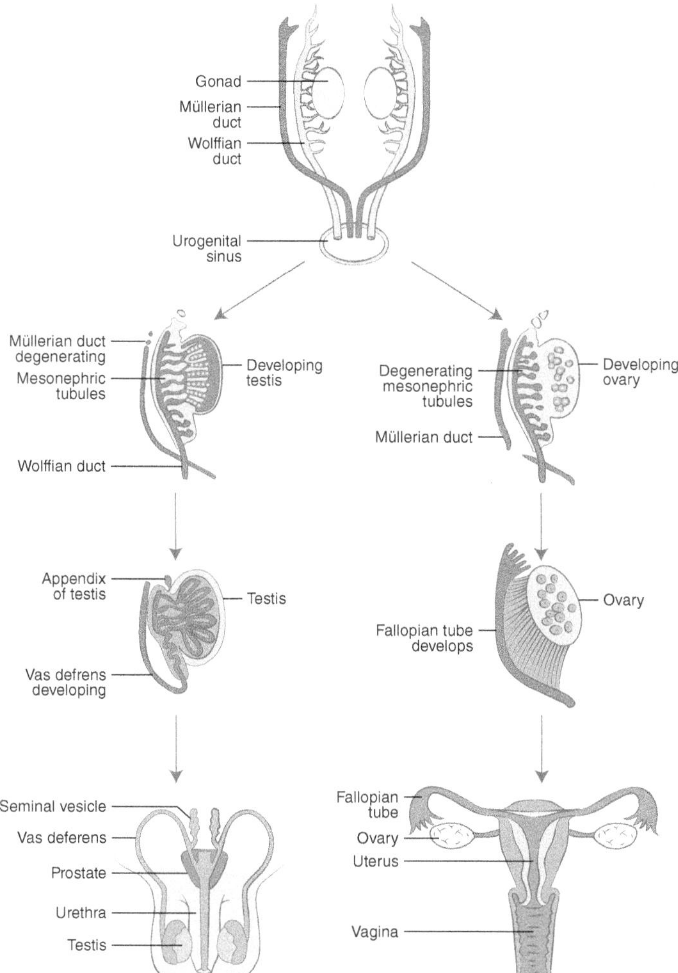

Figure 21.2 Overview of sexual/gonadal differentiation.

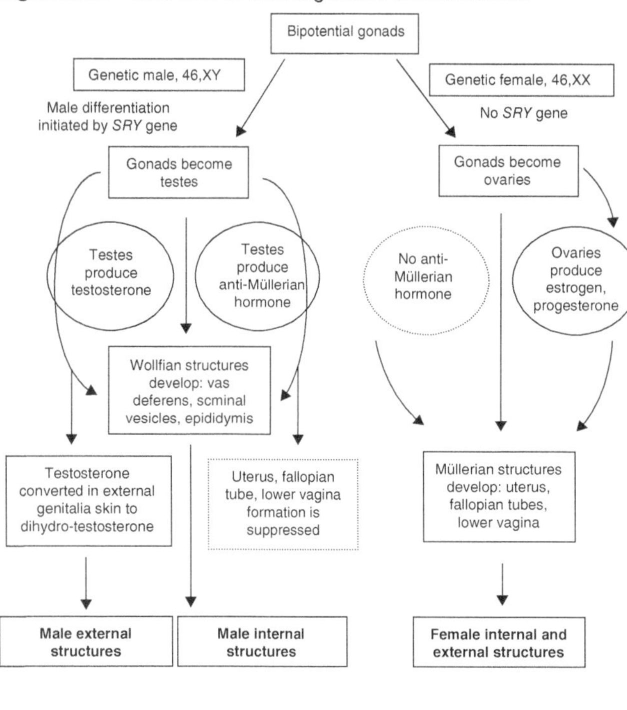

Symptoms and clinical features

Children born with a DSD do not typically present as medical emergencies. However, the quality of life ramifications are significant. Untreated or inadequately managed DSDs can remain a lifelong barrier to social relationships or potentially compromise mental wellness as an individual born with a DSD faces struggles with identity or a sense of belonging. The most critical facet of DSD diagnosis and treatment is the way an individual may be at risk for other conditions such as cancers, immune compromise, metabolic issues, and other chronic illnesses. While understanding a DSD does not serve as a blueprint for treatment, it does provide potentially life-saving information about secondary conditions resulting from the DSD.

Management

A multidisciplinary team including geneticists, radiologists, endocrinologists, urologists, surgeons, and neonatologists. It is important to remember that clinical care needs to be complemented by behavioural and developmental health professionals as the child ages through infancy, adolescence, and adulthood. Management involves three facets: health, appearance, and fertility.

Health is the most important concern. DSDs can present health risks either from the condition itself or the surgical procedures used in sex rearing, fertility preservation, or any cosmetic surgeries. DSD cases lack uniformity and surgery must be broached on an individual basis.

Appearance refers to any procedure or treatment that aims to manage the physical deviation from typical sex development caused by a DSD. Surgical options are the most effective at correcting DSD issues, but these solutions depend on the severity of each individual case.

Fertility is often compromised in individuals born with a DSD, but there are experimental and new approaches to fertility preservation that should be discussed with the parents. It should also be noted that many surgical procedures to address other aspects of DSDs often result in infertility.

The future

Ongoing work is needed to help assign sex for some infants alongside better understanding of the factors and processes involved in gender identity development. A better evidence-base is also required to address the timing and techniques of any interventions, including in relation to preservation of fertility.

22 Congenital adrenal hyperplasia

Background

In 1865, Italian anatomist Luigi DeCrecchio first studied a female patient with male genitalia lacking testes, an internal female reproductive system, and enlarged adrenal glands. In 1950, a disturbance in the normal feedback mechanism in adrenal glands causing a lack of cortisol was identified. In 1963, congenital adrenal hyperplasia (CAH) was subdivided into closely related enzyme abnormalities, with the most common being 21-hydroxylase deficiency, alongside other abnormalities in 11 beta-hydroxylase, 17 alpha-hydroxylase, and others. In 1978, the discovery of location of the gene responsible for 21-hydroxylase, short arm of the sixth chromosome, provided a better understanding of genetic transmission.

Aetiology

CAH comprises of a group of disorders which ultimately impair adrenal hormone production and is the most common cause of ambiguous genitalia of the newborn. 90–95% of cases are due to 21-hydroxylase deficiency. Broadly, classic and non-classic forms of this exist, affecting 1 in ~15 000 and 1 in ~1000 newborns, respectively.

Genetics

All forms of CAH are inherited in an AR manner, with affected individuals therefore likely having both parents as carriers. Carriers themselves rarely show features of CAH.

Pathophysiology

Glucocorticoids, mineralocorticoids, and sex hormones are produced by the adrenal cortex. A classic negative-feedback mechanism controls cortisol production, dependent on adrenocorticotrophic hormone (ACTH). Aldosterone, responsible for salt-control, is under control by the renin-angiotensin-aldosterone system. Cholesterol is the building block for all endocrine glands that produce corticosteroids. Cortisol and aldosterone production require several steps governed by enzymes (Figure 22.1). 21-hydroxylase deficiency is the most common enzyme deficiency that causes CAH, comprising 90–95% of cases. This enzyme converts 17-hydroxyprogesterone to 11-deoxycortisol and progesterone to deoxycorticosterone, which are precursors for cortisol and aldosterone, respectively. Adrenal androgens are produced in excess due to the accumulation of 17-hydroxyprogesterone and continuous ACTH release from a lack of cortisol. These excess androgens are converted by the liver to testosterone, which leads to virilisation of individuals (develop male characteristics). CAH can be categorised into classic and non-classic forms. The classic form can be subcategorised into salt-wasting and simple virilising - these reflect the degree of mineralocorticoid deficiency (aldosterone). The non-classic form is the mildest.

Figure 22.1 Pathophysiology of the most common cause of congenital adrenal hyperplasia.

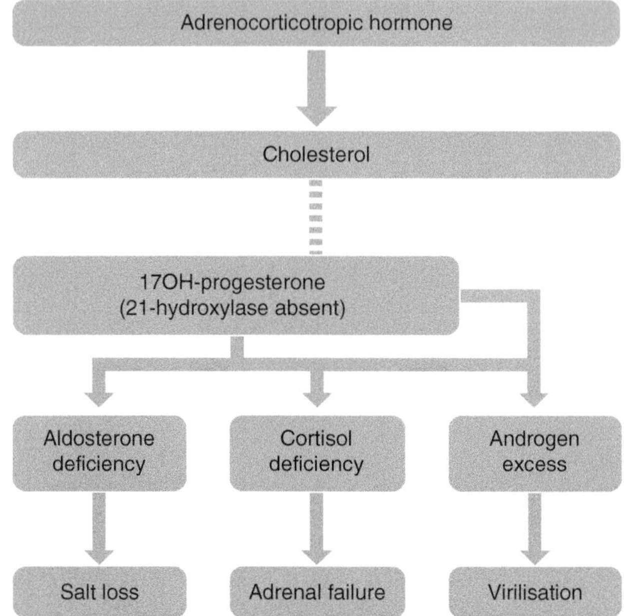

The most common enzyme defect (21-hydroxylase) is shown. The dotted line indicates several enzymatic steps from cholesterol to steroid hormone production. Accumulation of 17OH-progesterone acts as a substrate for increased androgen production. Hypersecretion of adrenocorticotropic hormone occurs from the negative feedback effect of cortisol deficiency.

Symptoms and clinical features

- **Classic cases:** Classic CAH can be life-threatening. The salt-wasting form, if not treated or identified, can cause shock, coma, and even death. Female infants (Table 22.1) are diagnosed at birth usually by observing ambiguous genitalia – internally; however, they have ovaries and uterus but may display virilised external genitalia (an enlarged clitoris). Male infants may have enlarged penises. They tend to show signs of early puberty before their peers, including a growth spurt and pubic hair. If not identified at birth, frequent vomiting, dehydration, shock, diarrhoea, and arrhythmias can follow. These result from the lack of aldosterone, and therefore hyponatraemia, hyperkalaemia, and hypoglycaemia can present shortly after birth.
- **Non-classic cases:** For non-classic form, signs and symptoms may not be evident until later in life. In both males and females, patients can suffer from acne and similarly show early signs of puberty. Decreased fertility can also commonly affect individuals. Adolescent and young adult females may have male characteristics - a deepened voice, facial hair, and infrequent or absent menstruation (Table 22.1). In both forms, hyperpigmentation can occur due to increased production of ACTH. Melanocyte-stimulating hormone is a by-product of ACTH, thus leading to increased pigmentation of the skin. Furthermore, though patients have earlier growth spurts, their final heights are 1-2 standard deviations below their estimated.

Clinical Genetics and Genomics at a Glance, First Edition. Edited by Neeta Lakhani, Kunal Kulkarni, Julian Barwell, Pradeep Vasudevan, and Huw Dorkins.

Table 22.1 Clinical features of congenital adrenal hyperplasia.

Age	Sex	Presentation
Postnatal period	F	Ambiguous genitalia
	M/F	Loss of salt
Early childhood	M	Virilisation, rapid growth
Late childhood	F	Early pubic hair, rapid growth
Adolescence and young adulthood	F	Hirsutism, infertility, acne, irregular menses, delayed menarche, hyperpigmentation, short final height
	M	Infertility, testicular masses, hyperpigmentation, short final height

Diagnosis

In some countries, newborns are screened for 21-hydroxylase deficiency (i.e. classic CAH). Diagnosis is usually confirmed by raised concentrations of serum 17-hydroxyprogesterone and testosterone. Hyponatraemia, hyperkalaemia, and hypoglycaemia indicate a salt-losing crisis. An exaggerated 17-hydroxyprogesterone response from short-acting ACTH stimulation (synacthen) may be observed. Specific *CYP21A2* alterations can be identified through genetic analysis. Risk determination for future children can be performed after diagnostic confirmation. Underlying causes of ambiguous external genitalia should be identified promptly for sex assignment. CAH can be reliably established through karyotype analysis showing XX chromosomes, fluorescence *in situ* hybridisation, an increased 17-hydroxyprogesterone concentration, and a pelvic ultrasound showing a uterus. X-rays can help confirm the diagnosis (advanced bone age).

Management

During childhood, management focuses on gender assignment, genital surgery, and optimising growth and development. CAH has significant cardiovascular and metabolic morbidity in later adult life. CAH has significant cardiovascular risks compared to non-CAH individuals. Preventing metabolic syndrome, bone loss, and focusing on fertility are goals with older age. Clinical trials have shown promising results using modified-release hydrocortisone preparations, which aim to replicate the dynamics of endogenous cortisol.

The future

In the future, genetic studies linked with clinical phenotyping hope to characterise long-term implications of genetic findings. New treatment approaches minimising glucocorticoid exposure are being researched. Alternative analytes to 17-hydroxyprogesterone are being determined to improve sensitivity and specificity of newborn screening programmes. Clinical trials have shown promising results using modified-release hydrocortisone preparations, which aim to replicate the dynamics of endogenous cortisol.

23 Androgen insensitivity syndrome

Background

Androgen insensitivity syndrome (AIS) was first described by John Morris in 1953. Lyon and Hawkes then reported a gene in the mouse that was associated with testicular feminisation in 1970. In 1989, the human androgen receptor (*AR*) gene was localised to Xq11-12 and Brown et al. were the first to demonstrate AR gene mutations caused AIS. In the same year, the sequence of intron-exon boundaries was reported for the human *AR* gene, which further provided a molecular background.

Aetiology

AIS can be categorised based on androgen sensitivity, creating three subgroups with differing phenotypes in 46 XY individuals. Complete AIS (CAIS) occurs in approximately 1 in 20 000 to 1 in 65 000. Partial AIS (PAIS) has an estimated incidence of 1 in 30 000. Mild AIS (MAIS) is rarer; its incidence has not been determined.

Genetics

AIS's inheritance is an x-linked manner. Diagnosis is via karyotyping initially, followed by molecular genetic testing for known *AR* variants. The *AR* gene makes the androgen receptor protein. Affected 46,XY individuals are almost always infertile, hence there is an important role in genetic counselling.

Pathophysiology

AIS can be classified as a 46,XY disorder of sex development (46,XY DSD). Gonad development (Figure 23.1) is critical from 8 to 14 weeks of gestation and depends on both androgens and a normal androgen receptor. Androgens exert their effects via the androgen receptor and is, responsible for the normal male phenotype. Endogenous androgens, namely testosterone and dihydrotestosterone (DHT), allow masculinisation. DHT is particularly important for the development of the penis, scrotum, and prostate. Testosterone stimulates Wolffian duct structures to differentiate into the seminal vesicles, vas deferens, and epididymis. Both hormones require the presence of the androgen receptor within target tissues. The androgen receptor is activated through ligand-dependent activation. When either hormone binds to the androgen receptor, it dimerises and translocates into the nucleus after conformational changes. Here, it initiates transcription (Figure 23.2). Any event that could lead to the impairment of the normal androgen receptor may result in under-virilisation of the male embryo through insufficient androgen.

Figure 23.1 Pathophysiology of CAIS.

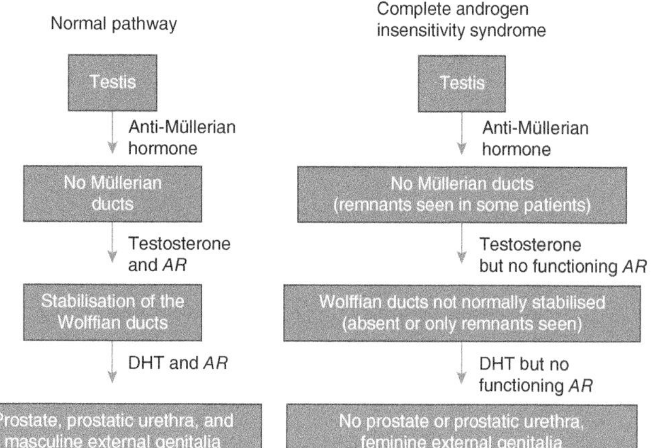

Figure 23.2 Ligand-gated *AR* activation.

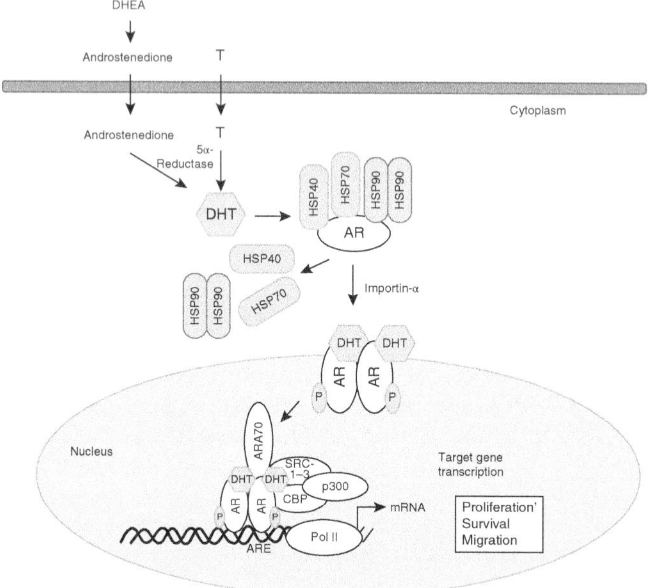

Symptoms and clinical features

Individuals normally have female external genitalia but internally male. These could incidentally present before puberty as inguinal canal masses (e.g. hernias). Common features include primary amenorrhoea, normal breast development, and a lack of axillary or pubic hair (Figure 23.3).

PAIS can display various phenotypes (Figure 23.4), which are dependent on under-virilisation severity, i.e. activity of the androgen receptor. Wolffian duct structures can be fully or partially developed. The spectrum ranges from a predominantly female phenotype, mild clitoromegaly, labia fusion and pubertal pubic hair development to a predominantly male phenotype, hypospadias, micropenis, and cryptorchidism.

Being the mildest subgroup with male external genitalia, individuals may manifest pubertal gynaemastia and oligospermia.

Diagnosis

AIS is suspected through clinical, radiologic, laboratory findings and family history. Diagnostic features of AIS include the following: female external genitalia, ambiguous genitalia or

Clinical Genetics and Genomics at a Glance, First Edition. Edited by Neeta Lakhani, Kunal Kulkarni, Julian Barwell, Pradeep Vasudevan, and Huw Dorkins.

Figure 23.3 Clinical features of CAIS.

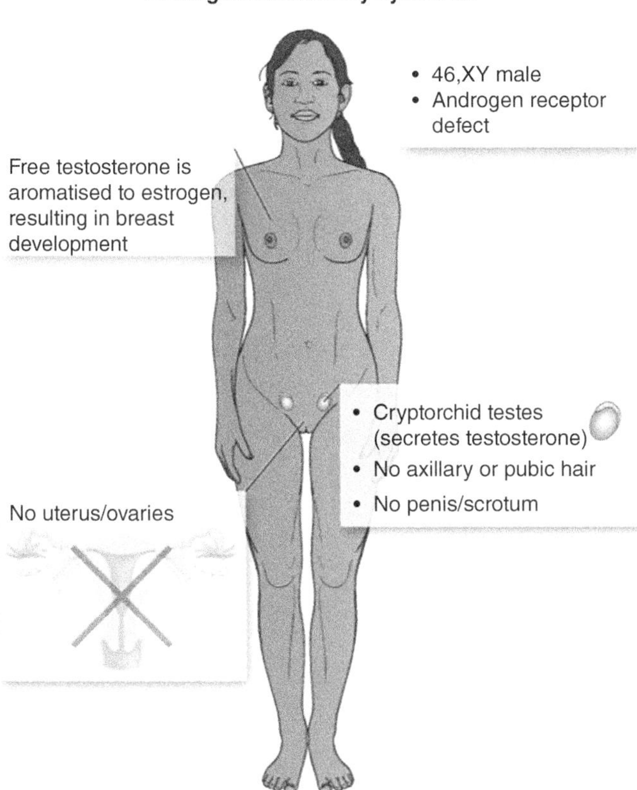

Figure 23.4 Clinical features of AIS and subgroups.

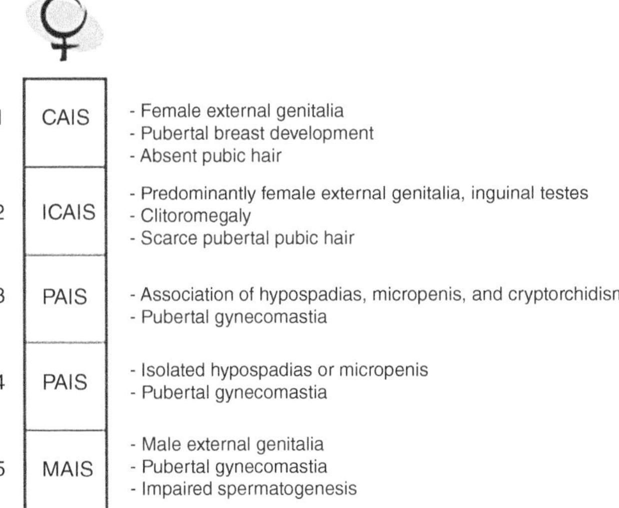

under-virilised genitalia combined with a 46,XY karyotype, high levels of FSH and/or LH, and normal/high levels of testosterone and DHT. CAIS patients are difficult to identify from normal female newborns at birth. At puberty, therefore, the lack of pubic and underarm hair along with absence of menstruation (Figure 23.3) may help with indication. Abdominal testes through needle biopsy can confirm the diagnosis along with hormone level evaluation. PAIS can be suspected through the presence of ambiguous genitalia and confirmed through poor breast development and similarly a needle biopsy with confirmation of testicular tissue and hormone testing. Under-virilisation – i.e. a micropenis, development of feminine features like gynaecomastia, and a high-pitched voice – could indicate MAIS. Molecular genetic testing can involve testing a single gene, *AR* or consideration of multi-gene panels to rule out differential diagnoses. Ultrasonography could show impaired development of Wolffian duct structures. Prenatal testing through amniocentesis and chorionic villus sampling are employed also.

1 CAIS
- Female external genitalia
- Pubertal breast development
- Absent pubic hair
2 ICAIS
- Predominantly female external genitalia, inguinal testes
- Clitoromegaly
- Scarce pubertal pubic hair
3 PAIS
- Association of hypospadias, micropenis, and cryptorchidism
- Pubertal gynecomastia
4 PAIS
- Isolated hypospadias or micropenis
- Pubertal gynecomastia
5 MAIS
- Male external genitalia
- Pubertal gynecomastia
- Impaired spermatogenesis

Management

Management for AIS is broken down into three categories: surgery to reconstruct external genitalia, gonadectomies to reduce risk of neoplasia, and hormone therapy. The efficacy and aim of these management strategies vary depending on subgroup. In CAIS patients, oestrogen replacement therapy supplements removal of the testes after puberty or prepubertal gonadectomies, both of which aim to prevent testicular malignancy. Recently, gonadectomies are becoming controversial given the low occurrence of testicular malignancy and other viable treatments such as vaginal dilation aiming to prevent dyspareunia. PAIS individuals are treated similar to CAIS cases but prepubertal gonadectomies are more common to prevent clitoromegaly during puberty. PAIS patients with male or ambiguous genitalia are typically referred to experts for assistance in sex rearing. PAIS individuals raised male undergo orchiopexy and hypospadias repair or even mammoplasties for gynecomastia, while those raised female sex may require oestrogen and androgen replacement therapy after gonadectomies. Like other DSDs, surveillance and follow-ups are essential to prevent complications. Bone health is assessed through monitoring bone mineral density with DEXA scans. Genetic counselling is important for carriers, as most affected individuals are infertile.

The future

In the future, genetic diagnosis and treatment of AIS may become much more precise and effective than what exists today. It is important to encourage DNA storing of affected individuals to provide the most complete data set for future studies. Gene therapy and genetic testing are two key areas that stand to benefit from robust DNA banking of AIS-affected individuals.

24 Klinefelter syndrome

Background

In 1942, Dr. Harry Klinefelter and colleagues from the Massachusetts General Hospital (Boston, USA) published a case series of nine men who were unable to produce sperm, had enlarged breasts, lacked body and facial hair, and had underdeveloped testes. The underlying genetic basis of Klinefelter syndrome was identified in the late 1950s.

Aetiology

This affects 1 in 650 live male births, making this the most common sex chromosome disorder and the most common genetic cause of infertility.

Genetics

The basis of Kleinfelter syndrome is the presence of an extra copy of the X chromosome, commonly by non-disjunction (i.e. 47,XXY), hence it is not inherited. Mosaic Klinefelter (46,XY/47,XXY) is also not inherited and occurs due to an error in cell division during foetal development; some cells therefore have one X chromosome (i.e. 46,XY) and others have an extra X chromosome (i.e. 47,XY). More cell line variations with additional X chromosomes, e.g. 48,XXXY and 49,XXXXY have been reported, although are much rarer (Figure 24.1).

Figure 24.1 Clinical features of Klinefelter syndrome.

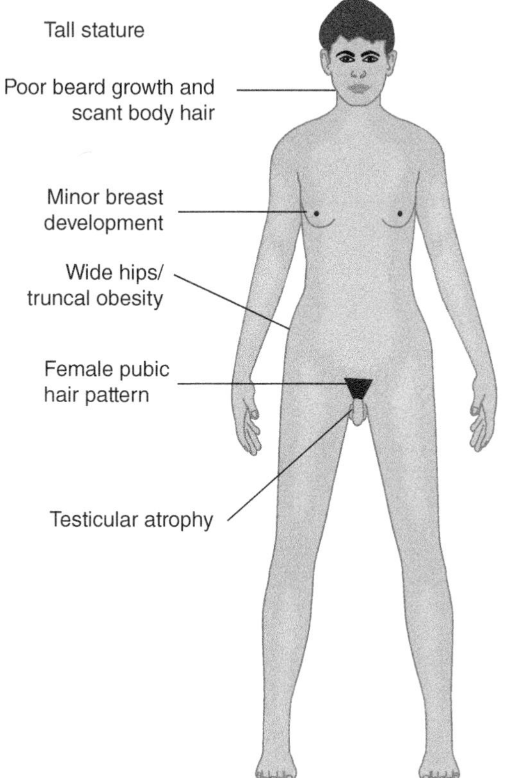

Pathophysiology

The extra X chromosome is usually retained due to a non-disjunction event (a failure of homologous chromosomes separating) (Figure 24.2). This can occur in both the mother and father, creating either a XX egg or a XY sperm, respectively, during meiosis II. When these combine with their counterpart, they yield XXY offspring. Males effectively have a copy of the genes from the extra X chromosome(s), disrupting their development and particularly affecting sexual characteristics. This extra X chromosome material leads to testicular hyalinisation and fibrosis, causing primary gonadal failure or *hypergonadotropic hypogonadism*. This results in reduced production of testosterone, which is responsible for the clinical features observed.

Symptoms

In the postnatal period, individuals may be easily fatigued, with fluctuant emotions. They may have passive, introverted personality types. In childhood, patients may face language and learning problems, with some children having difficulties in socialising with others alongside a delay in global speech. At puberty, body image issues, anxiety, and depression are often present. ADHD and autism spectrum disorder are also associated. Infertility is a major concern upon entering adulthood.

Clinical features

Signs and symptoms can vary with age (Table 24.1). Patients usually appear as normal males until they reach puberty, when they develop characteristic features to suggest the diagnosis. Additional dosage of the *SHOX* gene of the X chromosome leads to tall stature and a reduced upper/lower segment ratio. Gynaecomastia and small testicles are common.

Diagnosis

- **Blood tests:** Used to assess hormone levels, specifically testosterone and gonadotrophins (LH and FSH). The typical pattern patients will have a low testosterone, with raised LH and FSH. As part of the feedback response due to reduced testosterone, the pituitary gland is stimulated to secrete higher levels of LH and FSH.

Figure 24.2 Chromosome pattern.

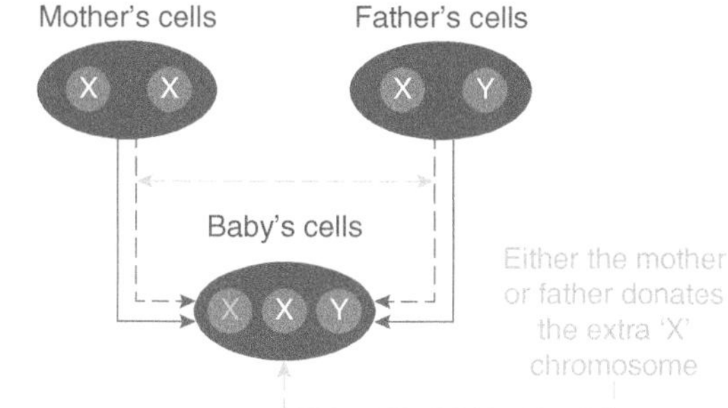

Clinical Genetics and Genomics at a Glance, First Edition. Edited by Neeta Lakhani, Kunal Kulkarni, Julian Barwell, Pradeep Vasudevan, and Huw Dorkins.

Table 24.1 Clinical features of Klinefelter syndrome.

Age	Presentations
Postnatal period	Micropenis Hypospadias Simian transverse palmar crease Cryptorchidism
Childhood	Hypotonia, leading to constipation and abnormal posture Tall stature Delay in developmental milestones
Puberty	Small testes Lack of facial, pubic, and underarm hair Gynaecomastia Sexual dysfunction Truncal obesity
Adulthood	Infertility Low libido Fatigue

Figure 24.3 Karyotype showing an extra X chromosome.

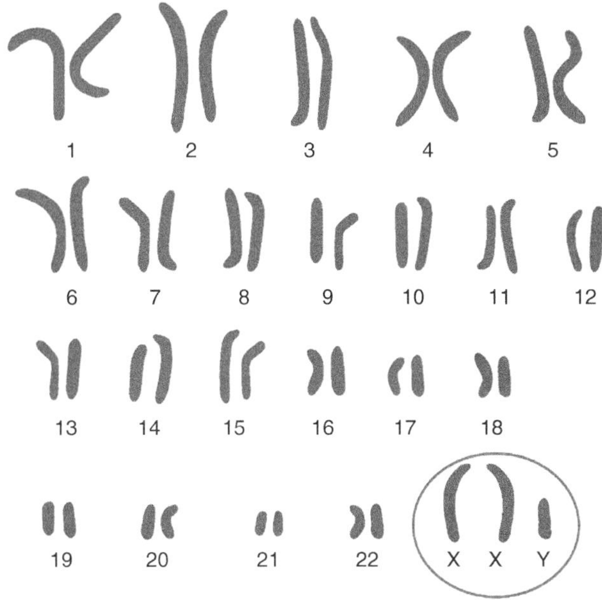

- **Chromosomal analysis or karyotyping:** Can confirm the diagnosis (Figure 24.3).
- **Amniocentesis and chorionic villus sampling:** Performed during pregnancy to karyotype (around 10% of overall diagnosis).

Management

- The fundamental chromosomal abnormality cannot be altered; therefore, the aim of management is to offer symptom control and prevent long-term complications. This varies between patients depending on the severity of symptoms and the age of diagnosis.
- Testosterone injections are used to improve many symptoms and are generally well-tolerated. They are required from the start of puberty and the dose can be changed to maintain appropriate levels.
- Fertility problems can be addressed through IVF techniques.
- Gynaecomastia may require breast surgery for cosmesis and the higher risk of breast cancer.
- Regular follow up helps address complications and adjust testosterone therapy. An MDT approach encompassing speech and language therapy, educational support, physiotherapy, and occupational therapy is essential

The future

To address infertility, some centres cryopreserve pre-pubertal testicular tissue. This tissue could theoretically be used to derive sperm cells in the future.

25 Turner syndrome

Background

Eponymously named after Illinois endocrinologist Henry Turner, Turner syndrome is a disorder of sexual development (DSD) discovered in 1938 that exclusively affects females. It is also referred to as Ullrich-Turner syndrome or Bonnevie-Ullrich-Turner syndrome (in acknowledgement of European doctors who detailed earlier cases). Soviet endocrinologist Nikolai Shereshevsky believed the condition to be caused by a combination of congenital malformations of internal development and underdeveloped gonads and anterior pituitary gland to be the cause.

Aetiology

Occurs with 1 in 2500 live female births, but only 30% of cases are diagnosed at an early age. Turner syndrome is more common among pregnancies that do not survive (stillbirths and miscarriages) to term.

Genetics

Affecting girls, Turner syndrome results from a missing or partially missing X chromosome (i.e. 45,X). It is not usually inherited. In some cases, two X chromosomes are present but one is incomplete. Alternatively, in mosaics, some cells in the body have two X chromosomes, whereas others only have one.

Pathophysiology

The severity of the condition varies depending on both, the degree and frequency of chromosome loss. The most severe cases are monosomy X (45,XO), meaning the entire second sex chromosome is absent, while more mild cases involve partial loss. This is usually the result of a random chromosomal non-disjunction during meiosis II (Figure 25.1). Moreover, cells can be independently affected (mosaicism). Due to this variable loss, phenotypes are diverse. Various systems, organs, and tissues can be affected through this chromosomal loss, known as the 'gene dosage effect'.

Figure 25.1 Non-disjunction during meiosis II, causing Turner syndrome (monosomy X).

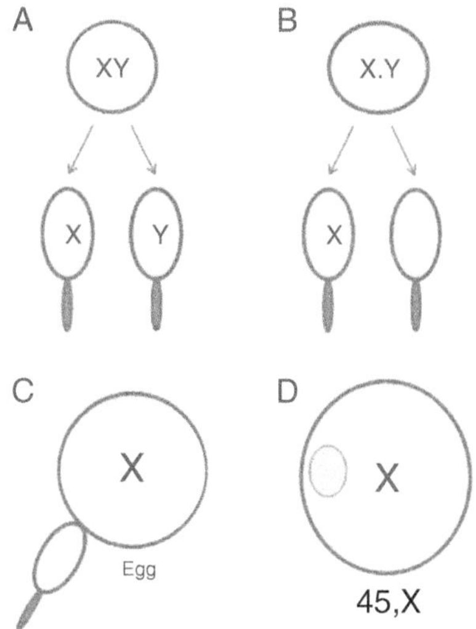

Symptoms

Patients often do not experience puberty naturally and have missing ovaries or otherwise compromised reproductive systems. Features of cardiovascular disorders may be evident, such as malformation of the heart or major veins and arteries. Due to the associated developmental issues, patients are prone to osteoporosis. Individuals are also more likely to develop the features of autoimmune and endocrine disorders, such as type II diabetes mellitus and thyroid problems, the latter occurring in as up to 30% of cases. Infertility is common with 85% of patients born with total germinal cell loss and only 10–15% of those patients containing enough germinal cells to undergo pubertal responses, and an even fewer 5% able to have menstrual cycles.

Clinical features

Hallmarks of Turner syndrome are short height, ovarian development issues, and cardiac defects.

A webbed-like neck is often present (Figure 25.2). Short stature occurs in over 90% of cases, typically resulting in 20–22 cm shorter height than population averages. Spontaneous growth in patients is usually marked by moderate intrauterine growth delay and depressed childhood growth leading to separation in growth

Figure 25.2 Clinical features of Turner syndrome.

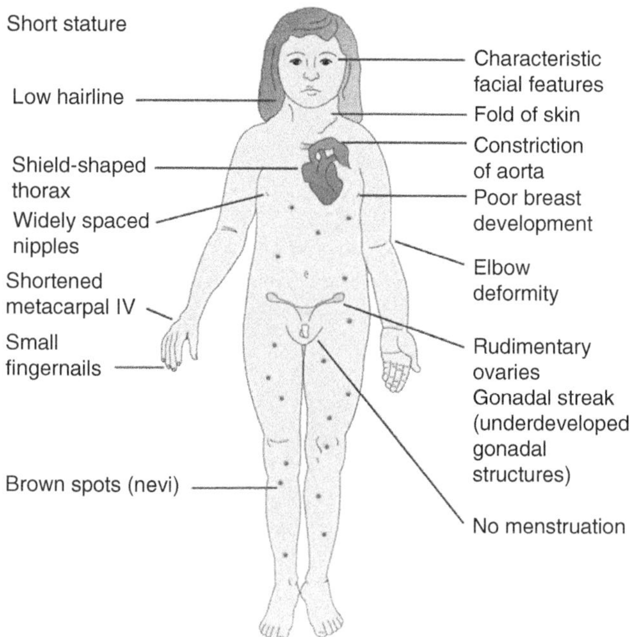

Clinical Genetics and Genomics at a Glance, First Edition. Edited by Neeta Lakhani, Kunal Kulkarni, Julian Barwell, Pradeep Vasudevan, and Huw Dorkins.

trajectories from peers as puberty development is stunted or absent, and bone maturation is delayed.

Other physical manifestations include a 'shield chest' (due to widening of the thorax) and cubitus valgus. Less frequent presentations include dorsal wrist angular deformities ('dinner fork sign'). Congenital cardiac defects affect 40% of patients - a major contributor to early mortality. Cardiovascular abnormalities include a narrow aorta, bicuspid aortic valves, and anomalous pulmonary venous returns.

Diagnosis

The most indicative symptoms of Turner syndrome are the physical presentations of short stature and webbed neck. A karyotype is used to confirm diagnosis (Figure 25.3). Diagnosis can be made during pregnancy via chorionic villous sampling or amniocentesis and analysing foetal chromosomes, but most cases are not diagnosed until later in life. While most cases are diagnosed before the features of diabetes or osteoporosis appear, it is important to note the broad spectrum of severity and the need to diagnose and treat the associated conditions.

Figure 25.3 Karyotype of Turner syndrome (45,XO).

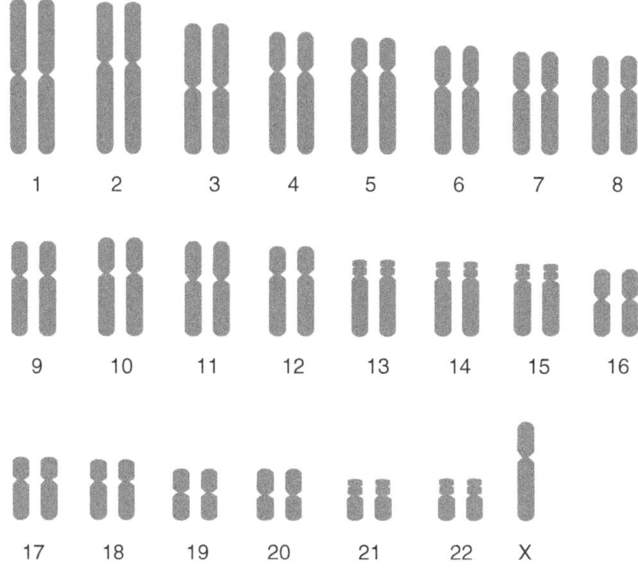

Management

Fundamentally, management involves growth hormone and oestrogen replacement therapy. Treatment varies depending on the severity of individual cases, via a MDT approach. It is possible to improve physical development via growth hormone and oestrogen hormone therapies during childhood. Hormone therapies are the primary treatment and other options seek to ameliorate symptoms rather than combat causes for underlying issues. Infertility is common, but *in vitro* fertilisation is possible with donor eggs (cryopreservation). Most females with Turner syndrome remain infertile, but oestrogen therapy can allow individuals to undergo puberty and lead largely normal lives. Gonadectomies are suggested to mitigate risks of cancers where Y chromosome material is thought to be present.

The future

Recent studies have found that chromosomal imbalance leads to epigenetic changes. Expression- and methylation-based pathways are correlated with Turner syndrome's phenotypes. Clarifying these pathways could benefit future patients by looking to increase life expectancy and offer targets for early pharmaceutical intervention.

26 Diabetes mellitus

Background

Diabetes comes from the Greek '*to pass through*', and mellitus from the Latin '*sweetened with honey*'. Ancient Egyptians described features similar to diabetes mellitus around 3000 years ago, but the term *diabetes* was only first used by the physician Aretaeus of Cappadocia in the second century AD. Later, in 1675, *mellitus* was added by Thomas Willis, a physician who rediscovered the urine's sweet taste. A major turning point in the history of diabetes was the discovery and use of insulin by Banting and Best in 1921. The first oral hypoglycaemic agents were marketed in 1955.

In 1974, the first cases of Maturity-onset diabetes of the young (MODY) were reported as mild hereditary familial diabetes – a distinct entity from Type 2 diabetes mellitus (T2DM).

Aetiology

Around 415 million people worldwide have diabetes – i.e. around 1 in 11. Nearly 50% of cases are undiagnosed. Type 1 diabetes accounts for 5–10% and is autoimmune in aetiology. Around 90–95% of patients with diabetes have T2DM, a polygenic condition caused by both insulin resistance and a defect in insulin secretion, often associated with what is termed 'metabolic syndrome' and high BMI. MODY is associated with monogenic defects in β-cell function with few or no defects in insulin action. It is estimated to affect 1 in 23 000 children and 1 in 10 000 adults.

Genetics

MODY was previously categorised as having onset < age 45, AD inheritance, and lack of β-cell autoimmunity. However, recent changes to diagnostics have recategorised MODY as presenting < age 25, familial history of diabetes for two consecutive generations, and the preservation of β-cell functionality resulting in lack necessity for insulin treatments. Currently, 14 gene alterations, 6 of which are responsible for encoding proteins that are linked to the MODY 1–6 subtypes, have been identified (all AD inheritance). There are 11 subtypes of MODY, but types 7–11 are recent discoveries and less fully understood than types 1–6. Prevalence and treatment strategies vary depending on subtype.

Pathophysiology

Type 1 diabetes is an autoimmune condition causing destruction of the pancreatic β cells resulting in absolute insulin deficiency (Figure 26.1). It presents in children and young adults. Infiltration of the pancreatic islets by activated macrophages, cytotoxic, and suppressor T lymphocytes and B lymphocytes that are highly selective for the β cell population. Approximately 70–90% of β cells must be destroyed before the onset of clinical symptoms. Type 1 DM is a polygenic disorder with genetic factors accounting for about 30% of the susceptibility to the disease. Type 2 diabetes is characterised by insulin resistance coupled with relative insulin deficiency. The mechanism of insulin resistance in Type 2 diabetes remains unclear. The consequence of prolonged hyperinsulinaemia is the development of insulin deficiency. The different forms of MODY are due to either insufficient insulin production or its release from β cells through monogenic alterations. These alterations often affect transcription factor genes (see Figure 26.2).

Symptoms

Patients with MODY may exhibit blurry vision, frequent infections like skin or yeast, or hyperglycaemia. However, patients may be asymptomatic. As discussed in other sections, MODY is hereditary. Patients with a family history of MODY may not have obvious symptoms, but other clinical features will be present. Other symptoms include frequent urination, weight loss, and fatigue; however, these symptoms are typical of many types of diabetes.

Figure 26.1 β-cell.

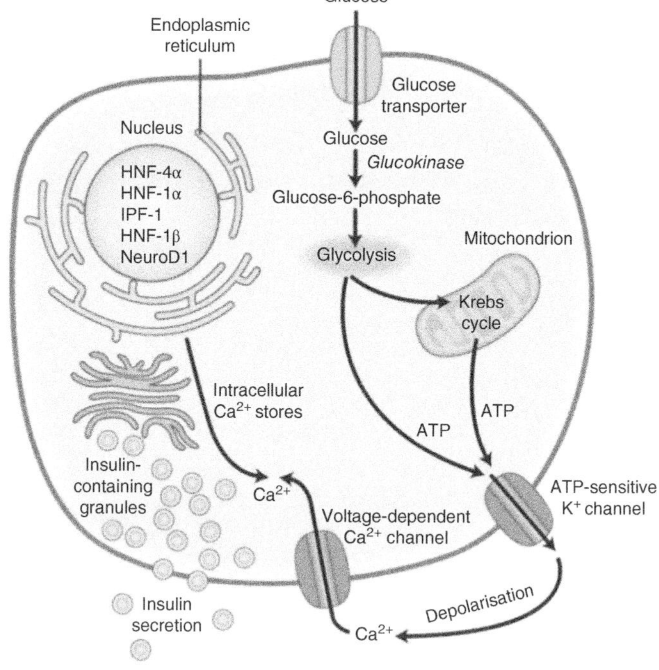

Clinical Genetics and Genomics at a Glance, First Edition. Edited by Neeta Lakhani, Kunal Kulkarni, Julian Barwell, Pradeep Vasudevan, and Huw Dorkins.

Figure 26.2 Transcription factor network in MODY.

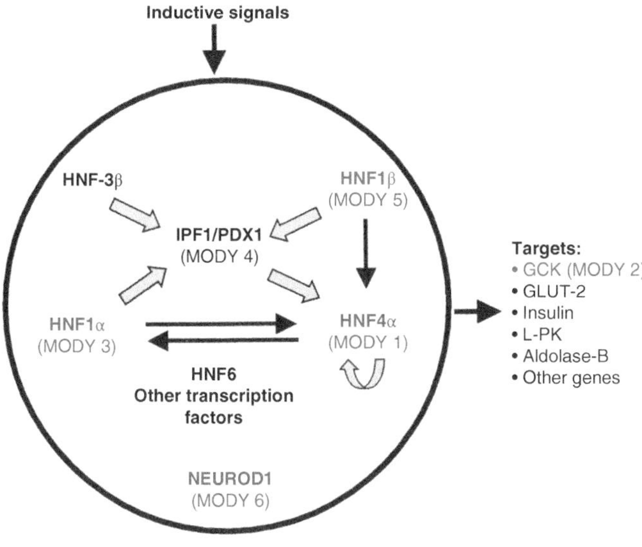

Clinical features

A family history of diabetes, particularly MODY, is a strong indicator. Patients will also exhibit insulin independence, endogenous insulin production, lack of autoantibodies targeting pancreatic antigens, and absence of ketoacidosis. While these features are uncommon in type 1 diabetes, they share similarity with type 2 diabetes, but MODY will not typically be accompanied by obesity or other insulin resistance features common in type 2 diabetes. The clinical features and absence of key markers of type 2 diabetes are the best indicators of monogenic diabetes.

Diagnosis

The diagnosis of diabetes is made either in the light of symptoms or on routine 'screening' (see Figure 26.3). In symptomatic individuals (e.g. polyuria, polydipsia, and unexplained weight loss), the diagnosis can be made based upon the WHO 2006 criteria (Box 26.1) (see Figure 26.4). Diabetes should not be diagnosed in individuals with no symptoms based on a single glucose reading; this requires confirmatory testing. At least one additional glucose test result on another day with a value in the diabetic range is essential.

Patients that are at higher risk of developing overt diabetes should be educated regarding lifestyle measures in an attempt to delay or halt its onset. They should be under regular surveillance to monitor their glucose status, with repeat blood testing at least every one-two years. Those at higher risk for developing type 2 diabetes should be offered screening. If between the age of 40 and 75, a risk assessment should be made, accounting for symptoms or risk factors.

MODY diagnosis based on clinical features is difficult, but the distinguishing feature of MODY is the preservation of β-cell functionality. A potential indicator for MODY over type 2 youth-onset diabetes is weight. Obesity is commonly observed in type 2 diabetes

Figure 26.3 Diagnostic algorithm.

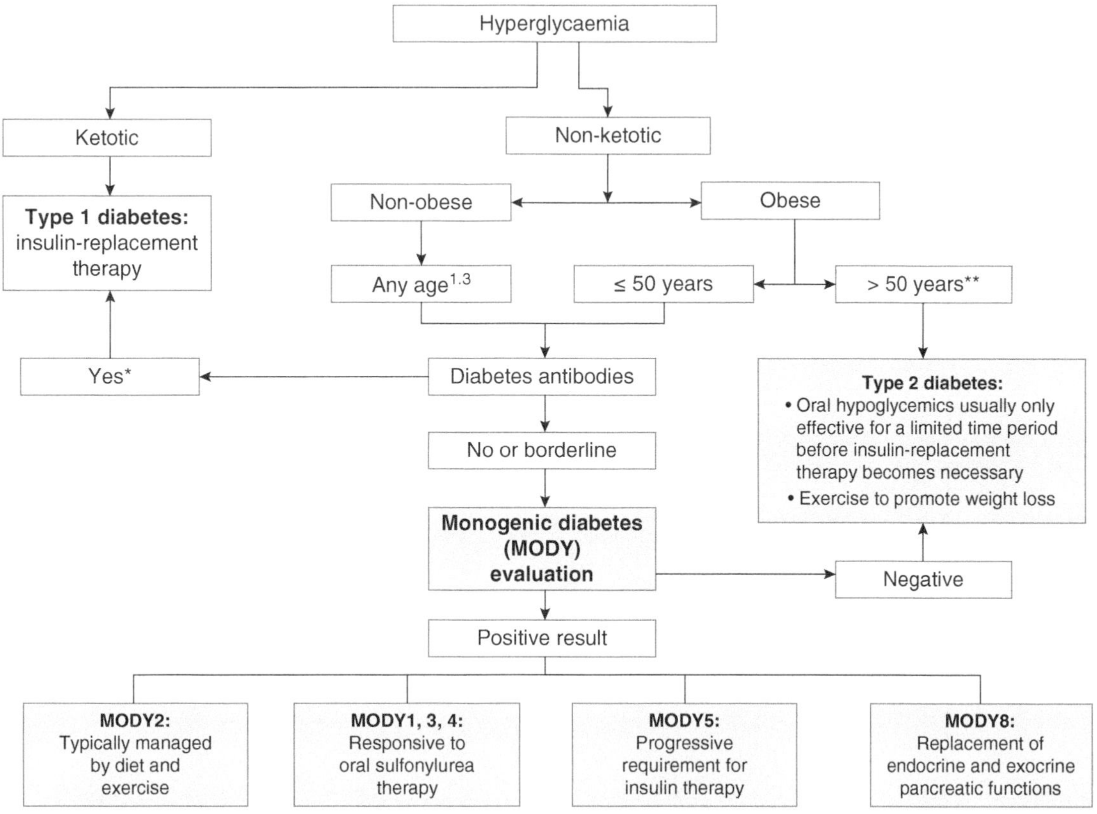

* False positive rate of 10% **Proportion of MODY cases expected to be very low.

Box 26.1 WHO criteria

WHO criteria (2006)	WHO HbA1c criteria (2011)
In presence of symptoms: • Random plasma glucose ≥11.1 mmol/l *or* • Fasting plasma glucose ≥7.0 mmol/l *or* • 2 hour plasma glucose ≥11.1 mmol/l 2 hours post 75 g OGTT	• HbA1c≥48 mmol/mol (6.5%) value with symptoms and plasma glucose≥11.1 mmol/l *or* • HbA1c≥48 mmol/mol (6.5%) values in asymptomatic patient
In asymptomatic individuals, at least one of the above criteria fulfilled on two separate occasions	Not to use in children and young people, type 1 DM symptoms within 2 months, pregnancy, drugs causing hyperglycaemia or blood conditions affecting Hb

but is not typically present in patients with MODY. MODY is caused by genetic alterations and obesity is not believed to be an indicator or risk factor for MODY. Diagnosis confirmation and subtype identification is obtained via genetic testing. Patients for consideration of MODY are generally not obese but have hyperglycaemia, β-cell functionality preservation, lack of evidence of β-cell autoimmunity, or other features not consistent with insulin resistance, and similar familial diabetic history. Direct sequencing of known MODY-causing genetic alterations can have sensitivity rates of 100%, but the expensive nature of genetic testing should be reserved for strongly probable MODY cases. Most MODY subtypes can be determined via the genetic examination of pancreatic β-cells.

Management

MODY treatment depends on the subtype, but upon initial diagnosis, blood glucose level monitoring with ketones is mandatory. Insulin can be administered. Patients should be referred to monogenic diabetes specialists to create treatment plans for the specific MODY subtype the patient has. Treatments for the subtypes draw from oral antidiabetic drugs (OAD), insulin, dietary changes/restrictions, or no medication at all. The treatment will depend on the subtype of MODY and which genes have been affected (Table 26.1).

The future

The genetics of MODY are being further studied with the hopes of creating a predictive modelling system that can determine when people with MODY-causative gene mutations will develop diabetes. Moreover, the study aims to identify a new type of diabetes with MODY-like properties that exist in people with no mutations of the genes currently understood to cause MODY. Other efforts into more extensive and targeted genetic testing of MODY affected individuals is ongoing with the hopes of reducing misdiagnosis of MODY as other types of diabetes and better understanding the comorbidities arising from ethnicity or other genetic factors. Ongoing research also continues evaluating the polygenic nature of other forms of diabetes, including how single nucleotide polymorphisms (SNPs) can modify the risk of type 1 and 2 diabetes.

Figure 26.4 Stratification between different subtypes of diabetes.

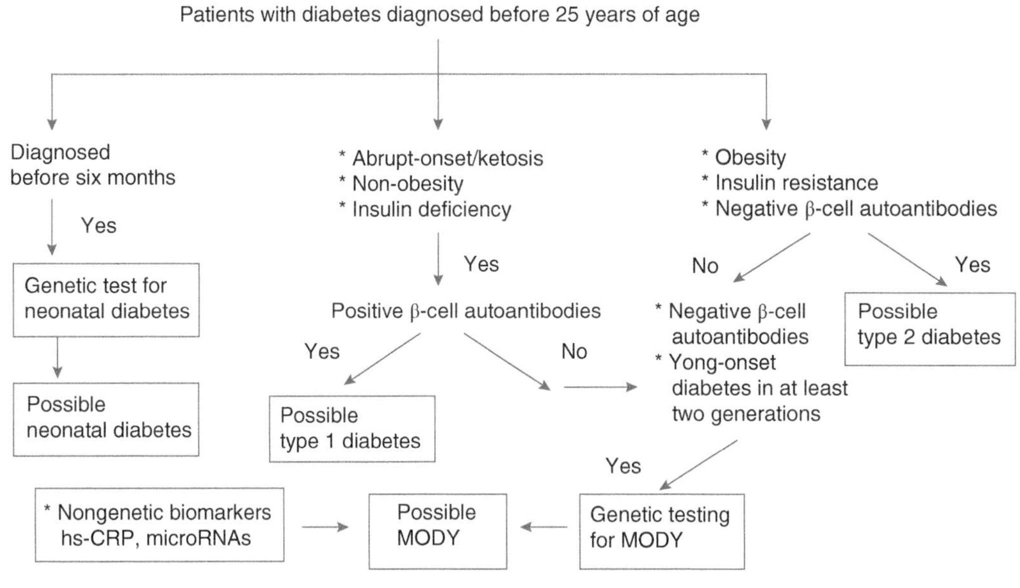

Table 26.1 Subtypes of MODY.

Type	Mutation	Prevalence	Features
MODY 1	*HNF4A*	5–10%	Sensitive to sulphonylureas Neonates macrosomic + hypoglycaemic
MODY 2	*Glucokinase (GCK)*	30–70%	Mild fasting hyperglycaemia No microvascular complications + managed with diet alone
MODY 3	*HNF1A*	70%	Severe hyperglycaemia + microvascular complications can occur Sensitive to sulphonylureas
MODY 4	*Insulin promotor factor 1* gene (*IPF-1*)	<1%	Older onset
MODY 5	*HNF1B*	5–10%	Associated with renal cysts, genital tract malformations + gout
MODY 6	*Neurogenic differentiation 1/B2* gene	Very rare (<1%)	Diagnosis >40 years, few require insulin

27 Diabetes insipidus

Background

Diabetes insipidus (DI) was identified approximately 200 years ago, several thousand years after diabetes mellitus. Thomas Willis noted the difference in taste of the urine from polyuric patients compared to healthy subjects. The name was derived from the French *insipide*, meaning *tasteless*. Since then, our understanding of DI has advanced: using posterior pituitary extracts to treat a proportion of DI patients, synthesising ADH, and the cloning of genes that encode for responsible pathways involving aquaporins and ADH.

Aetiology

DI is rare, affecting around 1 in 25 000 individuals. Causes are outlined in Table 27.1. There are four types of DI: central, nephrogenic, gestational, and primary polydipsia. Congenital links have been found in the first two forms. Central DI is the most common type of DI. Note that 'central' DI is now termed 'arginine-vasopressin (AVP) deficiency', and 'nephrogenic' DI as 'AVP resistance' (AVP-R).

Genetics

Nephrogenic DI has an x-linked recessive inheritance, and results from alterations in *AVPR2* (approx. 90% inherited cases). Approx. 10% cases are either AR (or more rarely AD), due to alterations in *AQP2*. Cranial DI is inherited in an AD manner, caused by alterations in the *AVP* gene.

Table 27.1 Causes of diabetes insipidus.

Cranial	Idiopathic
	Hypothalamic or stalk lesion
	Craniopharyngioma, sarcoidosis, head injury, postpituitary surgery, basal meningitis, histiocytosis
	Genetic
	Dominant
	Recessive: DIDMOAD (Wolfram) syndrome (diabetes insipidus, diabetes mellitus, optic atrophy, deafness)
Nephrogenic	**Primary**
	Genetic: sex-linked recessive, cystinosis
	Secondary
	Metabolic: hyperglycaemia, hypercalcaemia, hypokalaemia
	Drug therapy: lithium, demeclocycline
	Heavy metal poisoning

Pathophysiology

Antidiureric hormone (ADH), kidney function, and thirst regulate water balance. ADH (also known as vasopressin) is produced by the posterior pituitary gland. It is released into the bloodstream via the hypophyseal portal system (Figure 27.1). After targeting the kidney, ADH binds to V2-receptors located on collecting tubules. This triggers the Gs-adenyl cyclase signalling cascade, increasing cAMP, and phosphorylates aquaporin-2 (AQP2) water channels. This embeds the channels onto the cell membrane. AQP2 channels allow water flow into the collecting duct cells from the lumen, thereby concentrating urine through water retention (Figure 27.2). DI results from either an ADH deficiency or a lack of response from the kidney - the causes of central and nephrogenic DI, respectively.

Symptoms

Patients typically present with excessive dilute urination (polyuria), with high urine volume (>2 l) a day and excessive thirst (polydipsia), regardless of cause. In extreme cases, urination can be >20 l a day. Patients may complain of dry mouth and eyes, lightheadedness, headaches, weight loss, and a lack of concentration.

Figure 27.1 Pathophysiology of diabetes insipidus.

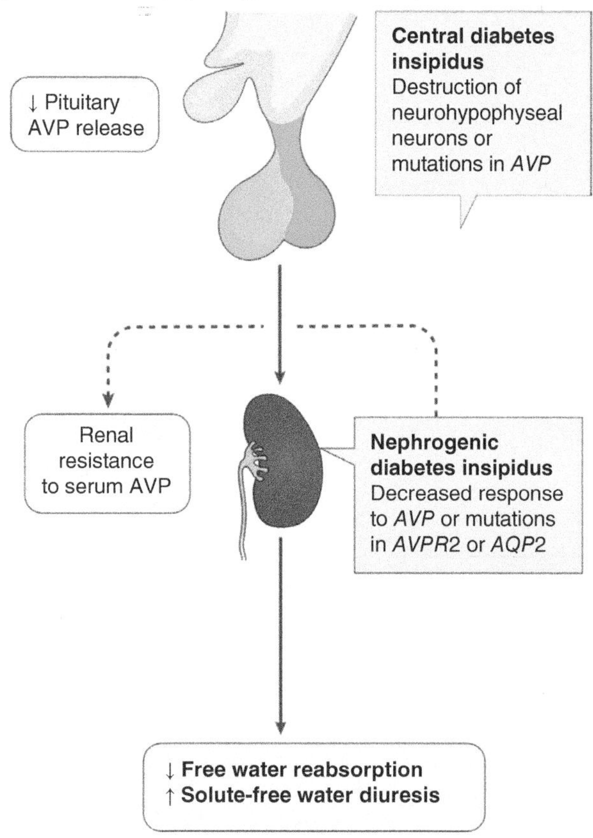

Clinical Genetics and Genomics at a Glance, First Edition. Edited by Neeta Lakhani, Kunal Kulkarni, Julian Barwell, Pradeep Vasudevan, and Huw Dorkins.

Figure 27.2 Signalling pathway of AQP2 translocation.

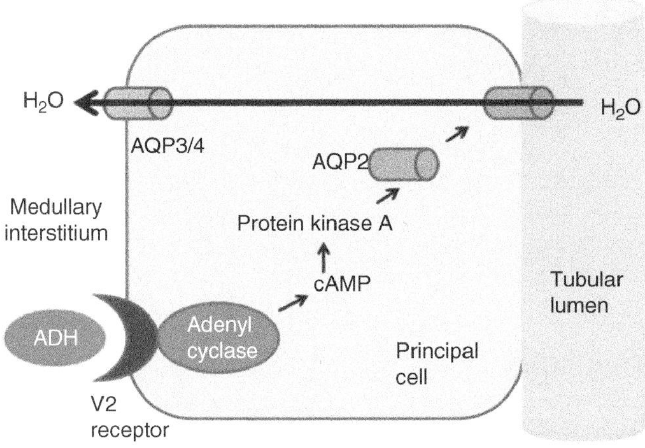

Figure 27.3 Water deprivation test.

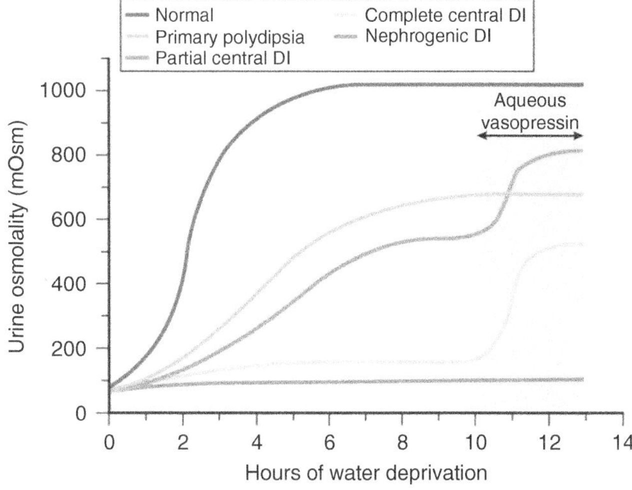

Clinical features

Due to dehydration, patients may also be tachycardiac, tachypnoeic, and hypotensive. If left untreated, patients may develop restlessness, agitation, and seizures due to hypernatraemia.

Diagnosis

DI is confirmed by demonstration of high urine volumes, high serum osmolality, and low urine osmolality. The clinical diagnosis is obvious with complete ADH deficiency due to the presence of extreme thirst and passing of large quantities of pale urine. DI is confirmed if serum osmolality is >295 mosmol/kg, serum [Na+] > 145 mmol/l, and urine osmolality <300 mosmol/kg. In partial DI, the diagnosis may be less clear-cut. In this situation, a water deprivation test can be useful (Figure 27.3). Patients with frank DI will have severe thirst and lose significant weight as a result of water loss. The test should be stopped if excessive weight loss occurs or symptoms are too severe. DI is excluded if patients concentrate urine osmolality >600 mosmol/kg and serum osmolality remains <300 mosmol/kg. In the second part of the test, synthetic ADH (DDAVP) is given. In cranial DI, DDAVP leads to reduced urine volume and increased urine osmolality, whilst in nephrogenic DI, there is no response.

Management

- Patients with confirmed *cranial* DI should be investigated for pituitary disease and managed as appropriate. Cranial DI responds well to DDAVP (desmopressin) administration and results in a good clinical improvement. Desmopressin can be given intranasally, orally, sublingually, or parentally. Overtreatment with DDAVP can lead to dilutional hyponatraemia, commonly characterised by headache and reduced cognitive ability, and, less commonly, seizures if there is a sudden drop in sodium. Signs of undertreatment with DDAVP are excessive thirst and polyuria. Rarely, patients with DI have an impaired thirst mechanism if there is hypothalamic involvement, termed hypodipsic DI. This can be seen in hypothalamic infiltrative disorders and requires specialist care because of the risk of severe hypernatraemia and dehydration.
- In *nephrogenic* DI, the underlying cause should be considered and reversed where possible. If symptoms persist, patients should drink according to thirst and keep up with their water loss. Specific measures to treat nephrogenic DI include the use of low salt, low protein diet, diuretics, and NSAIDs.

The future

Recently, an assay for copeptin has been made widely available. Copeptin is the C-terminus of precursor of vasopressin and provides a reliable diagnostic marker. This may yield promise for testing with higher diagnostic specificity.

28 Fabry–Anderson disease

Background

Fabry–Anderson disease, often referred to as just Fabry disease, is a rare lysosomal storage disease. It was first described in 1898 by Anderson and Fabry, but the enzyme deficiency was not defined until the 1960s.

Aetiology

Fabry disease is rare, with population estimates ranging from 1 in 80 000 to 1 in 120 000 live births. Alongside Gaucher's disease, it is one of the most prevalent metabolic storage disorders.

Genetics

Inheritance is XLR. Fabry disease arises from a defect in the gene for α-*Gal A* (alpha-galactosidase A), found on the long arm of the X chromosome. More than 200 alterations have been identified in the α-*Gal A* gene, with most associated with the classic phenotype, with multisystem involvement. Unlike other X-linked disorders, Fabry disease causes significant medical problems in many females, but the signs and symptoms usually begin later in life and are milder than those seen in their affected male relatives. Some females who carry an alteration in one copy of the α-*Gal A* gene never have any of the signs and symptoms of this condition.

Pathophysiology

Deficiency of α-*Gal A* leads to an inability to catabolise glycosphingolipids with terminal α-galactosyl residues. Glycosphingolipids are constituents of the plasma membrane and intracellular organelles and often circulate in association with apolipoproteins. In the absence of sufficient α-*Gal A*, these lipids accumulate progressively in the lysosomes of many cell types, particularly endothelial cells. The resulting accumulation of substrate leads to a progressive multisystem disease, predominantly affecting the kidneys, skin, heart, and central nervous system.

Symptoms and clinical features

- Fabry disease may be classified into either a *classic* form or a *cardiac* variant.
- Classic Fabry disease is a multisystem disorder involving the skin, eyes, kidneys, heart, and neurological system. The progressive glomerular damage results in proteinuria and non-visible haematuria. Renal function slowly declines over the years with secondary hypertension. End-stage renal disease (ESRD) usually develops by the fourth decade of life.
- Glycosphingolipid accumulation within the heart and coronary vessels leads to progressive coronary occlusive disease, ischemic cardiomyopathy, conduction abnormalities, and valvular heart disease
- Both the peripheral and central nervous system can be affected, leading to autonomic dysfunction, hypohydrosis, and paraesthesia. Glycosphingolipid accumulation can also result in cerebrovascular accidents.
- Angiokeratomas are small dilated veins of the upper dermis that become covered by hyperkeratotic epidermis. They usually present early in the disease and tend to cluster on the lower trunk and extremities and appear as clusters of small, dark red spots.

Diagnosis

- Clinical examination is often sufficient to help secure a diagnosis. Confirmation of diagnosis requires the demonstration of reduced or absent α-*Gal A* activity in serum, leukocytes, skin, or other tissue.
- Serum levels of globotriaosylceramide (Gb3 with GL-3) may be elevated.
- Urine may contain glycosphingolipid-laden epithelial cell aggregates containing oval fat bodies.
- Renal biopsy demonstrates characteristic glomerular changes with secondary tubular and vascular abnormalities. Numerous inclusions contained in lysosomes, especially within podocytes. These have a characteristic lamellated appearance and are known as myelin bodies.

Management

- In general, management involves managing symptoms and preventing renal function from deteriorating. Neuropathic pain can be managed with agents such as gabapentin, carbamazepine, and opioids. Antihypertensive and antiplatelet therapies are useful in reducing overall cardiovascular risk.
- The introduction of enzyme replacement therapy using recombinant human α-*Gal A* (agalsidase α and β) has transformed the treatment of Fabry disease. Studies have demonstrated that treatment with enzyme replacement for greater-than or equal to six months results in reduced plasma and urine glycosphingolipid levels, less neuropathic pain, and improved cerebral blood flow. Deteriorating renal function is also stabilised in most patients with mild–moderate chronic kidney disease (CKD) on treatment.
- Renal replacement therapy may be required for patients with ESRD. Renal transplantation is an effective treatment for advanced kidney disease but does not ameliorate the extra-renal manifestations. α-*Gal A* treatment should be continued in allograft recipients.
- Genetic counselling is necessary for affected individuals. In X-linked recessive disease, all daughters of affected males are carriers, and sons of affected males will not carry the gene for Fabry disease. It is usual for mothers of affected individuals to be considered carriers, and their siblings to therefore be at risk.

The future

An area being evaluated for potential future therapeutic agents is the use of small molecules that rescue and enhance the activity of mutant α-*Gal A* enzymes with residual activity.

Clinical Genetics and Genomics at a Glance, First Edition. Edited by Neeta Lakhani, Kunal Kulkarni, Julian Barwell, Pradeep Vasudevan, and Huw Dorkins.

Metabolic

Chapters

29 Introduction to the genetics of metabolic disorders

Introduction

The aim of this chapter is to provide a flavour of when to suspect a genetic metabolic condition (inherited errors of metabolism, IEM), what basic tests to undertake, and to detail five examples of different IEMs to highlight the principles of diagnosis and management.

There are many metabolic disorders, often presenting in broad and non-specific ways. The clinical variability in features often mimic common conditions, thus making detection difficult. The NHS newborn screening programme screens for six metabolic disorders. This number will expand greatly when the NHS newborn whole genome sequencing screening pilot launches in 2023. Even those screened can be missed, especially if due to milder alterations. The classical presentation for IEMs includes:

- The acutely unwell child
  - Particularly if acutely unwell after a period of starvation (restricted intake, sleep, fasting), intercurrent illness, or stress
  - Fluctuating/progressive neurological deterioration especially encephalopathy
  - Multi-system involvement, organomegaly, hepatic dysfunction
- A child with developmental delay, with or without dysmorphism

It is useful to think of metabolic disorders as being caused by:

- One of the main three body fuels: fats, carbohydrates, and proteins
- Rarer processes involving: metals, porphyrins, pyrimidines, purines, peroxisomes, lysosomes

Underlying biochemical patterns suspicious of a metabolic disorder include:

Hypoketotic hypoglycaemia, lactic acidosis, metabolic acidosis, ketosis, hyperammonaemia

A basic screen when an IEM is suspected includes:

- Ammonia (this is a tricky test to undertake, as it often needs to reach the lab fast and on ice)
- Blood gases
  - Glucose
  - Ketones (and urine ketone if possible)
  - Lactate and acidosis
  - Anion gap

The blood gas is the key starting point for diagnosing IEMs, as modern blood gas machines include nearly all of the basic components of the IEM screen (whereas in the past, one would have to send separate samples to the laboratory to get accurate individual results, for example for ketones).

Key principles in investigating IEMs

Carbohydrates are the primary body fuel. In hypoglycaemia, the body tries to release glucose from glycogen stores, but the glycogen reserves only last so long (one or two days at most, much shorter if exercising). If there is a problem with accessing reserves, or once they are depleted, the body switches to alternative fuel breakdown for energy: fats or proteins. This key theory drives many modern-diets, like keto diets (low-carb).

Low glucose and ketones

When glucose is severely low, this could be due to a problem with carbohydrate, fat, or even protein metabolism.

Normally, if glucose reserves are very low, the body will try to break down fatty acids or ketogenic amino acids, resulting in ketone bodies. Thus, once severely low glucose is detected, the next step is to determine the ketone levels. If they are low, this suggests the body is unable to correctly switch to alternative fuels, hence a fat or protein (fatty oxidation or ketogenic amino acid) metabolism issue (though there are always exceptions to this principal).

In states of severe hypoglycaemia, first exclude common causes such as sepsis or poor feeding; the history is key. If the low glucose is postprandial (after a meal), this could be related to glucose over-utilisation states (i.e. hyperinsulinism).

Ammonia

Ammonia is a neuro-toxic by-product of amino acid breakdown. Defective amino acid metabolism can be reflected in raised ammonia. Ammonia is converted to urea for clearance via the urea cycle. The end-product of fatty acid oxidation, acetyl co-A, is needed to facilitate the first step of the urea cycle. Raised ammonia could therefore reflect either a fatty acid metabolism disorder (not enough acetyl co-A being produced to facilitate ammonia clearance), or an amino acid metabolism disorder. Lastly, if there is significant liver damage, the urea cycle can be affected and ammonia raised.

Clinical Genetics and Genomics at a Glance, First Edition. Edited by Neeta Lakhani, Kunal Kulkarni, Julian Barwell, Pradeep Vasudevan, and Huw Dorkins.

Lactic acidosis

In simple terms, lactate builds up primarily as an end product of anaerobic respiration (anaerobic glycolysis) during tissue hypoxia (which is common in shock and periods of vigorous exercise). Lactate also builds up when lactate clearance is impaired. Lactate forms lactic acid, which leads to a metabolic acidosis (and low pH). High levels of lactate alone are not specific for IEMs (with many other causes including shock, liver failure, excessive training, sepsis, and drugs), hence they must be considered in the context of the glucose, ketones, ammonia, pH, and overall clinical picture.

As a general rule, in non-metabolic causes of hyperlactataemia, ketone levels are normal, whereas in IEMs, ketone levels are abnormal. If non-metabolic causes are excluded, then hyperlactataemia could indicate a fatty oxidation, carbohydrate, or rarely an amino acid metabolism defect.

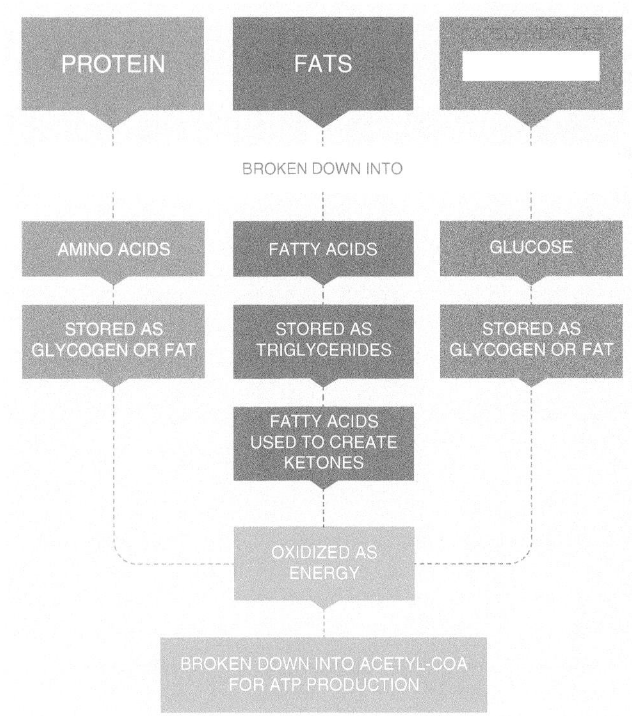

Screening IEMs

Six IEMs are part of the NHS newborn screening programme (via the bloodspot on day five). Note that as a screening programme, cases can still be missed. The six conditions are: phenylketonuria (PKU), medium-chain acyl-CoA dehydrogenase deficiency (MCADD), maple syrup urine disease (MSUD), isovaleric acidaemia (IVA), glutaric aciduria type 1 (GA1), homocystinuria (HCU).

30 Overview of disorders of amino acid metabolism

Background

Amino acids (AAs) are the building blocks of proteins, important in repair and growth. There are 20 'standard' amino acids coded for directly by DNA, and 2 others formed via an additional synthetic step. Dysfunction in their synthesis, transport, or breakdown results in over 50 amino acid metabolism disorders. Many of these cause symptoms early-on in life, thus six are included in the UK NHS newborn 'heel-prick' screening test: PKU, homocystinuria, maple syrup urine disease, isovaleric acidaemia, glutaric aciduria type 1, and MCADD.

Although humans can code for all 20 AAs directly from DNA, such AAs produce proteins, rather than being released as single AAs for use in other important bodily processes. Eleven stand-alone AAs are obtained via chemical reactions of compounds and are deemed 'non-essential AAs', whereas eight AAs (nine in infants) can only be obtained via diet and are deemed 'essential AAs'. Foods that contain all essential AAs are termed 'complete proteins' such as meat, poultry, eggs, dairy products, soy, quinoa, buckwheat, and dates.

When AAs are broken down, the ammonia nitrogen at one end of the amino acid is split off, incorporated into urea, and excreted in the urine. Defects in this process lead to a sub-set of amino acid metabolism disorders called 'urea cycle defect disorders', for example; OTC, citrulinemia, and arginemia. Another group of amino acid metabolism disorders involve defects in either the transport of amino acids from the GI tract to the blood, or reabsorption from the urine to the kidneys; examples include cystinosis and Hartnup disease. Other examples of common AA metabolism disorders include PKU and homocystinuria (HCU). In this chapter, we consider HCU as an example condition.

Epidemiology

The most common form of HCU affects approximately 1 in 200 000–335 000 individuals worldwide. Rates are higher in some countries, including Ireland (approximately 1 in 65 000), Germany (approximately 1 in 17 800), Norway (approximately 1 in 6400), and Qatar (approximately 1 in 1800).

Genetics

Amino acid metabolism disorders including HCU are generally inherited in an AR fashion, though OTC is the common exception, as it is X-linked recessive.

Pathophysiology

HCU is a multi-systemic connective tissue disorder caused by a deficiency of the enzyme cystathionine beta synthase or related enzymes. This leads to an inability to breakdown methionine (an essential amino acid), and the build-up of toxic homocysteine. Other causes of HCU include vitamin B deficiencies (B2: riboflavin, 6: pryidoxine, 9: folate, 12: cobalamin) (Figure 30.1).

Symptoms

Symptoms are often not present in the first year of life. Children usually present with learning difficulties,

Clinical features

Patients with homocystinuria have a marfanoid habitus (long, tall, thin, with long fingers). The chest is often either protruding outwards (pectus carinatum) or inwards (pectus excavatum). Visual problems included severe short sightedness and downward lens dislocation (as opposed to upwards lens dislocation in Marfan syndrome). Other features include vascular problems, weak bones, osteoporosis, and bone/joint problems.

Diagnosis

Although genetic testing is available, routine biochemical testing is first line in HCU, as it is relatively easy, quick, and cheap to test for serum or urinary amino acids to look for raised methionine in the presence of homocysteine. Despite the precision of genetic testing (even in single gene disorders), testing can lead to unclear results (variants of unknown significance), false negatives (failure to find the causal variant), or false positives (detecting what is wrongly felt to be a pathogenic variant).

Biochemical testing does require careful sample collection and interpretation, since there are several other causes of increased homocysteine in the urine (homocystinuria) such as vitamin B deficiencies (B2: riboflavin, 6: pryidoxine, 9: folate, 12: cobalamin), and re-methylation defects.

Management

As with many amino acid metabolism disorders, the management approach includes:

1 Decreasing amino acids in the diet (low protein diet) with the help of a specialist dietitian.

2 Taking medication to help clear the relevant amino acid. In HCU, betaine helps remove excess methionine.

Monitoring homocysteine levels is important. Where the underlying cause is due to deficiency of vitamin B6, pyridoxine replacement helps.

If HCU is diagnosed early and lifelong treatment is adhered too, then most children live healthy, long lives.

The future

Novel strategies to treat homocystinuria remain in development, ranging from functional replacement of the abnormal cystathionine beta synthase to improved clearance of homocysteine, alongside reducing its toxicity.

Clinical Genetics and Genomics at a Glance, First Edition. Edited by Neeta Lakhani, Kunal Kulkarni, Julian Barwell, Pradeep Vasudevan, and Huw Dorkins.

Figure 30.1 Methionine metabolic pathway.

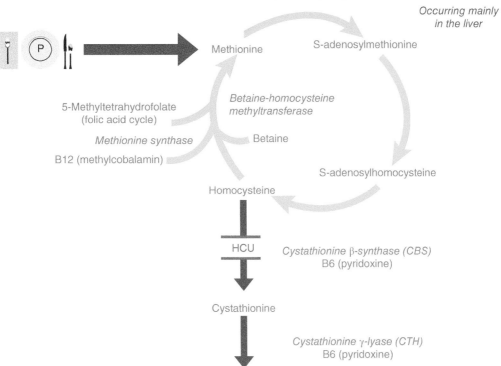

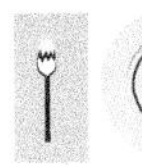
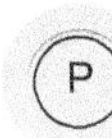

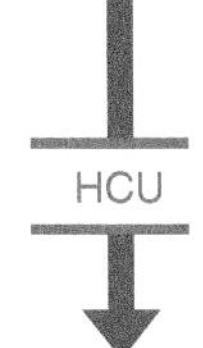
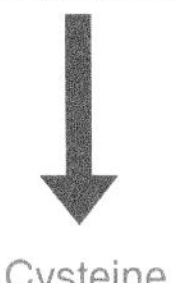

31 Overview of disorders of carbohydrate metabolism

Background

Defects in production or breakdown of carbohydrates can lead to many different carbohydrate metabolism problems, including galactosaemia, glycogen storage and fructose metabolism disorders. To understand these, it is important to remember the different types of carbohydrates.

In this chapter, we will explore one type of carbohydrate disorder (GSD I (von Gierke disease) type a) as a paradigm to the glycogen storage disorders (GSDs). Several other GSDs exist, including GSD II (Pompe disease) and GSD V (McCardle disease). GSDs are rare genetic conditions caused by deficiencies in enzymes involved in glycogen synthesis or breakdown. They vary in presentation.

Epidemiology

GDS I (von Gierke disease) occurs in 1 in 100 000 individuals.

Genetics

GSD I is an AR- inherited disorder. Carriers for GSD I are healthy.

Pathophysiology

During periods of fasting, the main mechanism for supplying the body with glucose is glycogenolysis (glycogen breakdown), primarily in the liver; see Table 31.1 for types of carbohydrates. In GSD Ia, an important enzyme in converting glycogen to glucose – glucose-6-phosphotase (G6P) – is deficient, hence patients experience marked hypoglycaemia, liver glycogen build-up (leading to hepatomegaly), and other complications.

Symptoms

If untreated, GSD I can present in the neonatal period with severe hypoglycaemia (which manifests neonatally as irritability or non-specific symptoms similar to an infection), or more commonly in infants aged between 3 and 4 months with hypoglycaemia, an enlarged protuberant abdomen (due to hepatomegaly), and growth failure. Hypoglycaemia is seen after even short periods of fasting (2–4 hours).

Infants with GSD I are often described as having doll-like faces (with a round face, full cheeks, a short nose, and a relatively small chin), with thin extremities and short stature.

Clinical features

One may suspect that if the body is unable to breakdown glycogen as fuel, it would switch to fat or protein breakdown instead, but both these processes are impaired in GSD I. The build-up of G6P prevents normal fat breakdown, so fats accumulate in the liver and kidney (leading to nephromegaly), hyperlipidaemia, and hypertriglyceridaemia. Hyperlipidaemia can manifest as xanthomas (yellow fatty deposits, plaques on the skin). G6P is broken down to lactate (hence lactic acidosis) and urate (hyperuricaemia). Hypoglycaemia can lead to seizures.

Long-term complications of untreated GSD I include growth failure, osteoporosis, delayed puberty, gout, renal disease, pulmonary hypertension, hepatic adenomas (with potential for malignant transformation), polycystic ovaries (in virtually all females), pancreatitis (secondary to hypertriglyceridaemia), and cognitive dysfunction.

Diagnosis

Diagnosis should be suspected in neonates or infants who present acutely unwell with profound hypoglycaemia, hepatomegaly, and growth failure. Further laboratory investigations should confirm lactic acidosis (which in this case is a by-product of alternative fuel breakdown), hyperlipidaemia (both raised triglycerides and cholesterol due to impaired fat metabolism), and hyperuricaemia (related to high levels of G6P).

The next step in diagnosis is molecular genetic confirmation (looking for biallelic variants in the causative genes *G6PC1 [formerly G6PC]* or *SLC37A4)*. This is preferred to biochemical enzyme-level tests, as these require a liver biopsy (but may be required if genetic testing is inconclusive).

Management

The dietician plays a central role in management, in not only preventing hypoglycaemia but ensuring optimal nutrition for growth and development. Hypoglycaemia is prevented by small and frequent meals with high complex carbohydrates (throughout the day and just before bedtime) with frequent snacking between meals. Complex carbohydrates release glucose more slowly into the bloodstream as opposed to simple sugars (mono- and disaccharides). Uncooked cornstarch is a particularly useful complex carbohydrate, as it is slowly digested. Overnight glucose infusion via a nasogastric tube prevents hypoglycaemia during sleep.

In the long term, it is important to lower levels of harmful by-products, thus allopurinol is prescribed to bring down uric acid levels, and lipid-lowering medication is used in some circumstances to prevent atherosclerosis and pancreatitis.

A MDT approach, including nephrology management to avoid end-stage renal disease (ESRD) and hepatology/immunology input, is required. Normal growth and puberty is expected in treated children, although long-term complications can still develop such as hepatic adenoma and proteinuria. Most affected individuals live into adulthood, but those untreated die young.

Clinical Genetics and Genomics at a Glance, First Edition. Edited by Neeta Lakhani, Kunal Kulkarni, Julian Barwell, Pradeep Vasudevan, and Huw Dorkins.

Table 31.1 Disorders of carbohydrate metabolism.

Monosaccharides (one sugar)	Disaccharides (two sugars)	Oligosaccharides (a few sugars, 3–10)	Polysaccharides (many sugars)
Glucose (dextrose)	Sucrose (fructose + glucose) = Table sugar / Fruit sugar	Oligosaccharides often combine with other molecules (proteins/lipids) to form:	Glycogen (storage carbohydrate in animals)
Fructose	Maltose (glucose + glucose) = Malt sugar		Starch (storage carbohydrate in plants)
Galactose	Lactose (glucose + galactose) = Milk sugar	Glycans (e.g. glycoproteins, glycosamines, glycolipids etc.)	Cellulose (carbohydrate providing structural support in plants)
Ribose/Deoxyribose		Fructans (e.g. fructosamine)	

The future

Despite dietetic management, the condition is still very serious and dangerous as constant consumption of glucose is needed. Individuals who miss a cornstarch meal may suffer a seizure, and patients often worry about going to sleep and not waking up again.

The future is exciting with the world's first gene therapy for GSD currently under trial in the largest centre for glycogen storage diseases in Connecticut Children's Hospital, USA. The gene therapy, DTX401 (AAV8G6PC), targets the liver and provides a working copy of the gene to allow for glucose to be stored to glycogen. Early results in limited patients have seen some discontinue conventional treatment. The study is ongoing and in phase 3 as of late 2022.

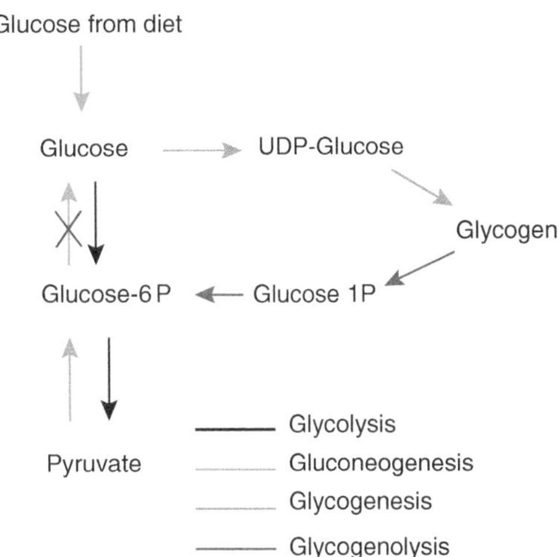

32 Overview of disorders of lipid metabolism

Background

Inborn errors of lipid metabolism are numerous and include fatty acid oxidation and metabolism disorders. There are two main types: those related to lipid synthesis (lipogenesis) and those related to lipid breakdown (lipolysis) leading to overaccumulation/lipid storage diseases (lipidoses). Lipids can either be produced within the body or ingested, hence defects can also occur with lipid digestion, absorption, and transportation. However, most inborn errors of lipid metabolism tend to occur with lipid synthesis and breakdown.

Lipids are metabolised by lysosomes, the 'cell-recycling centre'. Lysosomes turn unwanted cell materials into reusable substances, hence lipid metabolism disorders fall under the lysosomal storage disorders umbrella. Lysosomes also process polysaccharides (including glycogen and mucopolysaccharides), proteins (including glycoproteins and collagen), peptides, and nucleotides (DNA and RNA), hence lysosomal storage disorders also encompass other conditions including mucopolysaccharidoses. More information on the different types of lipids and their importance can be found in Table 32.1. In this chapter, we consider Fabry Disease as an example condition.

Epidemiology

The incidence of Fabry disease is approximately 1 in 50–117 000 males. As genetic testing becomes more ubiquitous and milder phenotypes emerge, the incidence is becoming less uncommon than once thought (as with many genetic conditions). Recent screening studies in newborns in Italy and Australia have the incidence at 1 in 3–4000, with the majority having milder, late-onset phenotypes.

Genetics

Fabry disease is a X-linked disorder, with males classically affected and female carriers generally asymptomatic or having mild manifestations. Fabry disease is caused by pathogenic variants in the *GLA* (alpha galactosidase) gene.

Pathophysiology

Glycosphingolipids (a subset of glycolipids or sphingolipids) are important in the cell membrane for cell–cell interactions and signalling, especially in the central nervous system. There are three main glycosphingolipids: cerebrosides (that give rise to cerbrosidoses like Krabbe disease and Gaucher's disease), globosides, and galacatasides (that give rise to galactasidoses; Tay-Sach and Fabry disease). In Fabry disease, deficiency of the enzyme alpha galactasidase A (α-Gal A) leads to build up of galactosides (lipids) in the lysosome.

Table 32.1 What are the different types of lipids and why are they important?

Lipids are a category of molecule unified by their inability to mix well with water. Different types of lipids include fats (triglycerides), oils (fats that are liquid at room temperature), phospholipids (important in cell membranes), sphingolipids (important in neural tissue membranes), glycolipids (cerebrosides, globosides, and gangliosides; important in cell recognition), glycophospholipids, lipoproteins (important in lipid transport), lipopolysaccharides, and steroids/sterols. Cholesterol (a lipid) is the commonest steroid in the body and is an important precursor for steroid hormone production (for example sex hormones), vitamin D and bile production, as well as being implicated in the development of atherosclerosis. Functionally, lipids are important in providing insulation, as structural components, as building blocks for hormones, and as energy sources.

Nearly all lipids contain a fatty acid chain, with fats containing three fatty acids per molecule. Oxidation of fatty acids is an important way for the body to produce energy during fasting (when glycogen reserves are depleted) or in periods of high energy demand. Fats contain twice as much energy per gram as carbohydrates (nine calories worth of energy per gram versus four), so are an efficient way to store energy long term. Not only do fats fare better than carbohydrates in energy density, but the body can store more fat than glycogen.

Glycogen (stored carbohydrates) reserves in the liver and muscle are limited, equating to ~2000 calories of energy (or 90–120 min of vigorous, sustained exercise), whereas stored fat reserves are virtually unlimited. Even in lean athletes, fat reserves can fuel 100 000 calories of continuous, vigorous exercise (over 100 hours of marathon running!). Although fats are good for long-term storage, if you need energy quickly, it is more efficient to burn carbohydrates than fats, as less oxygen is required.

Lipid breakdown to release energy

Fatty oxidation (the process by which energy is released from fats) occurs primarily in the mitochondria. A preliminary step to enable this occurs in the cytosol, where the addition of a coenzyme A group to the fatty acid forms fatty acyl-coA. Many different enzymes are involved downstream, coded by different genes, to enable the release of energy from the fatty acyl-coA. Disorders in this pathway include the coenzyme-A dehydrogenase deficiencies (VLCAD, LCHAD, MCADD, etc.) and carnitine-related disorders (primary carnitine deficiency, carnitine palmitotransferase deficiency I and II).

Separate to lipid catabolism for energy, lipid breakdown in the lysosome can be defective and lead to several lipidosis where harmful fats build up in tissues, for example Gaucher and Fabry diseases; the latter condition will be considered in more detail in this chapter.

Clinical Genetics and Genomics at a Glance, First Edition. Edited by Neeta Lakhani, Kunal Kulkarni, Julian Barwell, Pradeep Vasudevan, and Huw Dorkins.

Symptoms

It is little surprise that Fabry disease was first described by a dermatologist (Dr Johannaes Fabry) in 1898, as the first manifestations are often dermatological.

The classic form of Fabry disease presents in childhood or adolescence in males, often beginning with angiokeratomas (dark red-blue lesions, occurring anywhere in the body including the oral cavity, especially between the navel to knee, that worsen with age) and painful periodic crisis of extremities (acroparesthesias); these are described as an intense burning pain that last between minutes to days, and radiate proximally and to other areas such as the abdomen. Acroparasthesias often decrease with age, but can worsen in some people, so much so, that the patients may contemplate suicide. Lack/absence of sweating is common, which can manifest as overheating during exercise.

Clinical features

Corneal opacities are visible on slit lamp examinations; these are common in carrier females too. Cardiac manifestations, such as left ventricular hypertrophy, are often associated with intraventricular septal hypertrophy and are progressive. These may be present in females as well. These changes are secondary to glycosphingolipid infiltration in cardiac cells and can subsequently lead to cardiac dysrhythmia and other cardiac sequelae (hypertension, heart failure, angina). Cerebrovascular disease may also be present. Glycosphingolipid build up in the kidneys leads to gradual deterioration of renal function, and in untreated patients is the most serious cause of mortality. If untreated, this leads to death in males in the fifth decade, following cardiac complications. Other systems including gastrointestinal and respiratory, may be involved,

Diagnosis

- The constellation of angiokeratomas (which can be seen in other LSDs), intermittent acroparasthesias (which can mimic familial Mediterranean fever or other inflammatory arthritis conditions), unexplained left ventricular hypertrophy, unexplained stroke, visual changes, and renal disease, should make one suspect Fabry disease.
- First-line diagnostic testing is biochemical, via measuring α-Gal A enzyme levels. Levels less than 1% are consistent with classical Fabry disease. Reduced levels are consistent with atypical Fabry disease.
- Molecular genetic testing adds further confirmation and allows for screening of female carriers. Biochemical testing is not reliable in female carriers as some carriers have levels with in the normal range.

Management

- Management requires a MDT approach, with input from cardiology (cardiac surveillance), dermatology, nephrology, ophthalmology, genetics, and neurology.
- Acroparathesias can be managed with phenytoin, carbemazepine, and gabapentin.
- Fabrazyme®, an enzyme replacement therapy (ERT), replaces the deficient α-Gal A enzyme and has been licensed for over a decade. Galafold® (migalastat), a more recent drug, is a chaperone therapy that binds to the misfolded protein to help it fold into the correct shape for proper function. Galafold is only suitable for certain alterations (around a third of protein misfold types).
- There is emerging consensus that both drugs have limited impact in long term outcomes. Despite this, they are generally recommended to be started as soon as possible in all affected males and those females with significant disease.

The future

One may wonder why ERTs have limited value considering they tackle the underlying disease problem. However, ERTs cannot reach all parts of the body, particularly across the blood brain barrier (BBB), hence have limited value in preventing stroke complications. Also, the body may recognise the enzyme as being foreign, hence develop an immune response to the drug.

A new class of drugs called 'substrate reduction' therapies (SRTs) are in clinical trials; these do cross the BBB and are expected not to cause the immune response of ERTs. SRTs are drugs that block the production of the toxic by-products

Other drugs in development include more active forms of ERTs. Several gene therapies are under trial.

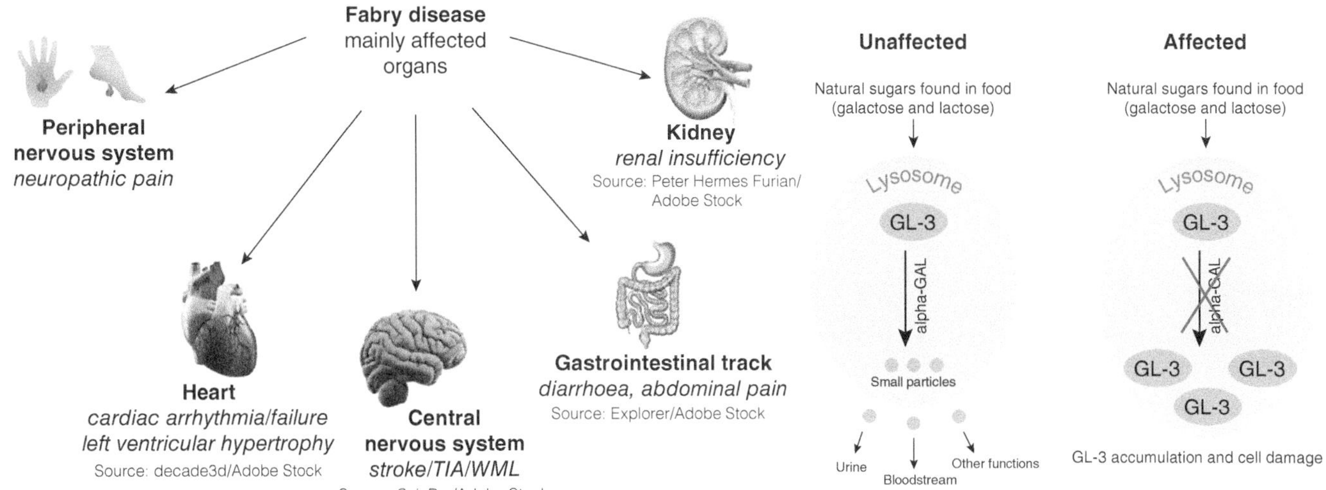

33 Overview of peroxisomal disorders

Background

Peroxisomal disorders are a group of variably presenting metabolic disorders caused by peroxisome dysfunction. These include Zellweger spectrum disorders, pseudo neonatal adrenoleukodystrophy, rhizomelic chondrodysplasia punctata (RCDP) disorders and hyperoxaluria. Zellweger syndrome was the first described peroxisomal disorder (in the 1940s). Zellweger spectrum disorders (ZSD) lie on a phenotypic continuum ranging from severe to mild (relating to previous diagnostic labels of Zellweger syndrome (severe ZSD), neonatal adrenoleukodystrophy (intermediate / mild ZSD) and infantile refsum disease (intermediate / mild ZSD).

Peroxisomes are cell organelles important in:

- the production of cholesterol, bile acids, and ether phospholipids (e.g. plasmalogens), thus contribute to phospholipid content of the brain white matter
- detoxification of glycolate (whose accumulation leads to excess calcium oxalate build up) and hydrogen peroxide.
- oxidation of beta-fatty acids
- peroxisomes are important in VLCFA breakdown.

Epidemiology

ZSDs are 'ultra-rare' with a prevalence of 1:133,000 in one US study and 1:500,000 in one Asian study. A rare disease by definition affects <1 in 2,000, whereas an ultra-rare disease affects <1 in 50,000.

Genetics

ZSDs are inherited in an AR manner. They are a heterogeneous group of conditions, with 13 *PEX* (peroxin) genes known to cause the conditions. There is one exception to the recessive rule, a variant in *PEX6* (p.Arg860Trp) causes a dominant form of ZSD.

Pathophysiology

The *PEX* genes encode for peroxins, important proteins in peroxisome biogenesis (especially in development of the peroxisome membrane and the peroxisome import machinery within the peroxisome matrix). Loss of function variants in *PEX* genes cause ZSD. Note *PEX5* and *PEX7* cause RDCP (Figure 33.1).

Symptoms

ZS often presents neonatally with floppiness (central hypotonia) and poor feeding, with or without seizures. The floppiness may manifest as exaggerated head lag, difficulty swallowing, and poor suck.

Clinical features

Affected individuals are often dysmorphic, with a high forehead, flat facial profile, and large anterior fontanelle. Cataracts or other visual abnormalities are sometimes present, including retinopathy. Hypotonia is severe, with associated hypo- or areflexia. Intellectual disability is often severe.

A hallmark sign is a stippled epiphysis of the patellae. Stippling is a rare skeletal sign, usually seen before the age of one year, with a limited list of differentials; stippling at the knees is pathognomonic for ZS, albeit with a limited window of detection.

Antenatal presence of ventriculomegaly and bilateral renal cysts can manifest. Liver disease can be severe.

Diagnosis

- Suspicion of ZS is raised through physical examination findings after a neonate presents with severe hypotonia.
- Radiological findings are contributory to a diagnosis, including a MRI head finding of polymicrogyria and knee radiographs of stippled epiphyses.
- Biochemical evaluation confirming raised very long chain fatty acids (VLFCAs) and low plasmalogens is also supportive (whereas in RCDP the plasmalogens are low, but VLCFAs are normal).
- Definitive diagnosis is made via molecular genetic testing. Since there are several potential causative genes, a panel-based approach is often a sensible starting point.

Management

Prognosis is sadly poor, with most infants dying in the first year of life. In survivors, retinopathy can often lead to blindness. Management is based around management of symptoms, often requiring gastrostomy for adequate nutrition, fat soluble vitamin supplementation, hearing aids, cataract surgery, and an MDT approach for other complications.

The future

Gene therapies for ZSD are somewhat behind other conditions; for example in GSD, the target gene therapy needs to only primarily reach one body organ (i.e. the liver), which makes producing a drug easier. However, in ZSD, the disorder affects all body cells, hence it is harder to address with a single agent that needs to reach all the tissues. However, successful retinal gene therapy to combat retinopathy-related blindness has been demonstrated in mouse models of ZSD in 2018.

Clinical Genetics and Genomics at a Glance, First Edition. Edited by Neeta Lakhani, Kunal Kulkarni, Julian Barwell, Pradeep Vasudevan, and Huw Dorkins.

Figure 33.1 Peroxisome biogenesis pathway.

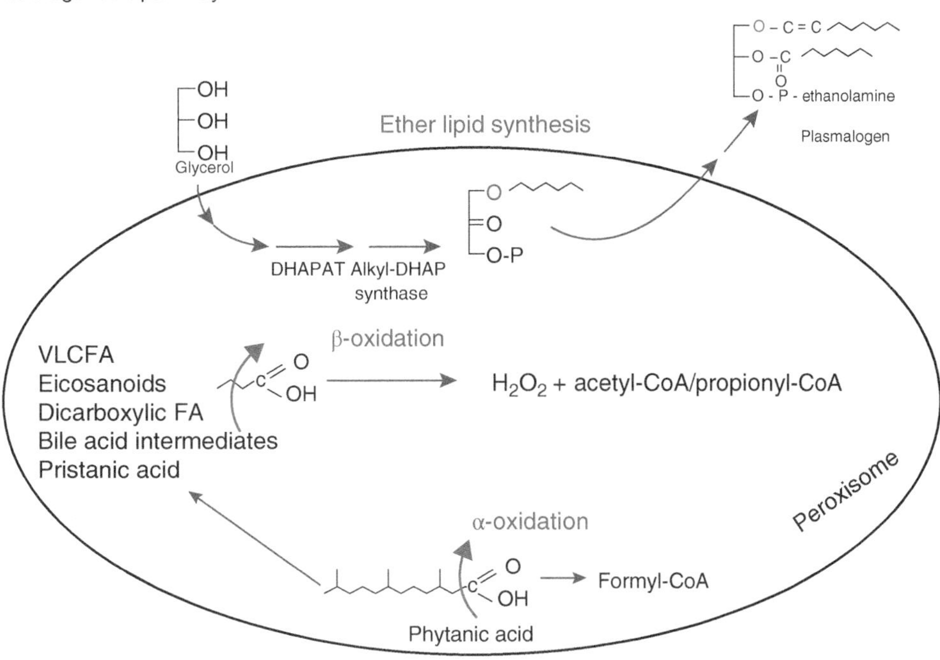

34 Overview of disorders of purine and pyrimidine metabolism

Background

Purines and pyrimidines are important nitrogenous bases. When combined with phosphates, ribose, or deoxyribose, they form nucleotides – the building blocks of DNA and RNA. Purine bases are guanine (G) and adenine (A). Pyrimidine bases are cytosine (C) and thymine (T). Defects in their production or breakdown lead to metabolic disorders.

For example, Lesch-Nyhan disease (LND) is a genetic disorder of purine nucleotide salvage, and orotic aciduria is a problem with purine production. LND was first discovered by medical student Michael Lesch and his mentor paediatrician Dr William Nyhan, when they came across a boy with a urine infection and developmental delay (whose brother also had developmental delay, bit his hands and chewed away his lower lips). They tested his urine and found raised uric acid and wondered if they had stumbled across a new disease. In this chapter, we will consider LND (also known as juvenile gout) further.

Epidemiology

LND affects 1 in 380 000 live births.

Genetics

LND is a X-linked recessive (XLR) inherited disorder, caused by alterations in the *HPRT1* gene (hypoxanthine guanine phosphoribosyl-transferase), on the X chromosome. Generally, in XLR disorders, males are more severely affected than females, as females have two copies of the X chromosome, whereas males only have one. In females, the additional X chromosome contains a working copy of the gene, providing protection from the disorder, thus in most XLR conditions females are asymptomatic or 'healthy carriers'. Likewise in LND, female carries are virtually always asymptomatic though some can develop mild symptoms of gout with age.

Pathophysiology

The HPRT enzyme is important in recycling purine nucleotides. Purines and pyrimidine bases are mainly made from amino acids though a minority are made from degraded DNA (the 'salvage pathway'). HPRT is important in the purine salvage pathway. If HPRT is defective, then degraded purine DNA/RNA is not recycled and instead forms its normal waste product, uric acid. The build-up of uric acid leads to gout. Other features of the condition include self-mutilation and neurological sequelae, though the mechanism for this is unclear.

Symptoms

LND is characterised by the triad of neurological dysfunction, cognitive/behavioural changes (especially self-mutilation), and hyperuricemia. Self-mutilation to the degree seen in LND is a distinguishing feature of the condition. Affected individuals may painfully bite fingers and lips, often leading to amputations. Patients are often aware they are compulsively and painfully harming themselves, but are unable to stop themselves.

One of the first symptoms parents notice are orange sand-like crystals (uric acid crystals) or 'gravel' in the nappy. The uric acid build up can lead to renal stones and therefore haematuria, renal flank pain, and urinary tract infections. Later, the uric acid can deposit in the joints can lead to gouty arthritis.

Neurological features such as hypotonia and developmental delay (especially motor) may not become apparent until 3–6 months of age. Uncontrollable self-injurious behaviour presents in 85% of males and starts around the age of three years. Behaviours such as repaying kindness with coldness or rage, spitting, aggression, and coprolalia (involuntary swearing) can manifest in early childhood, some even in the first year.

Clinical features

Within the first few years of life, neurological dysfunction can present with irritability, involuntary movements (like those seen in Huntington's disease), and a cerebral palsy-like picture due to basal ganglia damage. Patients may adopt a 'fencing stance' posture and are unable to walk without treatment. Although neurological features evolve in the first few years, after this they are not expected to progress. Affected males go onto suffer delayed growth and puberty, and often testicular atrophy. A third of patients can develop seizures and some require gastrostomy feeding. Rare (but often difficult to manage) features can include unexplained apnoea, unexplained emesis, and dystonic crisis.

Diagnosis

- Initial suspicion may be raised by uric acid crystals in the urine soon after birth, though blood tests for uric acid may be normal (as the body is good at clearing high serum uric acid).
- Diagnosis is more likely later when developmental delay occurs (between 3 and 6 months), especially in the context of a relevant family history, and is often only made when self-injurious behaviour manifests. Self-injury is also seen in other developmental disorders like Rett or Tourette syndromes, but is more severe here, as it can involve tissue damage. This degree of self-injury can be seen in Cornelia de Lange syndrome and familial dysautonomia too, though is different in LND, as self-injury in other conditions is usually in the form of head banging or non-specific mutilation, whereas in LNS it is commonly fingertip, cheek, and lower lip biting.
- Once LNS is suspected, HPRT enzyme levels from blood or skin fibroblasts of less than 1.5% of usual activity confirms the diagnosis.
- Molecular genetic testing can also be pursued and is helpful to identify carrier females (in whom the enzyme test is unreliable) and milder cases. This has led to a reconsideration of LND being part of a spectrum (albeit on the more severe end) of conditions caused by *HPRT1* gene alterations.

Clinical Genetics and Genomics at a Glance, First Edition. Edited by Neeta Lakhani, Kunal Kulkarni, Julian Barwell, Pradeep Vasudevan, and Huw Dorkins.

Management

An MDT approach to LND is key. Management is largely symptomatic:

- Allopurinol reduces uric acid levels and alleviates the gout and kidney-related problems, though does not resolve the neurological deficits and self-injury. This reinforces the unclear cause of neurological sequelae. It is important to avoid drugs that precipitate uric acid build up and to keep well hydrated to avoid renal stones.
- There is little in the way of medical treatment for the neurological complications, though baclofen and benzodiazepines can be used for spasticity.
- There is no drug to cure self-injury, though restraint can help. Many patients have their teeth removed to prevent injury.

The future

When originally diagnosed in the 1960s, patients with LND would often die before their fifth birthday, but with improved treatment can now live well into their fourth decade. There is still no cure. Gene therapy for LND has shown partial phenotype rescue as far back as in 1984. A retrovirus with a working copy of the *HPRT1* gene was inserted into human Lesch-Nyhan cell lines *in vitro*. However, *in vivo* experiments have yet to be successful. Technological advances have shown success *in vivo* for other conditions, but perhaps the rarity of LND has prevented the requisite funding for success thus far.

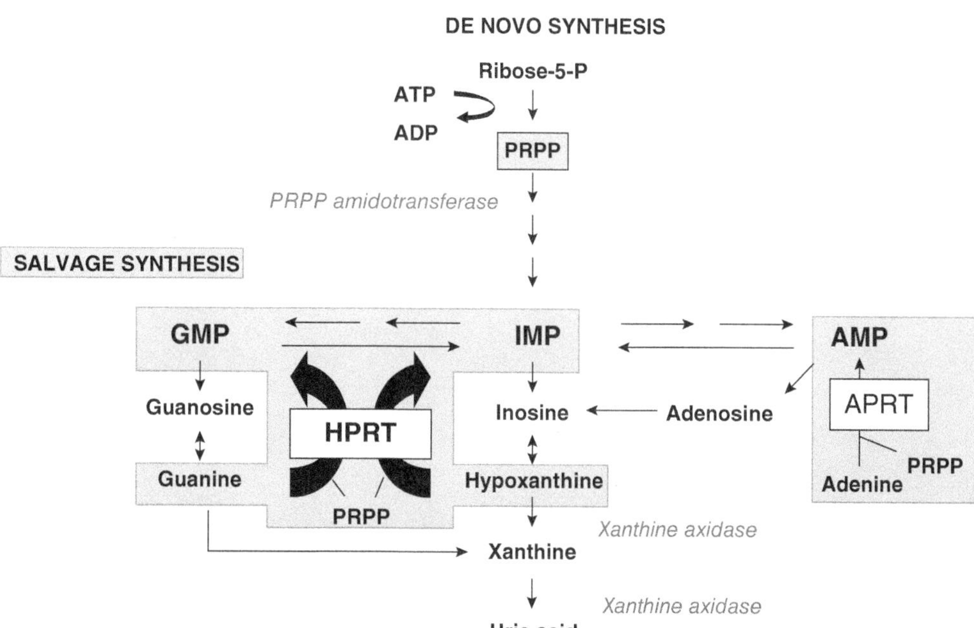

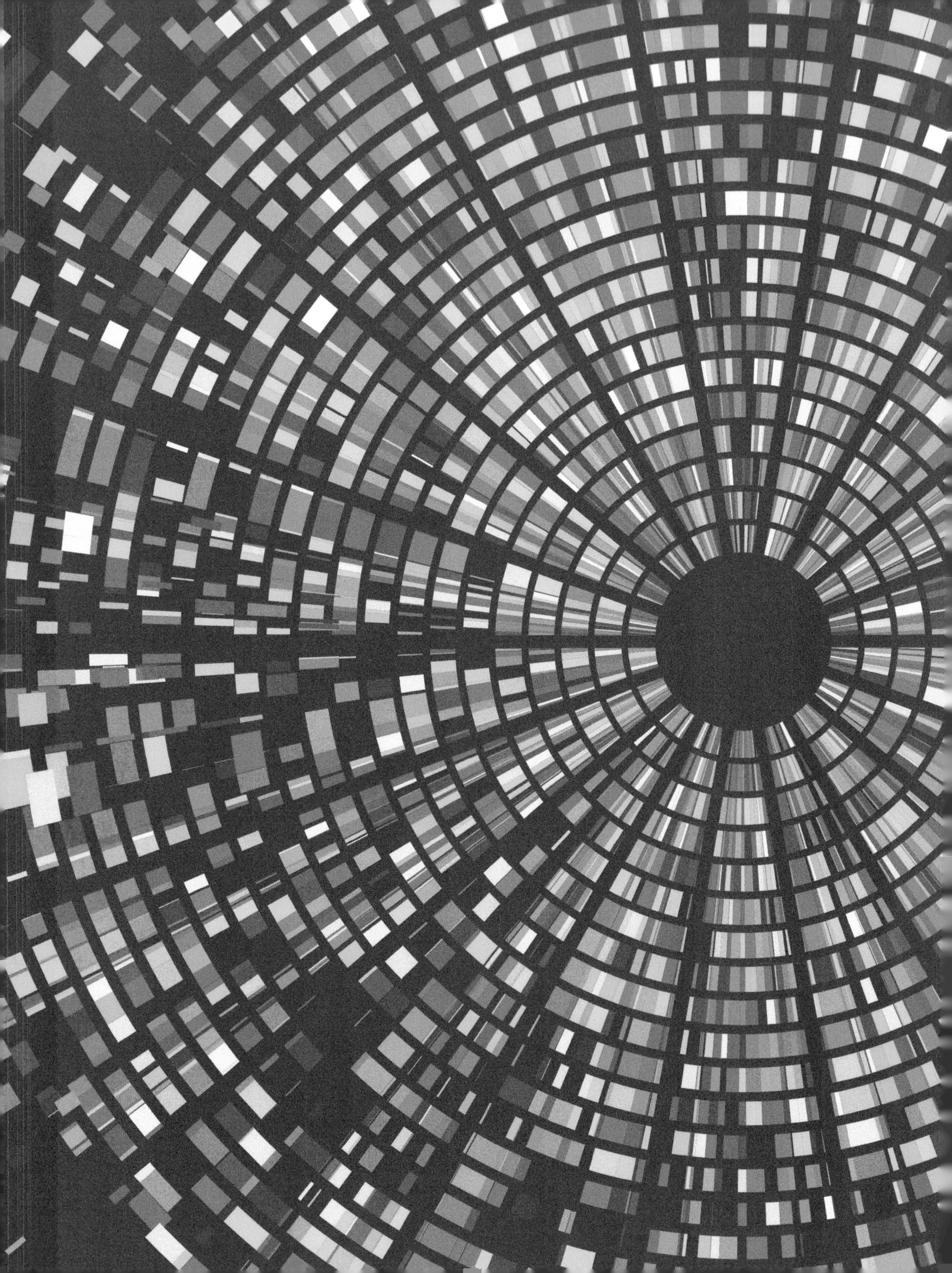

Gastroenterology

Part 6

Chapters

35 Inflammatory bowel disease

Background

'Inflammatory bowel disease' (IBD) includes both Crohn's disease (CD) and ulcerative colitis (UC). These are chronic inflammatory conditions, predominately affecting the gastrointestinal tract. CD may affect any part of the gastrointestinal tract from mouth to anus, whereas UC affects the colon. Age of onset is typically between 15 and 30 years of age.

Aetiology

Prevalence of CD is around 100–300 : 100 000 and UC is around 40–240 : 100 000. Both are commoner in Western populations. Numerous aetiologies have been suggested to be the cause of inflammatory bowel disease, ranging from infectious agents such as atypical mycobacteria, autoimmunity, refrigerators, and even toothpaste. None has been unequivocally proven. Currently, it is thought to be due to a combination of multiple genetic factors and environmental factors (such as smoking) coalesce to result in an aberrant immune response to antigenic material in the gut, giving rise to chronic inflammation increasing susceptibility.

Genetics

The role of genetics in susceptibility to inflammatory bowel disease, particularly CD, is accepted. Up to 17% of patients with CD report a positive family history. The concordance rate in monozygotic twins is approximately 50% for CD and 19% for UC. Over 200 different genetic loci contributing to susceptibility to IBD have been identified by GWAS. There is overlap in loci for both CD and UC, as well as other chronic inflammatory conditions and a susceptibility to infections such as leprosy.

Specific genes implicated in the susceptibility to IBD are summarised in Table 35.1.

Whilst most cases of IBD involve a complex interaction of multiple genetic and environmental factors, it is of note that certain rare monogenic disorders can predispose to IBD, including:

- **Chronic granulomatous disease:** This is a primary immunodeficiency disorder resulting from mut alterations ations in genes encoding components of NADPH oxidase. Up to 50% of patients are afflicted with a non-infectious granulomatous colitis that histologically is indistinguishable from CD.
- **Hermansky-Pudlak syndrome:** An AR disorder characterised by oculocutaneous albinism, bleeding diatheses secondary to platelet dysfunction, and pulmonary fibrosis. Up to one third of patients develop a granulomatous proctocolitis.
- **Glycogen storage disease type 1b:** A metabolic disorder resulting from mutations in the *G6PC* gene encoding glucose-6-phosphate translocase.

Table 35.1 Genes implicated in the susceptibility to IBD.

Gene	Details
NOD2	• First susceptibility gene for CD to be discovered. Three different variants, including two amino acid substitutions and one frameshift alteration increase susceptibility to ileal CD. Individuals heterozygous for one of the polymorphisms have a 2–4 times increased risk, for homozygotes or compound heterozygotes the risk is 20–40 times higher. • *NOD2* encodes a pathogen pattern recognition receptor that is highly expressed in innate immune cells. In response to MDP (a component of bacterial peptidoglycan), the NOD2 receptor initiates downstream intracellular signalling cascades resulting in induction of pro- and anti-inflammatory cytokine release by immune cells. • The three polymorphisms associated with CD impair the ability of the NOD2 protein to recognise MDP. • Other genes linked to IBD, which may affect the innate response downstream of pathogen pattern recognition receptors include ***TNFSF15, IRF5,*** and ***TPL2.***
ATG16L1, IRGM, and LRRK2	• Genetic polymorphisms in several genes with roles in autophagy have been associated with CD, including *ATG16L1*, *IRGM*, and *LRRK2*. • Autophagy is the process by which organelles are targeted to and degraded in lysosomes, which also has a key role in host defence against bacteria. • The CD-associated *ATG16L1* variant (resulting in an amino acid substitution) impairs anti-microbial autophagy in intestinal Paneth cells, a specialised type of intestinal epithelial cell with a critical role in host defence against microbes. • Risk-associated variation in the *IRGM* gene results in impaired regulation of gene expression, thereby affecting intracellular clearance of CD-associated adherent invasive *Escherichia coli* by autophagy.
IL-23R	• A rare coding variant in the *IL-23R* gene confers protection against both CD and UC. Other common variants increase susceptibility to disease. • IL-23 has a critical role in the generation of Th17 cells, a pro-inflammatory subset of T cells that produce high levels of IL-17 and have been implicated in a number of inflammatory and autoimmune disorders. • Other genes with important roles in the IL-23-Th17 axis such as ***IL-12B***, ***STAT3***, ***TYK2***, and ***JAK2*** have also been linked to IBD in genetic studies.

Clinical Genetics and Genomics at a Glance, First Edition. Edited by Neeta Lakhani, Kunal Kulkarni, Julian Barwell, Pradeep Vasudevan, and Huw Dorkins.

Table 35.1 Continued

Gene	Details
IL-10 and *IL-10R*	• Variants in the anti-inflammatory cytokine IL-10 and its receptor have been linked to CD and UC. • Rare loss of function mutations in the IL-10R cause a hyperinflammatory response resulting in early onset colitis. • Common variants in IL-10 are associated with adult-onset IBD, highlighting the importance of this pathway to disease pathogenesis.

Pathophysiology

IBD arises from an aberrant immune response to antigens in the gut, although the precise mechanisms remain poorly understood. Classically, CD has been considered a T-cell-mediated autoimmune condition. However, genetic and functional studies in patients have indicated a key role for the innate immune system in disease pathogenesis. Abnormal innate immune system function is understood to result in impaired clearance of bacteria in the gut. The persistence of antigenic material triggers the consequent adaptive immunological response and gives rise to the chronic inflammatory state seen in CD.

Symptoms and clinical features

Gastrointestinal symptoms of IBD include chronic abdominal pain and diarrhoea, weight loss, gastrointestinal bleeding, and malnutrition. There may be associated systemic symptoms such as fever and malaise. Malabsorption may lead to sequelae such as anaemia, metabolic bone disease, and kidney stones. Extraintestinal manifestations are common and may affect the joints, eyes, and skin. Patients with UC and colonic CD are at increased risk of colorectal cancer. There is an association between UC and primary sclerosing cholangitis (PSC), a condition characterised by progressive inflammation and fibrosis of the bile ducts, giving rise to symptoms of pruritus and jaundice.

Diagnosis

- **Colonoscopy and biopsy:** The gold standard investigation. Macroscopically, CD is characterised by mucosal oedema and erythema, aphthous ulceration, and discontinuous 'skip' lesions. Microscopically, transmural inflammation with non-caseating granulomas are the pathological hallmarks. In contrast, UC is characterised by continuous, non-granulomatous inflammation that is confined to the mucosal layers.
- **Stool culture:** Testing for Clostridium difficile is important to exclude infective causes of diarrhoea. Raised faecal calprotectin is supportive of a diagnosis, though not specific.
- **Imaging:** MR enterography and barium studies may also provide valuable information on areas not accessed during endoscopy such as the small bowel. Capsule endoscopy has an increasing role although is contraindicated in stricturing disease due to risk of capsule retention.
- **Genetics testing:** Not yet in routine use. Thiopurine methyltransferase genotyping is used in some centres to predict risk of myelosuppression with azathioprine.

Management

Acute exacerbations of IBD are managed with immunosuppressants such as steroids. Azathioprine and biological therapies (such as monoclonal antibodies directed against TNF such as infliximab and adalimumab) are options for refractory disease, particularly acute severe UC. Surgery may be required for complications such as perforation or obstruction. Azathioprine and anti-TNF agents are useful for maintenance of remission. Biological therapies, including vedolizumab (anti alpha4 beta 7 integrin) and ustekinumab (anti IL-12/23 shared p40 subunit), may also be used.

The future

An expanded range of therapies, especially biologics, will be available for the treatment of refractory IBD in the future. New monoclonal antibodies directed against new targets (such as ustekinumab, a monoclonal antibody directed against the p40 subunit of IL-23), alongside janus kinase inhibitors and sphingosine 1 phosphate receptor modulators, are currently being introduced into clinical practice. In the longer term, genotyping of individuals could be a useful diagnostic adjunct in individuals where histology is indeterminate and help identify individuals who are likely to respond to targeted therapies.

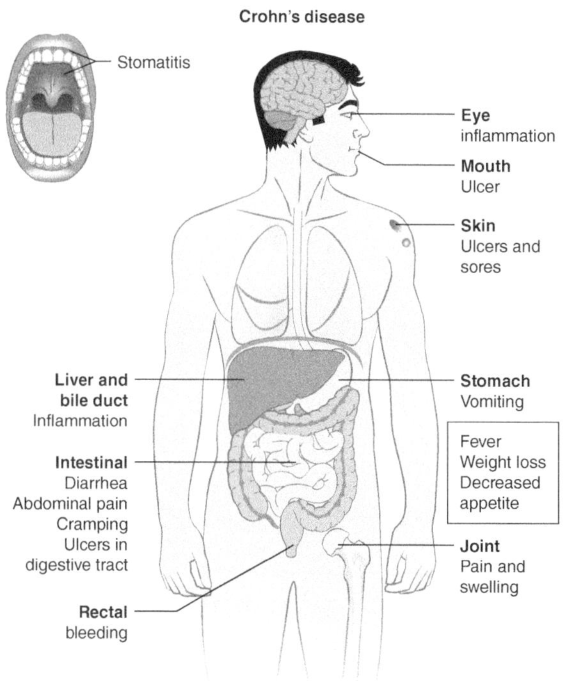

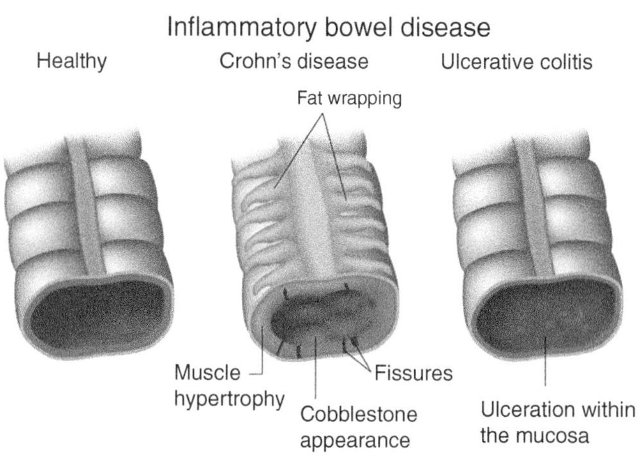

36 Wilson disease

Background

Wilson disease is a disorder in which there is impaired copper homeostasis, typically resulting in excess accumulation in the liver, brain, and eyes. Presentation of liver disease and associated neuropsychiatric features most commonly occurs during the teenage years.

Aetiology

Estimated prevalence is approximately 1 : 30 000. There is a clear genetic basis.

Genetics

Wilson disease is an AR disorder caused by alterations in the ATP7B gene located on chromosome 13q14.3. The gene encodes an ATPase that has a critical role in copper homeostasis and is highly expressed in liver and brain tissue. Over three hundred different alterations have been reported, the majority of which are missense alterations, although insertions, deletions, and splice site alterations have also been identified. The most commonly observed alteration in European patients is the missense H1069Q alteration. Patients with truncating alterations may have a younger age of onset of disease.

Pathophysiology

The protein encoded by *ATP7B* is localised to the intracellular transgolgi network, where it mediates the incorporation of free copper into the protein apoceruloplasmin to generate an apoceruloplasmin peptide that is released into serum. It is also localised to intracellular vesicles, facilitating intravesicular sequestration of copper within these vesicles, which can then be secreted via exocytosis. Alterations in *ATP7B* impairs the ability of the ATPase to both incorporate free copper into apoceruloplasmin and excrete it into bile. This results in accumulation of intracellular free copper and deposition in lysosomes, which causes oxidative stress, cellular injury, and cell death. Apoceruloplasmin devoid of free copper has a shorter half-life, giving rise to the reduced serum ceruloplasmin levels observed in the condition.

Symptoms and clinical features

Typical clinical features of Wilson disease relate to hepatic or neurological involvement. There is considerable heterogeneity in presentation, although onset is usually before 40 years of age. Children are more likely present with hepatic manifestations, whereas adults are more likely to present with neuropsychiatric symptoms (Figure 36.1).

Hepatic manifestations may include the typical features of acute hepatitis, acute liver failure, or chronic liver disease. Features related to decompensation such as encephalopathy, ascites, and jaundice may occur. Neurological manifestations include Parkinsonism, dysarthria, dystonias, tremor, ataxia, and psychiatric disturbance. Kayser-Fleischer rings (visible during slit lamp examination) are characteristic of the condition although only observed in up to 50% of patients without neurological involvement (Figure 36.2).

Diagnosis

- **Blood tests:** Initial diagnostic workup should include liver function tests and full blood count. Low serum ceruloplasmin is characteristic, although may be reduced in other conditions such as protein-losing enteropathy and end-stage liver disease of other causes.
- **Urine:** Raised 24-hour urinary copper excretion is a characteristic biochemical findings.
- **Liver biopsy:** If there is doubt regarding the diagnosis, this may be performed to quantify of liver copper content.
- **Genetic testing:** Sequencing the *ATP7B* gene may assist with diagnosis and screening of family members.

Management

The mainstay of treatment for Wilson disease is with copper chelating agents such as D-penicillamine. Oral zinc interferes with copper absorption and may be used as a maintenance therapy. A diet low in copper is usually advocated. For patients that present with acute liver failure or advanced liver disease, liver transplantation may be necessary.

The future

Editing of the *ATP7B* gene with gene therapy may be a promising therapeutic strategy in the future for affected patients and carriers.

Clinical Genetics and Genomics at a Glance, First Edition. Edited by Neeta Lakhani, Kunal Kulkarni, Julian Barwell, Pradeep Vasudevan, and Huw Dorkins.

Figure 36.1 System involvement in Wilson's disease.

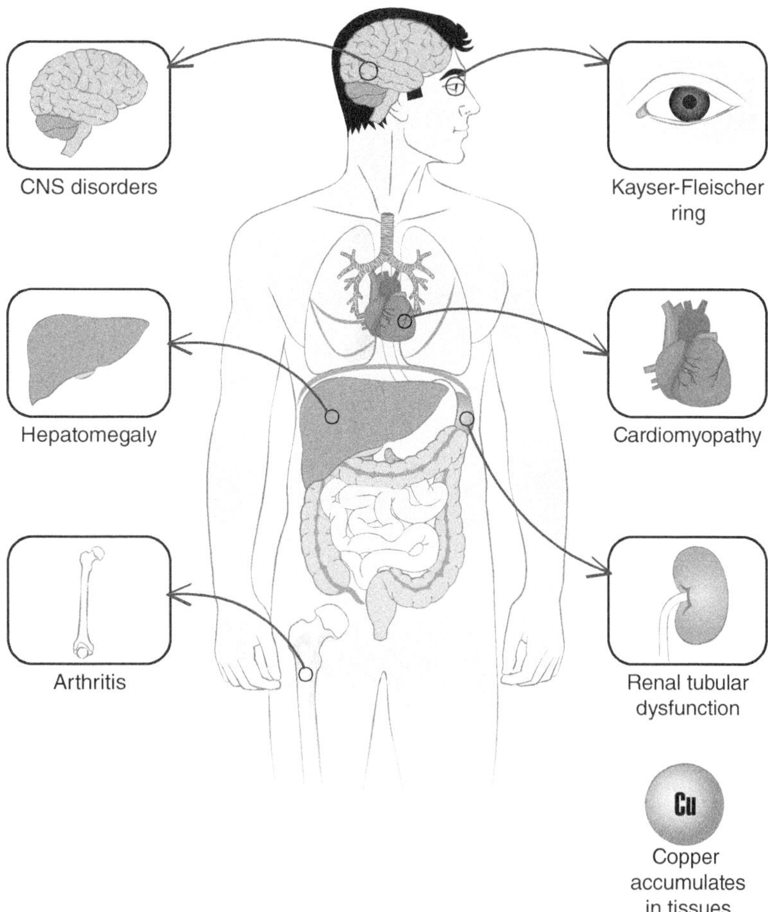

Figure 36.2 Kayser Fleischer rings.

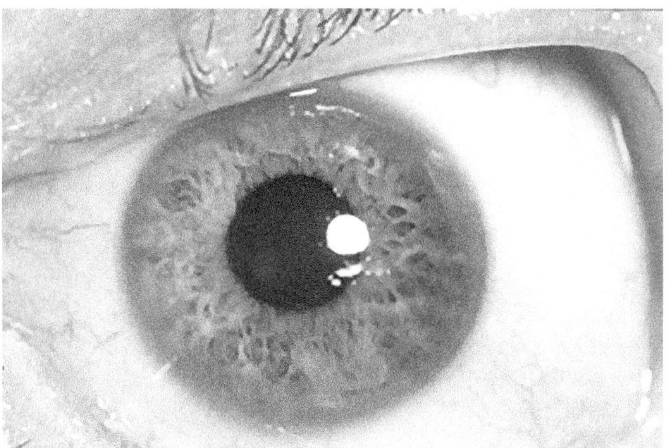

37 Hereditary haemochromatosis

Background

Hereditary haemochromatosis (HH) is characterised by iron overload, which can lead to liver fibrosis, cirrhosis, and hepatocellular carcinoma. Multiple organs may be affected. Age of onset is usually between 40 and 60 years in men and after the menopause in women (type 1 HH), although juvenile-onset (type 2) and intermediate (type 3) forms can also affect those below 20 years of age and between 30 and 40 years of age, respectively.

Aetiology

HH is a common genetic condition among individuals of Northern European lineage. It affects around 1 : 400 individuals. Despite a strong genetic component, there is incomplete penetrance. Estimates vary widely depending on the phenotypic criteria used to define the disease, but may be as low as 5% (or even 1% in one study). Other factors that may modify susceptibility to developing overt clinical disease include:

- Female sex – likely a protective effect of menstrual losses
- Presence of beta thalassaemia trait – associated with younger age of onset of disease
- *CYBRD1* polymorphisms
- Alcohol consumption
- Viral hepatitis infection

Genetics

Several known genetic alterations are known to cause HH. Types 1, 2, and 3 are inherited in an AR pattern, whereas type 4 is inherited in an AD manner.

- **Type 1 or 'classical' HH or HFE (Homeostatic Iron Regulator):** Approximately 90% of cases have alterations in the ***HFE*** gene, located on chromosome 6 in proximity to the HLA-A3 locus and encoding a protein involved in iron homeostasis. The most frequently observed alteration is a missense C282Y (>80% cases are homozygous). Others include H63D missense alterations, splice site alterations, and homozygous deletions.
- **Type 2 – *HJV* (originally named HFE2) and *HAMP*:** These genes encode haemojuvelin and hepcidin, respectively. Hepcidin normally regulates intestinal iron absorption by enhancing breakdown of the iron export channel ferroportin. Haemojuvelin acts to control hepcidin expression by acting as a coreceptor for the bone morphogenic protein (BMP) signalling pathway. Loss of function alterations in *HJV* and *HAMP* have been demonstrated in patients with Type 2 (juvenile) HH, a more severe form, with an earlier age of onset, and with cardiomyopathy and hypogonadism being the predominant clinical features (type II haemochromatosis).
- **Type 3 – *TFR2*:** Alterations in the gene encoding the transferrin receptor 2, located on chromosome 7q22, have been reported in familial and sporadic forms of Type 3 HH. Inheritance is AR, and individuals are homozygous or compound heterozygous for inactivating alterations. The clinical phenotype may be more severe than in Type 1 HH.
- **Type 4 – SLC40A1:** This gene encodes the iron export channel ferroportin, which is expressed at high levels in the basolateral surface of enterocytes and in macrophages and normally functions to facilitate iron absorption from the intestine into the bloodstream. The penetrance and presentation is highly heterogeneous between individuals, suggesting an important role for other genetic and environmental modifiers.
- **H-ferritin:** A point mutation in iron-responsive element of H-ferritin mRNA was reported in a Japanese family with AD iron overload. Ferritin normally functions to bind free ferrous iron and stores it in a non-toxic ferric state.

Pathophysiology

HFE is expressed in the intestinal crypt cells and liver Kupfer cells where it regulates iron uptake and efflux, although the precise molecular mechanisms by which it does so are still not fully understood. *HFE* forms complexes with β2-microglobulin, which binds with the transferrin receptor at the crypt cell surface. This system has been suggested to act as a sensor of iron. Under iron replete conditions, enterocytes downregulate expression of iron transporters such as divalent metal transporter 1 (DMT1) as a result of accumulation of intracellular iron. Mutation of *HFE* impairs the interaction of the transferrin receptor with transferrin, which may provide an inappropriate signal that iron levels are low. The overall effect is to increase total body iron, accumulating in the liver, heart, pancreas, anterior pituitary gland, and joints, and giving rise to the characteristic clinical features.

Symptoms and clinical features

HH may be identified incidentally in asymptomatic patients via blood tests. Early symptoms of the disease are usually non-specific and may include fatigue, altered skin pigmentation, arthralgia, and impotence. Later features include the development of chronic liver disease, cardiovascular complications such as features of conduction defects and congestive cardiac failure, and diabetes mellitus (Figure 37.1).

Diagnosis

- **Blood tests:** Initial investigations include blood tests such as serum ferritin and transferrin saturation, which are characteristically raised (this may be identified incidentally). Derangements in liver function tests may be observed.
- **Genetic testing:** *HFE* genetic testing for the *C282Y* and *H63D* alterations should be conducted.
- **MRI liver:** This is highly sensitive and can provide a quantitative estimate of iron concentration within the liver.
- **Transient elastography:** This may be useful to detect liver fibrosis.
- **Liver biopsy:** This may be required if there remains diagnostic uncertainty.

Clinical Genetics and Genomics at a Glance, First Edition. Edited by Neeta Lakhani, Kunal Kulkarni, Julian Barwell, Pradeep Vasudevan, and Huw Dorkins.

Figure 37.1 Systemic involvement of HHE.

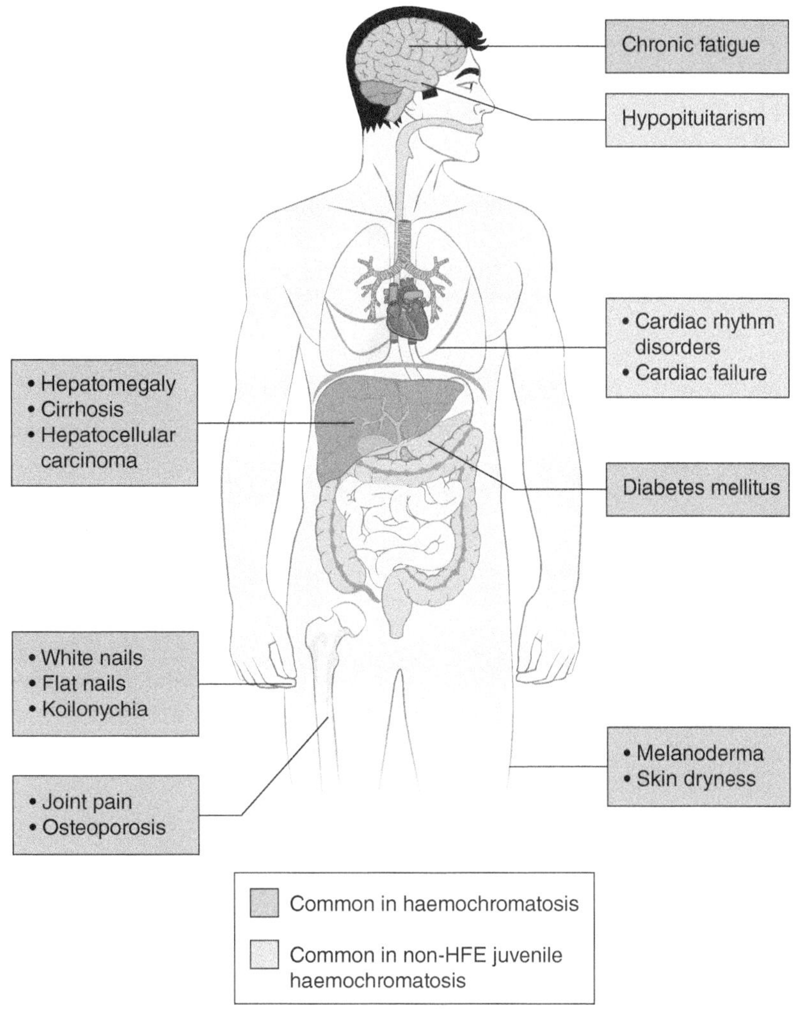

First-degree relatives of patients with HH should be screened for disease. Screening should include serum iron studies and, where a proband has a defined genetic alteration, screening could also include genetic analysis.

Management

Venesection is the cornerstone of management; typically one unit every 1–3 weeks. Iron chelation (desferrioxamine infusion) may be considered when venesection is not tolerated. Liver transplantation may need to be considered for patients with decompensated liver disease, although the risk of mortality due to cardiovascular complications and infections is high.

The future

In the future, novel therapies such as erythrocytapharesis (separation of erythrocytes from whole blood rather than venesection) may become available. Therapeutics targeting other molecules involved in iron regulation (e.g. hepcidin) are currently under development. Gene therapy could be a very promising treatment strategy in the future for selected patients.

38 Coeliac disease

Background

Coeliac disease is an autoimmune, gluten-sensitive enteropathy that results from an aberrant T-cell-mediated immune response to gliadin (a component of dietary gluten) in individuals with an underlying genetic susceptibility. Gluten is found in wheat, rye, and barley.

Aetiology

The disease primarily affects Caucasians, with prevalence estimates ranging from 1 : 100 to 1 : 500. There is strong evidence for a genetic predisposition to coeliac disease, although environmental factors may also influence its development.

Genetics

Up to 15% of first-degree relatives of affected probands are similarly affected, with a high concordance rate amongst monozygotic twins (approximately 70–100%). Approximately 40 different genetic loci have been identified as being disease associated in three different GWAS. Many of these regions are shared with other autoimmune conditions, particularly type 1 diabetes and rheumatoid arthritis. Implicated gene variants contributing to a genetic predisposition for coeliac disease are summarised in Table 38.1.

Genetic conditions associated with an increased susceptibility to coeliac disease include:

- **Selective IgA deficiency:** This is a deficiency in serum IgA in the presence of normal serum levels of IgM and IgG. It is a genetically heterogeneous condition resulting from alterations in the *IGAD1* and *IGAD2* loci on chromosomes 6p21 and 17p11, respectively. Individuals are reported to have a 10- to 20-fold increased risk of developing coeliac disease.
- **Down syndrome (trisomy 21):** Prevalence of coeliac disease up to 12%.
- **Williams syndrome (contiguous gene deletion in region 7q11.23):** Coeliac disease prevalence estimated at 3–10%.

Table 38.1 Gene alterations contributing to the susceptibility to coeliac disease.

Alteration	Details
HLA-DQA1 and ***HLA-DQB1***	• Strongly association with allelic variants of the human leukocyte antigen (HLA) class II genes *HLA-DQA1 and HLA-DQB1* located on chromosome 6p21. • Specific alleles encode the alpha and beta chains that make up the associated **HLA-DQ2** and **HLA-DQ8** heterodimer proteins which are associated with coeliac disease. • Over 90% of patients with coeliac disease are positive for DQ2 and the remaining 10% are positive for DQ8. • However, these alleles have a high frequency in the general population – 20–30 and 10% for DQ2 and DQ8, respectively. Hence, their presence is necessary but not sufficient for the development of disease. • The pathogenic effect of the DQ2 variant is likely to result from its high affinity for immunogenic epitopes from gluten, such as proline-rich gluten peptides that have survived gastrointestinal digestion.
CTLA4/ CD28 locus:	• This region on chromosome 2q33 has been associated with coeliac disease in both linkage and GWAS. • The proteins encoded by these genes are expressed on the surface membrane of T-cells and have important roles in control of T-cell activation and proliferation.
IL2/ IL-21 locus:	• A region on chromosome 4q27 is associated with susceptibility to coeliac disease. This locus contains the *IL-2* gene, which plays a critical role in T-cell activation and homeostasis, and *IL-21*. The IL-21 cytokine has effects on T, B, and NK cells. • Other cytokine and chemokine genes that have been linked to coeliac disease in genetic studies include ***IL12A, IL18RAP,*** and ***CCR3***.
BACH2:	• This gene is expressed in B cells, where it may influence class switch recombination and somatic hypermutation. • It is also expressed in T lymphocytes and may function to maintain them in a naïve state.
TNFAIP3 and ***REL***:	• Variants in loci containing these genes have been associated with coeliac disease in GWAS. • The proteins encoded function in the pro-inflammatory nuclear factor kappa B (NF-KB) pathway and may also influence intestinal permeability.

Clinical Genetics and Genomics at a Glance, First Edition. Edited by Neeta Lakhani, Kunal Kulkarni, Julian Barwell, Pradeep Vasudevan, and Huw Dorkins.

Pathophysiology

Tolerance to gliadin peptides is lost. Deamidation of glutamine to glutamic acid residues within gliadin peptides is catalysed by tissue transglutaminase in the lamina propria. If MHC DQ2 is present, the deamidated peptides are presented by antigen presenting cells to T-helper lymphocytes. These cells stimulate cytotoxic T cells, which result in cell death and villous atrophy and give rise to the characteristic pathological features of the disease.

Symptoms and clinical features

Patients present with gastrointestinal symptoms related to malabsorption, such as steatorrhoea, abdominal pain, weight loss and, in children, poor growth. Extra-intestinal manifestations include dermatitis herpetiformis (characterised by a blistering rash on extensor surfaces), other skin disorders, osteomalacia, arthritis, and neurological sequelae such as hypotonia, developmental delay, ataxia, and peripheral neuropathy. The clinical features characteristically improve with a gluten-free diet. There is an association with autoimmune disorders such as type 1 diabetes and thyroiditis, and an increased risk of malignancy, especially non-Hodgkin lymphoma.

Diagnosis

- **Serology:** Performed when a diagnosis of coeliac disease is suspected. Raised IgA anti-tissue transglutaminase (TTG) is characteristic, with estimated sensitivity >90% and specificity 95%. However, IgA anti-TTG may be falsely negative in individuals with selective IgA deficiency. In these situations, IgG anti-TTG and IgG deamidated gliadin peptide may be positive.
- **Duodenal biopsy:** Gold standard for diagnosis. Should be conducted if serological testing is positive or in cases with a high index of suspicion despite negative serology. Pathological hallmarks include villous atrophy and increased epithelial lymphocytes.
- **Genetics testing:** Negative findings for HLA-DQA1 and HLA-DQB1 alleles may be useful in excluding the diagnosis of coeliac disease.

Management

All patients should receive specialist dietary advice to help maintain a gluten-free diet. Consumption of high-gluten foods such as wheat and rye should be avoided. Up to 5% of patients may not respond to a gluten-free diet. In refractory cases, after checking compliance with the gluten-free diet and excluding complications such as intestinal lymphoma, immunosuppressive agents such as steroids may be considered. Associated vitamin deficiencies should be corrected and complications of disease such as osteoporosis should be treated appropriately. Pneumococcal vaccination is recommended.

The future

Agents that decrease intestinal permeability to gliadin are currently undergoing clinical evaluation. In the future, other therapeutic options could include coeliac-specific HLA and chemokine receptor inhibition.

39 Pancreatic cancer

Background

The majority of pancreatic cancers are adenocarcinomas that arise from exocrine cells.

Aetiology

Pancreatic cancer is the fourth most common cause of all cancer-related deaths in the United Kingdom (seventh worldwide). Incidence and mortality increase with advanced age. Pancreatic cancer results from a combination of hereditary and environmental factors, which trigger somatic alterations in oncogenes and tumour suppressor genes. Important environmental factors linked to susceptibility include smoking tobacco and obesity. Other medical conditions including diabetes and chronic pancreatitis also increase the risk.

Genetics

The development of pancreatic cancer involves both germline alterations and acquired somatic alterations. Up to 10% of pancreatic cancer patients report a family history of the disease. Familial clustering of cases of pancreatic cancer have been reported, and case control and cohort studies indicate odds of 1.76 for individuals with one affected first-degree relative in comparison to those without any family history.

Loss of function alterations in *BRCA2* are associated with an increased risk of pancreatic cancer. *BRCA2* is a tumour suppressor gene that has a role in DNA repair and is associated with susceptibility to a number of other cancers, including breast, ovarian, and prostate cancer. Deletion, insertion, and missense alterations have been reported. Germline alterations in *PALB2* (partner and localiser of *BRCA2*) have also been reported. This gene encodes a protein that interacts with *BRCA2* in the nucleus, thereby stabilising *BRCA2* and resulting in its accumulation.

Germline alterations in *p16/CDKN2A* are associated with increased susceptibility to pancreatic cancer and melanoma. This is a tumour suppressor gene with a critical role in the cell cycle. The p16 protein inhibits cyclin-dependent kinases 4 and 6 and prevents retinoblastoma phosphorylation, thereby acting as a brake on G1-S transition in the cell cycle.

Lynch syndrome, an AD condition resulting from alterations in DNA mismatch repair genes, is associated with an increased risk of pancreatic cancer, in addition to early onset of colorectal cancer.

Pathophysiology

As is with other cancers, pancreatic cancer results from activation of oncogenes and loss of function of tumour suppressor genes. Oncogenes commonly mutated in pancreatic cancers include *K-Ras* and *Notch*. *K-Ras* encodes a membrane protein involved in signal transduction and control of cellular proliferation and migration. Alterations result in a constitutively active form of *K-ras*, driving cells towards uncontrolled proliferation. *Notch* activation results in activation of the NF-KB transcription factor and may stimulate inflammatory cascades that aid in cellular activation, proliferation, and metastasis. Tumour suppressor genes commonly mutated in pancreatic cancer include *p53* and *p16*. This results in inhibition of apoptosis and uncontrolled proliferation, thereby further enhancing tumour growth. Loss of DPC4 is commonly observed and is associated with a worse prognosis after resection. This gene encodes the protein SMAD4, which may inhibit proliferation and angiogenesis.

Symptoms and clinical features

The most common symptoms include weight loss, jaundice, and abdominal pain, typically epigastric radiating to the back. Nausea, vomiting, diarrhoea, and dark urine are also frequently reported. Examination may reveal jaundice, hepatomegaly, and the presence of palpable masses in the right upper quadrant or epigastrium. Courvoisier's sign (a palpable, non-tender gallbladder in the presence of jaundice) indicates that the cause of jaundice is unlikely to be gallstones.

Diagnosis

To date, there is no national screening programme for pancreatic cancer.

- **Blood tests:** May reveal a cholestatic derangement with conjugated hyperbilirubinaemia and raised levels of the tumour marker Ca 19-9.
- **Abdominal ultrasound:** May reveal biliary duct dilatation and the presence of a pancreatic mass.
- **CT:** Has a sensitivity of up to 97% if a dedicated pancreatic protocol is used; characteristic findings include hypoattenuating masses.
- **Tissue diagnosis:** May be obtained by endoscopic ultrasound-guided fine needle aspiration, which has a sensitivity of up to 90%. Alternatives include CT-guided percutaneous biopsy.
- **Endoscopic retrograde cholangiopancreatography (ERCP):** Highly effective at visualising biliary tree obstruction due to pancreatic cancer and enables therapeutics such as stent placement to relieve biliary obstruction.
- **Genetic testing:** To date, there is no validated genetic test for accurately predicting pancreatic cancer risk. However, for some families with a strong family history of pancreatic cancer and

Clinical Genetics and Genomics at a Glance, First Edition. Edited by Neeta Lakhani, Kunal Kulkarni, Julian Barwell, Pradeep Vasudevan, and Huw Dorkins.

known germline *BRCA2* or *PALB2* alteration, early genetic screening may be appropriate in selected cases.

Management

The only curative treatment for pancreatic cancer is surgery, typically alongside adjuvant gemcitabine chemotherapy. However, this is only suitable for patients without distant metastases, evidence of encasement of the superior mesenteric artery, or direct involvement of the aorta or inferior vena cava. Unfortunately, patients often present late and fewer than one fifth of patients are usually suitable for surgery.

Options for patients with unresectable disease includes palliative chemotherapy and biliary stent placement. Patients should be supported by palliative care specialists and symptoms of pain and nausea managed appropriately.

The future

Further characterisation of abnormal signalling pathways may lead to novel therapeutic agents and individualised targeting of therapy. Certain DNA-based and whole-cell vaccines aiming to target the immune response have shown promise in initial studies.

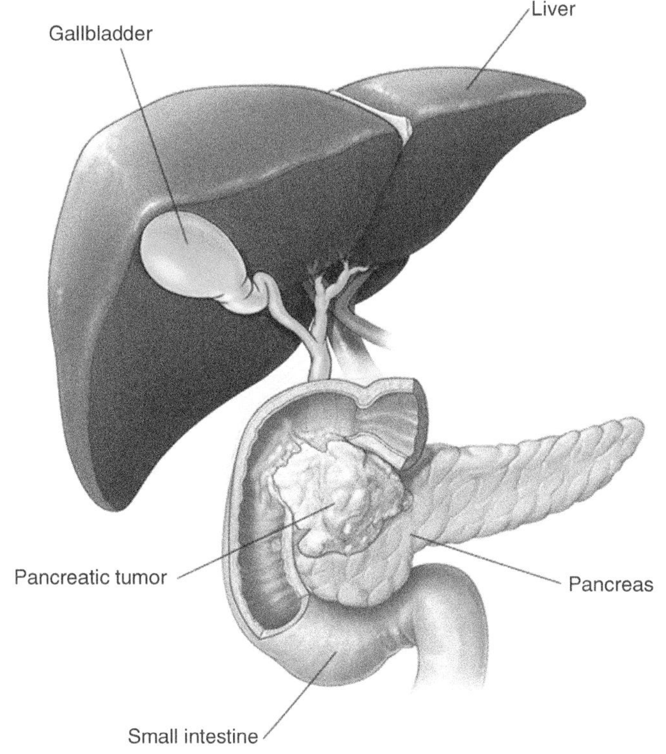

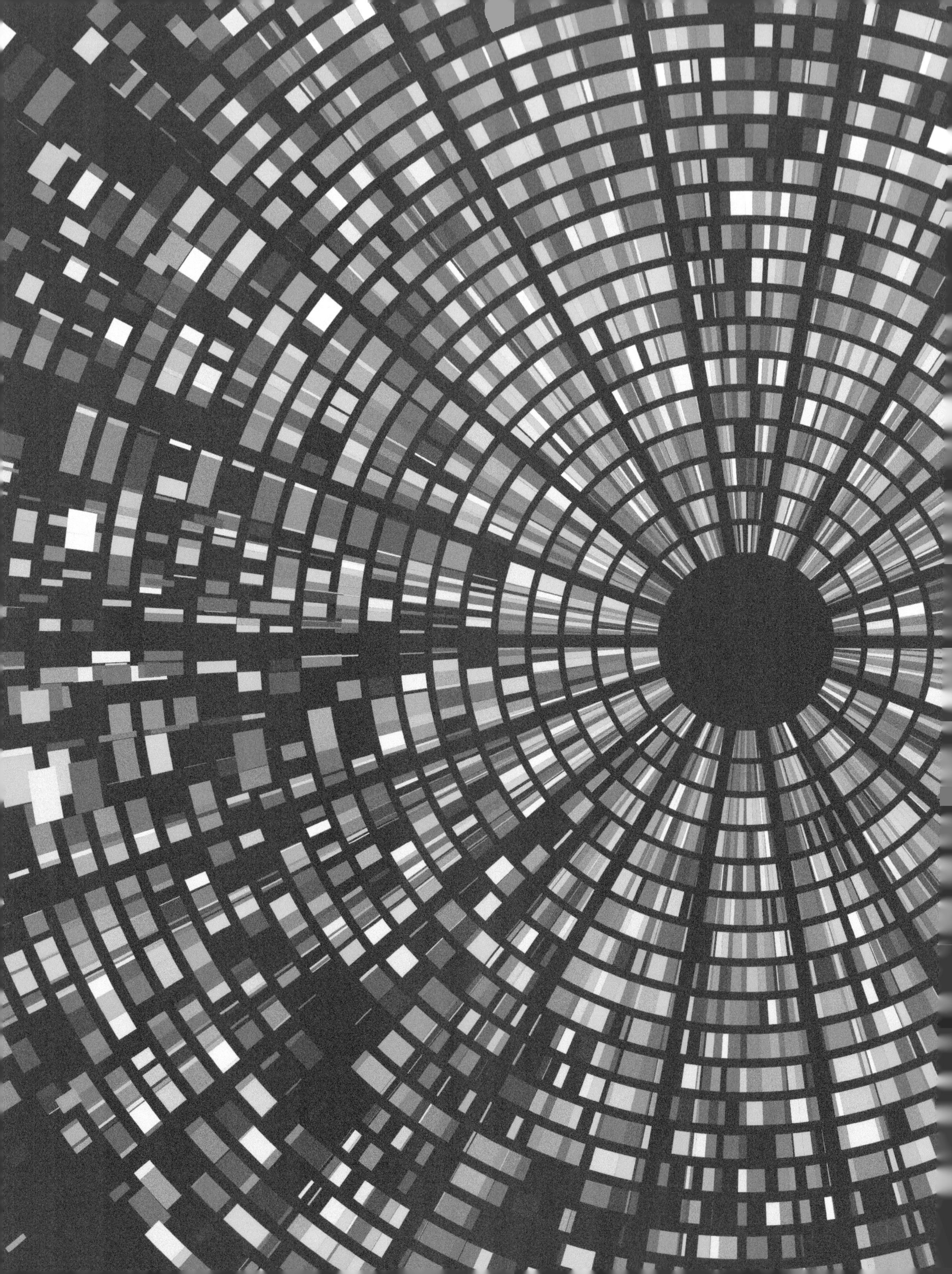

Haematology

Chapters

40 Malignant haematology

Background

Blood cancers, as with other malignancies, are acquired genetic disorders. They are broadly classified into lymphoid and myeloid disorders. The investigation of recurrent genetic abnormalities by metaphase and interphase cytogenetics and sequencing has been essential to understanding the varying molecular basis of these diseases.

Aetiology

Incidence of the leukaemias varies by type and country, ranging from 1 to 12 per 100 000, generally higher in males than females.

Genetics

Reciprocal chromosomal translocations define both lymphoid and myeloid disorders. Lymphoid diseases often show translocations in which there is over-expression of an oncogene, whereas in myeloid disorders, the translocations often result in the production of fusion proteins (Table 40.1). More recently, sequencing has shown specific gene alterations (Table 40.2) associated with specific disorders.

Pathophysiology

In many cases, these genetic abnormalities lead to the production of a constitutively active protein or over-expression of an oncogenic protein leading to dysregulation of signalling pathways with multiple consequences. The World Health Organisation (WHO) classification of haematological malignancies published in 2016 includes a growing number of classifications defined by genetic and molecular changes.

Lymphoid malignancies are derived from either B-cells or T-cells. Normal B-cells express or secrete antibodies with each cell having a unique immunoglobulin gene rearrangement and similarly normal T-cells express a unique T-cell receptor from T-cell receptor genes. The progeny of an individual B- or T-cell all have the same antibody or T-cell receptor rearrangement and constitute a clone. Diagnosis of lymphoid malignancies is supported by analysis of antibody or T-cell receptor genes to determine clonality. PCR techniques are used to assess for the presence of clonal immunoglobulin (IG) or T-cell receptor (TCR) gene rearrangements and are particularly useful in cases with diagnostic uncertainty.

Symptoms and clinical features

Patients with blood cancers may present with a variety of signs and symptoms, including fevers, night sweats, recurrent infections, trivial or recurrent bleeding, unexplained weight loss, lumps/swellings, persistent lymphadenopathy, shortness of breath, rash/itchy skin, joint pains, lethargy, pallor.

Table 40.1 Chromosomal translocations.

Disease	Translocation	Protein effect
Chronic myeloid leukaemia (CML)	t(9;22)(q34;q11.2)	BCR-ABL
Acute promyelocytic leukaemia (APL)	t(15;17)	PML-RARA
AML with recurrent genetic abnormalities	AML with t(8;21)(q22;q22.1);RUNX1-RUNX1T1 AML with inv(16)(p13.1q22) or t(16;16)(p13.1;q22);CBFB-MYH11 AML with t(9;11)(p21.3;q23.3);MLLT3-KMT2A AML with t(6;9)(p23;q34.1);DEK-NUP214 AML with inv(3)(q21.3q26.2) or t(3;3)(q21.3;q26.2); GATA2, MECOM AML (megakaryoblastic) with t(1;22)(p13.3;q13.3);RBM15-MKL1	Various
MDS with del (5q)	del(5q)	Various
Burkitt lymphoma	t(8; 14), t(2; 8) or t(8; 24)	*MYC* overexpression
Follicular lymphoma	t(14;18)(q32;q21)	*BCL2* upregulation
Mantle cell lymphoma	t(11;14)(q13;q32)	Cyclin D1 overexpression
ALK+ Anaplastic T-cell lymphoma	t(2;5)(p23;q35)	*NPM-ALK*
High-grade B-cell lymphoma with *MYC* and *BCL2* and/or *BCL6* rearrangements	Various	*MYC* overexpression and *BCL2* and/or *BCL6* dysregulation

Clinical Genetics and Genomics at a Glance, First Edition. Edited by Neeta Lakhani, Kunal Kulkarni, Julian Barwell, Pradeep Vasudevan, and Huw Dorkins.

Table 40.2 Gene alterations.

Diagnosis	Alteration	Importance
Myeloproliferative neoplasm (MPN)	*JAK2 V617F*	Diagnosis
MPN	*MPL* – exon 10/11	Diagnosis
MPN	*CALR* – exon 9	Diagnosis
AML	*FLT3* (ITD or TKD)	Prognosis, MRD
AML	*NPM1* – exon 12	Classification, prognosis, MRD
AML	*CEBPA* – biallelic	Classification
AML	*RUNX1*	Classification
Chronic neutrophilic leukaemia	*CSF3R*	Diagnosis
Hairy cell leukaemia	*BRAF V600E*	Diagnosis, treatment
Waldenströms macroglobulinaemia	*MYD88*	Diagnosis
AITL and Tfh lymphoma	*RHOA G17V*	
Histiocytic & dendritic neoplasms	*BRAF*	

Diagnosis

- Cytogenetics is used in the diagnosis of many haematological malignancies and also plays an important role in predicting clinical outcome for some conditions. The presence of defined cytogenetic changes in acute myeloid leukaemia (AML) and myelodysplasia (MDS) can lead to changes in management as some changes are associated with increased risk of relapsed disease and others with a better prognosis. The presence of *MYC* rearrangements together with *BCL2* or *BCL6* chromosomal translocations in diffuse large B-cell lymphoma (DLBCL), an aggressive lymphoid malignancy, is described as 'double hit lymphoma' and is associated with a worse prognosis than any of the translocations alone.
- The presence of gene alterations is of particular importance in the diagnosis of the myeloproliferative neoplasms, where they form an important part of the diagnostic criteria. For example, in AML, there are a growing number of alterations associated with prognosis, but standard testing includes *FLT3* and *NPM1* alterations as these will guide treatment decisions.

Management

Monitoring of minimal residual disease in AML is used to detect relapse early and can lead to initiation of treatment before the development of overt haematological relapse. Real-time quantitative PCR (RT-qPCR) assays have been developed to detect many common chimeric fusion genes and mutations. Diagnostic material is used to determine the most appropriate MRD marker for follow-up, with around 60% of cases having a suitable marker. These RT–qPCR assays have been standardised within Europe.

Exemplar conditions

Chronic Myeloid Leukaemia (CML)

The t(9;22) translocation, Philadelphia chromosome, in chronic myeloid leukaemia (CML) and the development of targeted kinase inhibitors, starting with imatinib, revolutionised treatment of the condition.

Management of CML is guided by regular RT–PCR of peripheral blood for detection of the *BCR-ABL1* transcript and assessment of the molecular response. In patients who do not respond to initial therapy or develop resistance to first-line therapy, direct sequencing of the kinase domain is carried out to detect the presence of mutations associated with TKI resistance and can be used to guide further therapy.

Recent studies have shown that therapy can be ceased in patients who achieve a deep molecular response. In around 40% at two years, there is no detectable return of the malignant cells and those with a return of detectable malignancy respond to re-initiation of treatment.

Burkitt Lymphoma

The translocation of *c-MYC* to an immunoglobulin gene locus is the hallmark of Burkitt lymphoma (BL); there are 3 clinical variants of the disease.

Endemic BL is found in equatorial Africa with a peak incidence in childhood (4–7 years of age); there is a strong association with chronic Epstein-Barr virus infection. Sporadic BL is found in Europe and Americas and also has a peak incidence in childhood (age 11) but also cases in adulthood with a median age of 30. Immunodeficiency-associated BL is seen in those with HIV infection, and occasionally other forms of immunodeficiency.

BL arises from a germinal centre or post-germinal centre B cell and occurs following a chromosomal translocation, which leads to the constitutive expression of *c-MYC* that encodes for the MYC protein transcription factor.

The future

The use of next generation sequencing (NGS) technologies is being investigated in MRD monitoring in both leukaemias without a currently standardised MRD assay, as well as lymphomas where the role of cell-free DNA is under investigation.

41 Non-malignant haematology

Background

A number of forms of haemoglobin are produced at various stages of development. Consequently, there are a number of haemoglobin disorders that arise from alterations that lead to either reduced or abnormal haemoglobin production, which can have a range of clinical consequences. In the developing world, infant mortality rates are very high due to a lack of treatment resources. This section will focus on the commonest two disorders: sickle-cell disease and α- and β-thalassemia.

Aetiology

Globally, haemoglobin disorder frequency ranges from 0.3 to 25 per 1000 live births. Global rates are difficult to accurately quantify but are predicted to rise over the coming years. Frequency is generally highest in regions where malaria is or was endemic, as the alterations confers protection to carriers against severe *Plasmodium falciparum* malaria (Figure 41.1).

- **Sickle cell anaemias:** Most common severe monogenic non malignant haematological disorder. Rates vary depending upon geography/ethnicity (commonest in sub-Saharan Africa, Middle East, Mediterranean, and southeast Asia). In some regions of sub-Saharan Africa/eastern Saudi Arabia/central India, prevalence of sickle-cell trait can be as high as 40%.
- **Thalassaemia:** Affects approximately 4.4 per 10 000 live births globally. Most frequently present in individuals of Mediterranean, south Asian, southeast Asian, and Middle Eastern origin. 1.5% of the global population are estimated to be β-thalassemia carriers, with 16–18% affected in the highest risk areas (Cyprus, Maldives) and 3–8% in medium-risk areas (India, Pakistan, Bangladesh, Malaysia, China). α-Thalassaemia incidence is overall generally higher than β, more so in southeast Asia than the Mediterranean, although β has more severe variants in affected regions, making this the more important public health problem.

Genetics

- **Sickle cell anaemias:** Inherited in an AR manner, this occurs due to the homozygous inheritance of an altered β-globin gene (chromosome 11), leading to either the substitution of valine for glutamic acid at amino acid 6 Hb(SS), or the co-inheritance of the sickle β-globin alteration and another β-globin mutation. HbS formed from 2 α-globin chains and 2 sickle-mutated β-globin chains is poorly soluble when deoxygenated leading to haemolysis, anaemia, and vaso-occlusion.
- **Thalassaemia:** Both main types are generally inherited in an AR manner, although note that the production of haemoglobin is polygenic. Carriers (trait) may get mild symptoms and rarely require treatment.
  - **α-thalassemia:** Caused by alterations in the *HBA1* and/or *HBA2* genes; >100 genetic variants have been identified to date, ranging from asymptomatic to fatal (Figure 41.2). Individuals have two copies of *HBA1* and two copies of *HBA2*; exact risk and phenotype depends on how many gene copies are deleted and which combination of the *HBA1* and *HBA2* genes are affected. Haemoglobin (Hb) Constant Spring (CS) is a particularly common structural variant associated with α-thalassemia in Asia. The *α(CS)* gene contains an alteration that abolishes the normal translation termination codon, so that polyribosomes 'read through' the normal translation termination site on alpha(CS) mRNA, translating an additional 31 residues from the normally untranslated 3′ extremity of the mRNA, until another in frame termination codon is reached. This 'read through' process disrupts normal α-globin mRNA stability, resulting in a highly unstable α(CS) mRNA that accumulates to only 1% of normal levels. The *α(CS)* allele thus functions as a severe *α-thalassemia* gene. It becomes clinically significant when inherited with *α-thalassemia* from the other parent and can lead to HbH or HbBarts.
  - **β-Thalassaemia:** Caused by alterations in the *HBB* gene. Most individuals are homozygous. >250 alterations have been identified to-date; most are single nucleotide substitutions with low frequency, several are more prevalent in certain areas. For example, IVS1-100 G→A, IVS1-6 T→C, and IVS1-1 G→A encompassed >90% of β-thalassemia variants in Cyprus.

Pathophysiology

Haemoglobin comprises four globin chains: foetal haemoglobin (HbF) has two α and two gamma chains (α2γ2), whereas adult haemoglobin (HbA) has two α and two β chains (α2β2). Genes in the α-globin and β-globin gene clusters (chromosomes 16 and 11) control globin-chain production.

- **Sickle cell anaemias:** Characterised by abnormally shaped red blood cells (RBCs), with a sickle/crescentic shape. Consequently, these do not last for as long as normal RBCs, resulting in increased haemolysis (anaemia) and microvascular occlusion (sickle crises/thrombosis).
- **Thalassemia:** Characterised by reduced levels of functional haemoglobin. The *HBB* gene is responsible for β globin, while the *HBA1* and *HBA2* genes are responsible for α globin. α and β are the commonest types, with other rarer variants including β- thalassemia intermedia, α-thalassemia major, and haemoglobin H disease.
- **α-Thalassaemia:** Impaired production of α-globin chains as a result of alterations to 1, 2, 3, or 4 α-globin chains.
- **β-Thalassaemia:** There is clinical heterogeneity seen in β-thalassemia as a result of the variation in alterations (β+ with reduced β-globin production and β0 with no β-globin production), and the co-existence of α-globin abnormalities. The clinical consequence of homozygous or compound heterozygous β-globin alterations arise from the relative excess of α-globin chains in the production of haemoglobin A and the development of α-globin tetramers, which are insoluble and precipitate within the cell. HbF levels are typically elevated.

Clinical Genetics and Genomics at a Glance, First Edition. Edited by Neeta Lakhani, Kunal Kulkarni, Julian Barwell, Pradeep Vasudevan, and Huw Dorkins.

Figure 41.1 Global distribution of haemoglobinopathies.

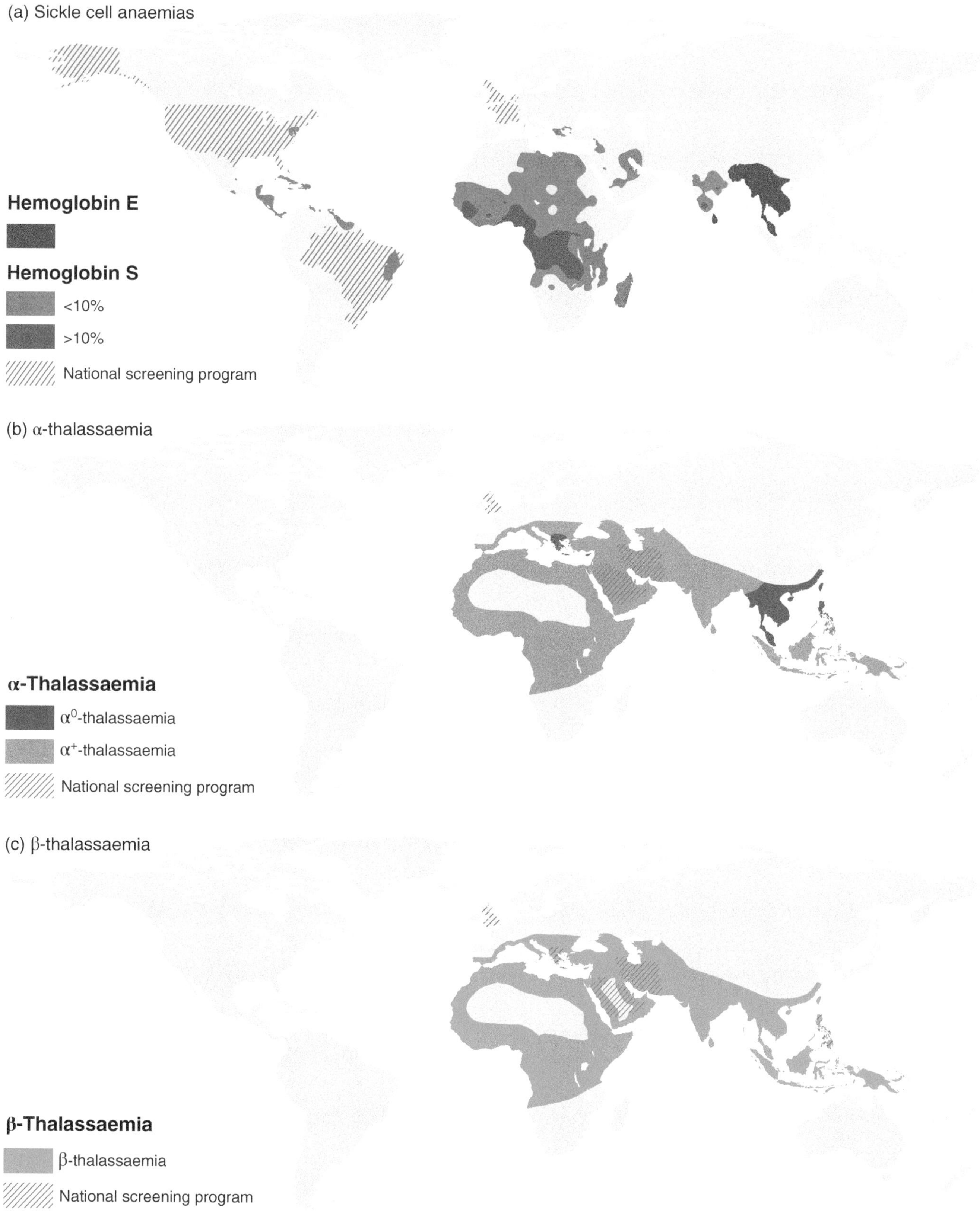

(a) Sickle cell anaemias

Hemoglobin E

Hemoglobin S

<10%

>10%

National screening program

(b) α-thalassaemia

α-Thalassaemia

α^0-thalassaemia

α^+-thalassaemia

National screening program

(c) β-thalassaemia

β-Thalassaemia

β-thalassaemia

National screening program

Source: F.B. Piel (2015). Global epidemiology of sickle cell disease and the thalassemias: new management challenges. Hematology Education; 9:147–154.

Symptoms and clinical features

- **Sickle cell anaemias:** Features can be varied and present from childhood. Chronic haemolytic anaemia (all patients) and recurrent infections (most patients) are the most common, alongside painful 'sickle-cell crises' and avascular necrosis of bone, the sequelae of splenic complications and chest pain in some patients. Patients may present with a range of symptoms and signs, including pain (bones, chest, abdomen), dactylitis, features of anaemia or infection (e.g. fevers, unwell, lethargy), and visual floaters.
- **Thalassaemia:** Patients often present in later childhood/early adulthood. Common presenting features include anaemia and

Figure 41.2 Genetics of α-thalassaemias.

Condition	Genotype	Phenotype
Hb Barts	--/--	Hydrops foetalis
Haemoglobin H	--/-α or --/αα^{CS}	Haemolysis, generally not transfusion dependent
α-Thalassaemia minor	-α/-α or --/αα	Hypochromia and microcytosis +/− mild anaemia
α-Thalassaemia minima	-α/αα	Asymptomatic with normal red cell indices

sequelae of iron overload (secondary to multiple blood transfusions). Other features include delayed growth, osteoporosis, and impaired fertility. In more severe cases, patients may have severe anaemia, poor appetite, pallor, dark urine, jaundice, and cardiomegaly.

- **α-Thalassaemia:** Clinical picture depends upon the number of alleles carrying alterations and whether the alterations lead to no production, reduced production, or the production of unstable variants.
- **β-Thalassaemia:** Signs and symptoms develop after six months of age as the levels of foetal haemoglobin fall (2 × α-globin chains and 2 × γ-globin chains) and are replaced by haemoglobin A production.
  - Those heterozygous for β-thalassemia are generally asymptomatic but have microcytic and hypochromic red cells and occasionally a mild anaemia. This is described as β-thalassemia minor or trait.
  - Homozygous or compound heterozygous β-globin alterations can lead to chronic haemolysis, severe anaemia, and expansion of bone marrow erythroid progenitors – intramedullary and extramedullary. Without treatment (transfusion, iron chelation), this can be fatal in <3 years.

Diagnosis

- **Sickle cell anaemias:** Blood films, haemoglobin electrophoresis, full blood count, and reticulocyte count aid diagnosis, alongside DNA-based assays. In acutely unwell patients, standard septic screening is required, including bloods (and peripheral cultures), oxygen saturation/arterial blood gas, and radiographs.
- **Thalassaemia:** Diagnosis is via genetic testing for *HBB, HBA1*, and *HBA2*. This is classified according to the haemoglobin chain affected (α or β) and the clinical consequences (major, intermedia, minor); it can also occur alongside a haemoglobin variant.
  - **α-Thalassaemia:** Identification of the alleles carrying alterations helps guide diagnosis:
  - **β-Thalassaemia:** Haemoglobin electrophoresis will show increased levels of haemoglobin A2 (2 × α-globin chains and 2 × δ-globin chains), except in rare cases with a co-inherited δ-globin alteration.

Management

- **Sickle cell anaemias:** Management focuses on controlling symptoms and includes analgesia to help during painful crises, hydroxyurea to help prophylactically prevent episodes of pain, antibiotic treatment/prophylaxis and vaccinations to treat/prevent bacterial infections, and blood transfusions as needed to deal with anaemia. L-glutamine (Endari) can help reduce the number of sickle-cell crises (patients >=5 years of age).
- **Thalassemia:** Management of thalassemia is with transfusion therapy, folic acid supplementation, and appropriate prevention of iron overload. Bone marrow transplantation can be curative.
- **Antenatal diagnosis and genetic counselling:** The UK has a sickle cell and thalassemia screening programme, which combines both antenatal and newborn screening. Newborn screening is carried out for all newborns as part of the heel prick test and screens for the following conditions: HbSS, HbS/ β-thalassemia, HbS/HPFH, HbSC, HbSD^{Punjab}, HbS/E, HbS O^{Arab}. Other conditions are likely to be detected if present, including β thalassemia major/intermedia, HbE/β-thalassemia, and HbH and are reported to the relevant clinician in order to facilitate management. The programme offers antenatal screening to detect significant maternal haemoglobinopathies and maternal conditions which require screening of the father, which may lead to potentially significant disease in the foetus. Screening varies depending upon the prevalence of haemoglobinopathies in the local population. The programme (alongside genetic counselling) has the following aims:
  - Support people to make informed choices during pregnancy and before conception (including recurrence risk assessment)
  - Improve infant health through prompt identification of affected babies
  - Promote greater understanding and awareness of the diseases and the value of screening.

The future

Haemoglobinopathies are a major global public health problem, with a high economic burden. Improving access to basic treatments, particularly in resource-poor nations, could save significant numbers of lives. For example, for sickle cell, some simple measures (e.g. antenatal diagnosis, antibiotic prophylaxis, transfusions) can markedly increase life expectancy. HbF induction and gene therapies are being investigated for thalassemia (for example beta-globin genes added to an affected individual's haematopoietic stem cells via a lentiviral vector, then reinfusing after chemotherapy, to increase HbA2 synthesis).

Immunology

Part 8

Chapters

42 Severe combined immunodeficiency

Background

Severe combined immunodeficiency (SCID) is a term used to describe a heterogeneous group of immunodeficiency disorders, occurring from birth, which affect both T- and B-cell immunity to varying degrees. It represents the most severe forms of primary immunodeficiency affecting adaptive immunity.

Aetiology

SCID is a rare condition, occurring in approximately 1 : 50 000 live births. There are multiple known genetic causes of SCID, some with distinct clinical phenotypes, along with as yet genetically undefined clinical cases.

Genetics

SCID can be classified based on the main lymphocyte compartments affected, as either 'T-B-' or 'T-B+ SCID'. Common to all forms of SCID is a severe deficit of mature T cells in the blood and tissues. X-linked common γ chain SCID accounts for 60%, JAK3 deficiency for 10%, IL7Rα deficiency for 1–2%, ADA deficiency for 20%. There are only 80 known cases of purine nucleoside phosphorylase (PNP) deficiency worldwide. AR forms are more commonly seen in communities with high rates of consanguinity. The most common or notable defects associated with SCID are summarised in Tables 42.1 and 42.2.

Pathophysiology

The link between the majority of the known forms of SCID is the inability to progress lymphocyte development beyond precursor stages (Figure 42.1). The two exceptions to this are ADA and PNP deficiency, which relate to metabolite toxicity. ADA and PNP are enzymes that are involved in the catabolism of purine nucleotides. Defects in these enzymes lead to the accumulation of toxic metabolites that inhibit further DNA synthesis. T cells are particularly affected. Lymphocytes need to produce diverse B- or T-cell antigen receptors (which are stimulated during lymphocyte development to allow progression to the next stage of maturation), but uniquely, without self-recognition. Failure of this stage is notably during VDJ recombination of the antigen-specific receptor gene segments, which produces the T-cell and B-cell receptors, and immunoglobulin.

Table 42.1 T-B- SCID (Markedly decreased numbers of both T cells and B cells).

Gene	Inheritance	Gene locus / OMIM	Specific features	Cellular defects	Pathophysiology
RAG1	AR	11p13 OMIM*179615	Omenn's syndrome as a presentation (hypomorphic variant, 'leaky SKID'): Partial RAG activity (development of some oligoclonal peripheral T cells containing receptors for self-antigens leading to auto-reactivity), hence later onset	Severe pan lymphopenia	RAG1/2 enzymes are involved in VDJ recombination. Alterations prevent formation of T-/B-cell receptors, so cells undergo apoptosis before maturation, leading to T-B-NK+ forms
RAG2	AR	11p13 OMIM*179616			
Artemis (*DCLRE1C*)	AR	10p13 OMIM*605988	Radiation sensitivity (impaired DNA repair)	May have normal B cells	DNA repair proteins, also involved in VDJ recombination, Deficiencies lead to multiple errors and unjoined breaks in DNA, and cell death
DNA ligase IV (*LIG4*)	AR	13q33.3 OMIM*601837		Markedly reduced T cells and B cells	
ADA1 deficiency	AR	20q13.12 OMIM*608958	Neurological and auditory abnormalities, lung and liver malformations	Progressive loss of T and B cells, low NK cells	ADA and PNP deficiencies cause build-up of metabolites toxic to lymphocytes). Higher turnover in early life as lymphocytes mature, hence more build-up Maternal ADA or PNP is protective in early neonatal period. Build-up dATP and S-adenosyl homocysteine (ADA deficiency), and dGTP (PNP deficiency)

Clinical Genetics and Genomics at a Glance, First Edition. Edited by Neeta Lakhani, Kunal Kulkarni, Julian Barwell, Pradeep Vasudevan, and Huw Dorkins.

Table 42.2 T-B+ SCID (Markedly decreased numbers of T cells, with normal numbers of B cells).

Gene	Inheritance	Gene locus	Cellular defects	Pathophysiology
Common γ chain	X linked	Xq13.1-13.3 OMIM*308380	Markedly low T and NK cells, but can have normal or elevated B cells	Defects in interleukin receptors of multiple cytokines required for lymphocyte development. T and NK cells fail to mature → lack of T cell and cytokine stimulation → (numerically normal) B cells unable to produce Ig
JAK3 deficiency	AR	19p12-13.1 OMIM*600173	Very low NK cells; normal or elevated B cells	JAK3 is an intracellular kinase responsible for producing signals in response to IL-2 activation. Prevents maturation of T and NK cells, (like common γ chain deficiency). Both associated with the T-B+NK- variant
IL7Rα deficiency	AR	5p13.2 OMIM*146661	Normal NK cells; normal or elevated B cells	IL-7 required for T cell maturation. Specific defects in receptor for α chains → prevent signalling through IL-7 pathway
CD3 deficiencies *CD3δ* *CD3ε* *CD3ζ*	AR	11q23.3 OMIM*186790 11q23.3 OMIM*186830 1q24.2 OMIM*186780	Normal NK cells and B cells	CD3 is a protein involved in T cell receptor signalling. Widely used as the main T-cell-specific marker in measuring lymphocyte subsets. Intact T-cell receptor complex is required for development of mature T cells
PNP deficiency	AR	14q13.1 OMIM*164050	Normal B cells with progressive loss of T cells	Haemolytic anaemia and progressive neurological features. *See ADA deficiency*

Figure 42.1 Disorders affecting different components of the immune pathway.

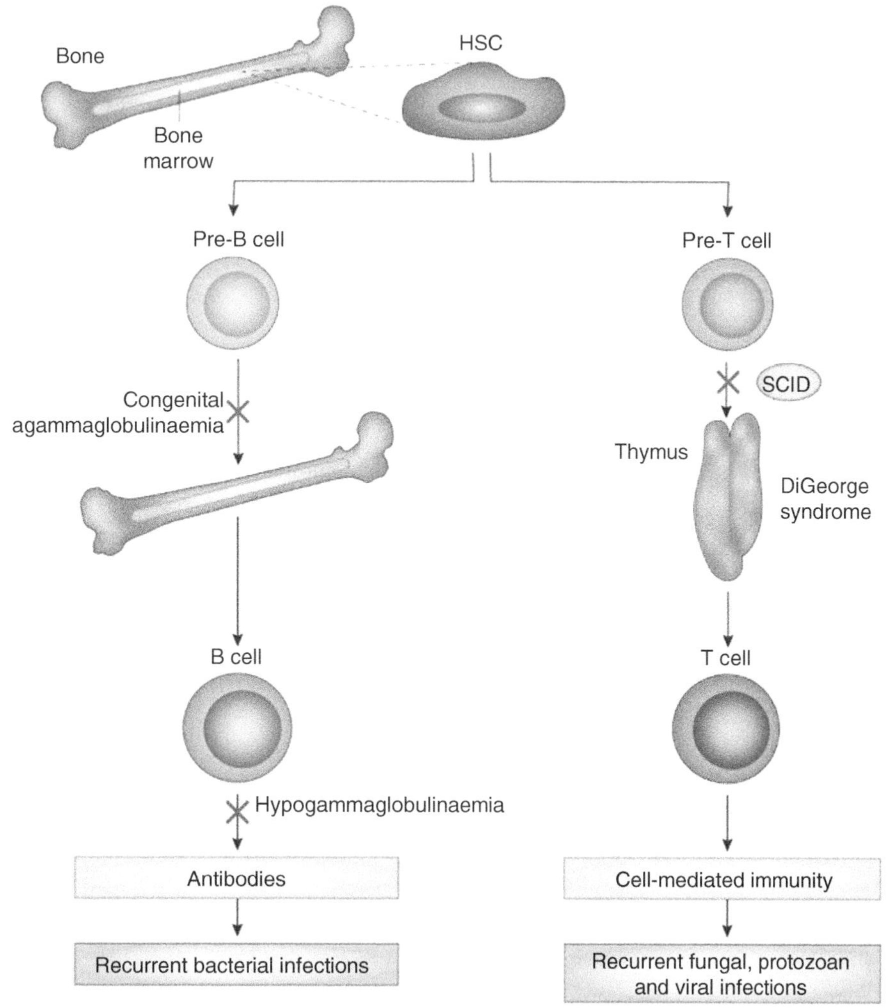

Symptoms and clinical features

All forms present within the first four years of life (majority in the first two years) with recurrent and often severe infections and failure to thrive. Due to its effect on the function of multiple immune cell types, SCID can present with bacterial, fungal, and viral infections, including opportunistic infections, such as *Pneumocystis jirovecii* pneumonia. There is a failure to clear usual childhood viruses, and there can be exaggerated reaction to BCG vaccine. Live vaccines should be avoided, as even attenuated strains can cause pathogenic infections. Hepatosplenomegaly may occur in some cases. Maternal T cells can cross the placenta and cause 'maternofoetal engraftment', mimicking graft versus host disease with a florid erythrodermic rash. Some specific clinical features include bone abnormalities, neurological and hearing impairment in ADA deficiency, neurological features in PNP deficiency, skin rashes in Omenn's syndrome and materno–foetal engraftment.

Diagnosis

- **Full blood count:** Lymphopenia is a key finding. A lymphocyte count of <2.8 × 10^{-9}/l in a neonate under two years old should trigger consideration of SCID.
- **Lymphocyte immunophenotyping:** First-line investigation to look at absolute number of CD4 and CD8 T cells, NK cells, and B cells. In materno–foetal engraftment, there may be normal numbers of T cells and further cytogenetics may be required.
- **Total immunoglobulins:** Checked at the outset.
- **Genetic testing:** The phenotypic pattern of T cells, B cells, and NK cells may give significant clues as to the gene(s) most likely to be affected. ADA and PNP levels should be checked.
- **Lymphocyte proliferation assays:** Useful in some cases, alongside responses to mitogens for cell function.
- **HLA typing:** Should be undertaken early, in case of need for haematopoietic stem cell transplantation (HSCT).
- **T-cell-receptor excision circle (TREC) analysis:** Provides an estimate of the number of T cells being released from the thymus into the circulation.

Management

SCID was the first primary immunodeficiency disease to be treated with HSCT and was one of the first conditions to undergo trials of gene therapy. All suspected SCID patients should be referred to a local immunology team urgently. Once diagnosis is confirmed, discussion with a paediatric immunology centre is undertaken. The SCID protocol should be initiated:

- Reverse barrier nursing;
- Antibiotic, antiviral and antifungal prophylaxis. Treat existing infections aggressively. Consider the possibility of opportunistic infections;
- Immunoglobulin replacement therapy for most patients;
- Live vaccinations are contraindicated in suspected SCID and relatives of SCID patients (until excluded);
- Blood products should be irradiated and CMV negative;
- Parenteral nutrition may be required.

HSCT remains the definitive treatment, with results having improved. With early treatment, survival is over 80%; however, delays in treatment and the presence of active infection reduce this.

ADA deficiency has been treated with pegylated-ADA replacement therapy, although this is generally viewed as a bridging method through to transplant. Post-transplant ADA levels can be monitored to indicate engraftment.

The future

Gene therapy was attempted in the past for SCID, although due to insertion of the new gene near an oncogene there was a high rate of leukaemia, and trials were suspended. However, modern gene insertion techniques reduce this risk (allow insertion of vectors away from oncogenes) and trials are ongoing. Neonatal blood spot tests for TRECs and KREKs (B-cell equivalent) have recently been introduced in some countries and may lead to early diagnosis (before symptomatic) of SCID and some other primary immunodeficiencies.

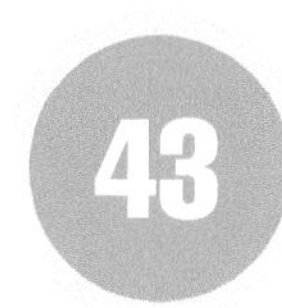

Common variable immunodeficiency

Background

Common variable immunodeficiency (CVID) is the commonest primary antibody deficiency to present clinically.

Aetiology

CVID overall affects approximately 1 : 25 000. It affects both genders equally. Up to 50% of patients have a family member with some form of antibody defect, including IgA deficiency and IgG subclass deficiency, who may be asymptomatic. Selective IgA deficiency is commoner than CVID (frequency around 1 in 700) and may progress to CVID, although most individuals remain asymptomatic. Heterogeneous condition, which groups together a number of monogenic and probably polygenic predisposing causes; 10% having an identified genetic defect (likely to increase with wider use of WGS), and 5–25% have a clear family history.

Genetics

Table 43.1 highlights the genetic basis of the various conditions.

Table 43.1 CVID - inheritance and features.

Alteration	Inheritance	Gene location	Details
ICOS deficiency (partial deletion)	AR	2q33.2	ICOS is a T-cell stimulatory receptor, which interacts with B cells, and is key for germinal centre formation and terminal B-cell formation
BAFF-receptor (BAFF-R) deficiency	AR	22q13.2	BAFF-R is a member of the TNF receptor family, which acts as a B-cell activator. BAFF-R deficiency tends to present as later onset CVID, but has also been described in some healthy individuals
NFκB-1 deficiency	AD	4q24	Functional haploinsufficiency of the canonical NFκB pathway, which responds to multiple receptors and is involved in many aspects of B-cell development and survival. Variable severity, even in same family
NFκB-2 deficiency	AD	10q24.32	Haploinsufficiency of the non-canonical pathway, which has a more limited set of receptors that activate it. Of note, 50% of these patients have pituitary insufficiency not seen in other forms of CVID
IKAROS deficiency	AD	7p12.2	Defect of a transcription factor causing haploinsufficiency and a progressive decline in immunoglobulins
CD21 deficiency	AR	1q32.2	Defect of the complement receptor 1 protein (CD21), with a number of compound heterozygous defects described. CD21 forms part of the B-cell co-receptor. Later onset of disease
CD81 deficiency	AR	11p15.5	Defect of the CD81 component of the B cell co-receptor, and is the only B cell receptor defect known to cause autoimmunity
CD19 deficiency	AR	16p11.2	CD19 is involved in modulating B-cell responses to antigen and in regulating antibody production
CD20 deficiency	AR	11q12.2	Loss of the B-cell regulatory protein CD20
CTLA-4 deficiency	AD	2q33.2	Severe early onset immunodeficiency and reduced CTLA-4 levels, resulting in dysregulation of regulatory T cells. Not all patients with defect and autoimmune disease meet the diagnostic criteria for CVID
LRBA deficiency	AR	4q31.3	Absence of the LRBA protein (part of the vesicle trafficking system to present CTLA-4 on the cell surface). Similar phenotype to CTLA-4 deficiency
Activated PI3-k delta syndrome (APDS)	AD	1p36.22	Gain of function mutation of the relatively ubiquitous PI3-kinase protein. Results in hyperphosphorylation of downstream mTOR and pushes cells towards senescence. Early onset immunodeficiency, often with a normal IgM and frequently early onset bronchiectasis and lymphoproliferation
TACI defects	AD or AR	17p11.2	Reported in selective IgA deficiency. TACI mutations are described in up to 2% of the healthy population, and so there is debate as to its degree of pathogenicity and the need for other mutations or triggers alongside TACI in the pathogenesis of CVID

Clinical Genetics and Genomics at a Glance, First Edition. Edited by Neeta Lakhani, Kunal Kulkarni, Julian Barwell, Pradeep Vasudevan, and Huw Dorkins.

Pathophysiology

The pathophysiology of CVID is complex, depending on the exact genetic defect (if known). The majority of cases relate to the interaction between T and B cells, required for antibody generation. ICOS, TACI, and BAFF-R are all directly involved in T- and B-cell interactions as cell surface receptors. APDS, NFκB, and IKAROS are involved in intracellular signalling to stimulate cell maturation and development. CTLA-4 and LRBA are involved in the interaction between T regulatory cells and B cells for ongoing stimulation, and act to downregulate immune responses. In their absence, self-peptides more readily induce responses causing the significant increase in autoimmunity. CD21/81/19 and CD20 defects are the 'pure' B-cell defects, where it is an absence of the B-cell receptor complex causing lack of antibody production. Therefore, in many cases of CVID, there is not a pure antibody deficiency, but a component of combined immunodeficiency.

Symptoms and clinical features

- **Recurrent bacterial infections:** This is the main presenting feature, most commonly of the sinopulmonary tract, alongside others (including conjunctivitis and GI infections, including recurrent/resistant giardiasis) (Figure 43.1). There is increasing evidence that some patients have persistent GI viral infection, such as norovirus. Some of the specific genetic forms of CVID have been shown to have an increased risk of opportunistic infections, and some can have severe or recurrent viral skin infections. Due to frequent respiratory infections, bronchiectasis is commonly seen.
- **Autoimmunity:** Can also be a presenting feature, most commonly as autoimmune cytopenias, including thrombocytopenia and haemolytic anaemia. These may be the trigger to identify the CVID. Autoimmune joint diseases, rashes, and enteropathies are also seen. CTLA-4 and LRBA deficiencies present with marked severe early onset autoimmune diseases including polyendocrinopathies.
- **Lymphoproliferative disease:** CVID patients have increased rates of benign (often virally driven) and malignant lymphomas.
- **Liver disease:** Can occur from a number of causes, including infective and inflammatory complications such as granulomatous disease or nodular lymphoid hyperplasia.
- **Granulomatous lymphocytic interstitial lung disease (GILID):** Can occur in some patients. It can be severe, and, if untreated, lead to respiratory failure. Inflammatory and autoimmune complications are seen more commonly in patients who have reduced number of class switched memory B cells.

Diagnosis

- Characterised by low IgG, with low IgA or IgM, and an absence of vaccine responses.
- Laboratory testing relies on total immunoglobulin measurement (usually with immunofixation and serum free light chains) as first line.
- If these are low, then proceeding to test for vaccination response is the next step. This is classically done to polysaccharide vaccines to test the T cell independent pathway, using Pneumovax II; however, other vaccine responses may be used if antibody testing is available. Isohaemagglutinins are rarely used in immunology in the United Kingdom.
- Class switched memory B cells are useful both diagnostically and prognostically for risk of inflammatory complications.
- It is important to note that CVID is a diagnosis of exclusion, and therefore, common causes of low immunoglobulins such as lymphoma/myeloma, drug-induced and protein loss should be considered.

The diagnostic criteria are outlined in Table 43.2.

Table 43.2 European Society of Immunodeficiency diagnostic criteria for CVID.

At least one of the following clinical features:
- Increased susceptibility to infection
- Autoimmune manifestations
- Granulomatous disease
- Unexplained polyclonal lymphoproliferation
- Affected family member with antibody deficiency

AND
- Marked decrease of IgG and marked decrease of IgA with or without low IgM levels (measured at least twice; <2SD below the age matched normal range)

AND at least one of the following:
- Poor antibody response to vaccines (and/or absent isohaemagglutinins); i.e. absence of protective levels despite vaccination where defined
- Low-switched memory B cells (<70% age matched range)

AND
- Secondary causes of hypogammaglobulinaemia have been excluded

AND
- Diagnosis is established after the 4th year of life (but symptoms may be present before)

AND
- No evidence of profound T-cell deficiency

Management

Multidisciplinary team involvement is vital to deal with both the immunological and organ-specific aspects of management:

- **Prompt aggressive treatment of infections:** Prolonged courses of antibiotics are a priority. Microbiological testing is important to track the organisms causing infection, which may aid if decolonisation is required. Testing for rare pathogens in the stool, including giardia and viral infections, may be required if there is diarrhoea. Most patients are commenced on prophylactic antibiotics. The majority of CVID patients do not require prophylactic anti-fungals or anti-virals, except in specific circumstances.
- **Intravenously or subcutaneous immunoglobulin replacement therapy:** If given correctly, this should raise the trough IgG level, but it does not replace IgA or IgM. Some centres will commence all CVID patients on immunoglobulin replacement therapy, whilst others will only do so if the infection burden is considered high enough. The dose of immunoglobulin should be adjusted to manage the infection burden, and higher doses may be required in bronchiectasis.
- **Respiratory function monitoring:** Most patients will have regular lung function testing and, if required CT, scanning to aid in detection of bronchiectasis or GILID. GILID presents similarly to sarcoidosis (note sarcoid should not be diagnosed in patients

with low immunoglobulins). GILID is treated mostly using steroids, but may require additional immunosuppression. Liver function monitoring and, if required, imaging and biopsy are used to identify the liver complications, and again these may necessitate immunosuppression.

- **Full blood count:** To monitor for cytopenias, which are managed as other autoimmune cytopenias. GI biopsy may be needed if a patient has diarrhoea or colitis symptoms to identify enteropathies, including celiac like enteropathies which may respond to a gluten-free diet.
- **Immunomodulators:** Rituximab and other classical steroid sparing DMARDs may be used. Both CTLA-4 deficiency and LRBA deficiency can be treated with Abatacept, a CTLA-4/immunoglobulin fusion protein, bringing significant improvement in lung disease and enteropathy.

The future

There is no gene therapy available for any of the CVID genotypes. This is not currently considered a transplantable condition. Different methods of delivering immunoglobulin replacement therapy, including rapid push and hyaluronidase facilitated therapy, are now available to help therapy adapt to patient lifestyles. Next-generation sequencing is being undertaken in increasing numbers patients to identify further genotypes; however, there is likely to be a significant polygenic or modifier gene effect in many cases.

Reference

1. Park MA, Li JT, Hagan JB, Maddox DE and Abraham RS. (2008). Common variable immunodeficiency: a new look at an old disease. The Lancet 372(9637): 489–502.

Figure 43.1 Clinical features.

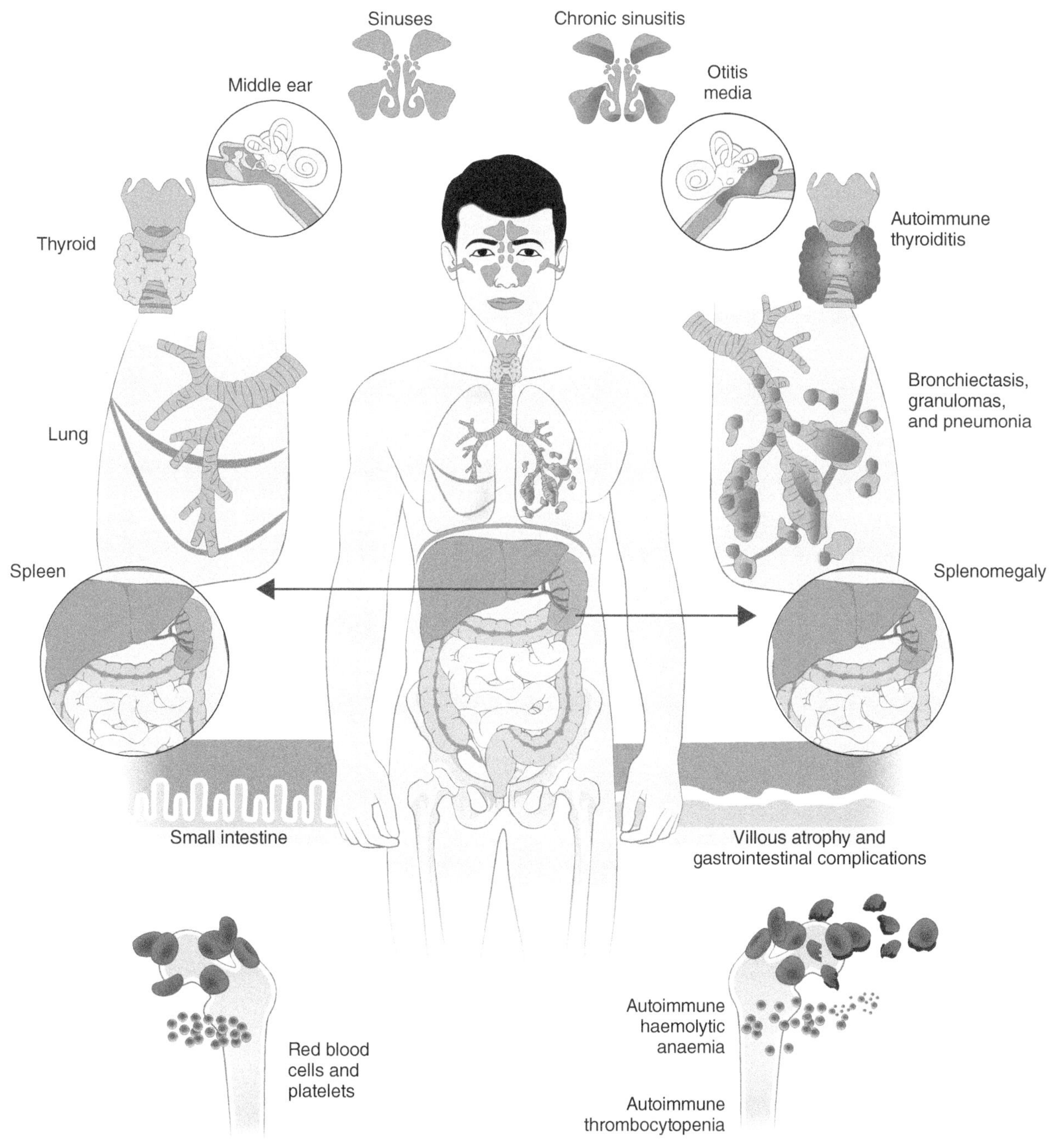

44 Congenital abnormalities affecting development of the thymus

Background

Congenital abnormalities affecting thymic development result in reduced numbers of T cells being produced. Two genetically defined conditions have been described, Di George/22q11 deletion syndrome (DGS) and CHARGE syndrome, both involving a constellation of features that includes thymic hypoplasia. In both cases, the degree of immunodeficiency associated with the condition is variable, depending on the numbers of T cells being produced by the residual thymic tissue.

Aetiology

DGS occurs in around 1 in 3000 live births, with males and females affected equally. There is a clear genetic basis, with the majority of cases arising from *de novo* mutations (Figure 44.1). Interestingly, in cases of inherited DGS/22q11 deletions, the clinical and immunological phenotypes can vary widely despite a common genetic basis. CHARGE syndrome occurs in around 1 in 10 000 live births. Males and females are equally affected. Approximately 70% of cases are associated with alterations in *CHD7,* with the majority of cases arising from *de novo* alterations. In the remaining cases, the genetic basis is currently unknown.

Genetics

Table 44.1 highlights the genetic basis of conditions affecting thymic development.

Table 44.1 Genetic basis of conditions affecting thymus development.

Condition	Inheritance	Alteration
Di George syndrome	AD	Majority are 22q11.2 microdeletions. Rarely alterations of *TBX1* or at a second DGS gene locus at 10p13-14
CHARGE syndrome	AD	Majority are *CHD7* gene alterations at 8q12.2 (encodes the chromodomain helicase DNA-binding protein 7). Association between *CHD7* alterations, CHARGE, and T-cell lymphopenia

Pathophysiology

- **DGS:** Arises from a failure of normal development and fusion of the third and fourth pharyngeal pouches, which gives rise to the characteristic features of conotruncal cardiac abnormalities, thymic hypoplasia, and parathyroid hypoplasia. *TBX1* encodes a protein (T-box 1) that acts as a transcription factor during embryonic development of the pharyngeal pouches and is required for the normal development of the structures associated with DGS. However, the genes that are regulated by T-box 1 have yet to be determined. Immune deficiency results from thymic hypoplasia, resulting in fewer T cells produced and released into the periphery. Further information on DGS can be found in the Paediatrics & Obstetrics section.
- **CHARGE:** Chromodomain helicase DNA-binding protein 7 (CHD7) is an ATP-dependent helicase enzyme that acts as a chromatin remodeller, with functions in a wide range of tissues, hence the broad range of abnormalities associated with CHARGE syndrome associated with *CHD7* alterations.

Symptoms and clinical features

Presentation and features are summarised in Table 44.2. The degree of immune deficiency in DGS varies widely, from mild to severe. Approximately 1% cases present as 'complete' DGS, with severe T-cell depletion (<50 naive T cells/ mm^3), levels more typically associated with severe combined immunodeficiency. In CHARGE, immune deficiencies mainly involve deficiency of T cells. As with DGS, presentation is a spectrum from mild to severe.

Table 44.2 Clinical presentation.

Condition	Features
Di George syndrome	• Significant variability • Classic triad of conotruncal cardiac defects, hypocalcaemia, and immune deficiency • Others include: facial dysmorphism, developmental delay, renal and palate abnormalities, and (later) development of autoimmunity • Due to the craniofacial features, DGS overlaps with velocardiofacial syndrome
CHARGE syndrome	• Clinical constellation of coloboma, heart abnormalities, choanal atresia, retarded growth or development, genitourinary abnormalities, and ear abnormalities/hearing loss • Immune abnormalities are common

Diagnosis

- **DGS:** Diagnosis is based on the clinical features, followed by cardiac evaluation and echocardiogram, evaluation of calcium and phosphorus levels, and evaluation of lymphopenia (full blood count), and T- and B-cell subsets (flow cytometry). Thymic shadow may be absent on chest X-ray, although this is not a reliable finding. Diagnosis should be confirmed by fluorescence *in situ* hybridization (FISH) analysis for 22q11.2 deletions, which are present in >90% of cases.
- **CHARGE:** Diagnosed by the constellation of clinical features (with two major and several minor features required for clinical diagnosis). Identification of mutations in *CHD7* is helpful in

Clinical Genetics and Genomics at a Glance, First Edition. Edited by Neeta Lakhani, Kunal Kulkarni, Julian Barwell, Pradeep Vasudevan, and Huw Dorkins.

confirming the diagnosis, but *CHD7* mutations are only found in about 70% of cases. Evaluation of T-cell numbers should be carried out to exclude the T-cell immune deficiency that may be associated with CHARGE syndrome.

Management

Management requires a multidisciplinary approach. Life expectancy of children with the most severe T-cell deficiencies who do not undergo transplantation is less than one year. The prognosis for those with less-severe immune deficiencies is variable and depends on the severity of the associated features (e.g. congenital cardiac abnormalities).

- **Immunological management:** Depends on the severity of the T-cell immunodeficiency. In milder cases, this primarily involves the use of antimicrobials to treat or prevent infections. More severe cases, where there is an associated antibody deficiency secondary to the T-cell deficit, may also require immunoglobulin replacement. The most severe cases (e.g. complete DGS) should be treated initially as for severe combined immune deficiency *(see SCID chapter)*.
- **Cultured thymic transplantation:** In recent years, this has proved beneficial in patients with complete DGS or CHARGE syndrome, although the technique is limited to a small number of centres worldwide.
- **Bone marrow transplantation:** May also be beneficial in those with an HLA-identical donor (although immune reconstitution in these cases is dependent on expansion of donor memory T cells within the transplant, rather than expansion and differentiation of pluripotent stem cells into naive T cells).

The future

Access to thymic transplantation for patients with complete DGS or CHARGE syndrome is currently limited to a small number of centres worldwide, but as access to this potentially lifesaving treatment widens, prognosis for these patients with the most severe forms of immunodeficiency should improve.

Figure 44.1 Disorders of thymic development.

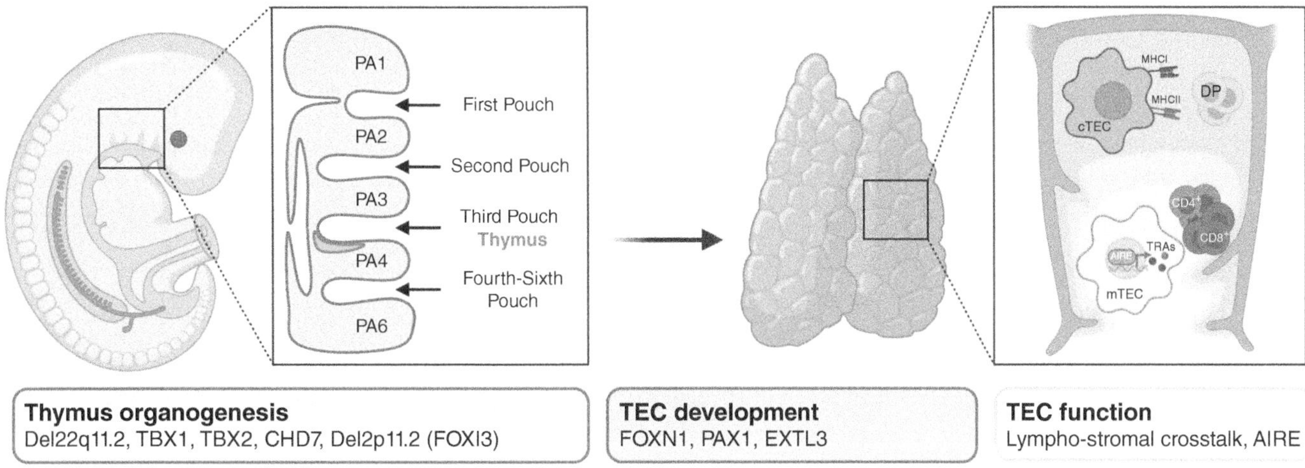

45 DNA repair defects

Background

Double-stranded DNA breaks can occur pathologically during exposure to ionising radiation, as part of normal cellular processes including in DNA replication, and during repertoire diversification in T- and B-lymphocyte development. Mechanisms exist to repair DNA breaks with either homologous or non-homologous end joining. Defects in these mechanisms can lead to either profound immunodeficiencies (see *Severe Combined Immunodeficiency* chapter), or the milder forms of immunodeficiency with specific syndromic features discussed here. The three commonest forms of DNA repair defect are ataxia-telangiectasia (AT), Nijmegen breakage syndrome (NBS), and Bloom syndrome (Table 45.1). In addition, there is the very rare ataxia-telangiectasia-like disorder (ATLD). DNA repair defects are associated with increased chromosomal instability and radiosensitivity.

Aetiology

AT occurs in approximately 1 : 100 000 births (may be as low as 3 : 1 000 000), without racial or gender predisposition. NBS is seen worldwide but is more frequent in Eastern Europe. There is no accurate information on incidence or prevalence. Bloom syndrome is rare in most populations but is seen most commonly in Ashkenazi Jews (in whom prevalence is 1 : 48 000). ATLD has fewer than 20 known cases worldwide.

Genetics

All forms of DNA repair defect exhibit AR inheritance

Table 45.1 Alterations in DNA repair defects.

Condition	Alteration	Details
AT	Ataxia-telangiectasia mutated (*ATM*) gene on chromosome 11q22.3	Four known disease-causing genetic complementation groups based on resistance to inhibition of DNA synthesis by ionizing radiation
NBS	*NBS1* gene on chromosome 8q21.3	
Bloom	Error in DNA helicase protein RecQ protein like 3 (*RECQL3*) gene (on chromosome 15q26.1	

Pathophysiology

The first step in sensing dsDNA breakages is with the MRN complex, which includes the non-phosphorylated form of the NBS1 protein, as well as MRE11 and RAD 50. Once the breakage is detected by the MRN complex, this activates the ATM protein, which can then initiate further signalling depending on the end outcome of the breakage, including:

- Direct or p53-mediated Caspase 2 activation with failure to repair;
- Phosphorylation of the NBS1 protein (acts as a cell-cycle checkpoint protein leading to cell cycle arrest or non-homologous end joining);
- Activation of the H2AX protein to lead directly to breakage repair.

ATM and MRN are not required for the Artemis-mediated dsDNA breakage repair seen in VDJ recombination; however, they are both required for immunoglobulin gene class switching and somatic hypermutation DNA repair. Reduction in function of the MRN complex or the ATM protein results in a decreased ability to sense and deal with DNA breakages, leading to increased alteration rates in all cell types, particularly lymphocyte progenitors (due to their high alteration rate to create antigen receptor diversity). AT, NBS, and ATLD show oligoclonal T- and B-cell populations. In AT, due to the importance of ATM in class switching, this results in the majority of B cells producing IgM, with little to no IgA, IgE, or IgG. In NBS, there is less impact on class switching, and therefore, the antibody deficiency is more variable, with some patients only having isolated isotype or IgG subclass deficiencies. In Bloom syndrome, there is a defect in RecQ helicase, which is responsible for ensuring that DNA, once unwound from duplexes, remains stable. Patients with Bloom syndrome commonly have reduced levels of serum immunoglobulins and impaired specific antibody responses.

Symptoms and clinical features

The classical history is of early onset ataxia and ocular telangiectasia. All patients with DNA repair defects have severe sensitivity to ionising radiation, and radiation exposure should be minimised. Malignancy risk is high; in AT and NBS, this is mostly lymphoid tumours. Of note, carriers and unaffected relatives of AT patients also have a significantly elevated risk of malignancy, especially breast cancer in women, possibly due to the role of ATM in phosphorylating BRCA1. Table 45.2 highlights the main clinical features. Heterozygotes appear to have increased rates of CLL.

Diagnosis

- **α-Fetoprotein:** Often elevated.
- **Variable hypogammaglobulinaemia:** Often with impaired polysaccharide responses.

Clinical Genetics and Genomics at a Glance, First Edition. Edited by Neeta Lakhani, Kunal Kulkarni, Julian Barwell, Pradeep Vasudevan, and Huw Dorkins.

Table 45.2 Clinical features of DNA repair defects.

Condition	Clinical features
AT	• Early onset cerebellar ataxia, normally presenting by end of the first year of life • Oculocutaneous telangiectasias (normally occurring by sixth year of life) • More generalised telangiectasia of the face and ears • Usually restricted growth and gonadal sterility • Frequent bacterial respiratory infections, with viral warts a common feature
NBS	• Classical 'birdlike features', microcephaly and mental retardation • Notable epicanthal folds, large ears, sparse hair • Propensity to respiratory infection
Bloom	• Short stature • Vitiligo • Infertility • Severe sensitivity to sunlight • Recurrent infections. • Very high rate of cancers.
ATLD	• Similar to AT • Ataxia of later onset and slower progression. Lack the telangiectasias

- **Low T-cell count:** With reduced function, low TRECs (as a measure of thymic output), and a skewed T-cell receptor V beta region repertoire. The thymus is often hypoplastic.
- **Genetic testing:** NBS is diagnosed with genetic testing of those with relevant clinical features (variable pattern of antibody deficiency, with low T-cell numbers and function, and evidence of a dysplastic thymus). Bloom syndrome is also diagnosed with genetic testing (usually low IgM, with reduced specific antibody responses to polysaccharide antigens, and commonly with T-, B-, and NK-cell functional defects).

Management

There is no specific treatment for any of the syndromes. Prognosis is poor due to the high rate of malignancy and difficulty in treating highly mutagenic cancers. The lack of availability of radiotherapy further limits treatment options. In NBS, malignancy is the leading cause of death. Lifetime incidence of malignancy in AT is 10–30%. However, in AT, there is a relentless progression of ataxia (most are wheelchair bound by the end of the first decade of life), which eventually leads to death in the early 20s in almost all cases. Due to the deterioration of bulbar function, PEG feeding may be required. In all cases, infections should be treated promptly and aggressively. In AT, ATLD, and NBS, immunoglobulin therapy can be given where there is evidence of an antibody deficiency; however, this only reduces the frequency and severity of infection, and does not alter disease progression. In Bloom syndrome, there is some evidence that immunoglobulin therapy is helpful in patients with documented antibody deficiency.

The future

Although these are single gene defects, gene therapy (using haematopoietic stem cells) would be limited by the activity of the mutated gene throughout the tissues of the body. Currently, there is investigation into a number of potential disease-modifying agents, including antioxidant agents and myoinositol, the initial results of which have been encouraging, but are not curative.

46 X-linked and autosomal recessive agammaglobulinaemia

Background

Agammaglobulinaemia is an absence or near absence of all major immunoglobulin isotypes. X-linked agammaglobulinaemia (XLA) was first described by Bruton in 1952. AR forms of agammaglobulinaemia also exist but are extremely rare. Collectively, they represent the most severe forms of predominantly antibody deficiencies.

Aetiology

XLA affects approximately 1 : 200 000 male births (~1 : 400 000 total live births) and accounts for ~90% of cases of primary agammaglobulinaemia. In almost one half of cases, there is no prior affected family member. The AR forms (accounting for the remaining ~10% of cases of agammaglobulinaemia) have each been identified in a few families only and are too rare for there to be accurate estimates of their prevalence.

Genetics

Primary agammaglobulinaemia is most commonly associated with alterations in Bruton's tyrosine kinase (BTK), an enzyme that is required for differentiation of pre-B cells into more mature forms, giving rise to an X-linked condition called X-linked agammaglobulinaemia (XLA). Table 46.1 highlights the inheritance and features of the two main subtypes.

Pathophysiology

BTK belongs to the Tec family of tyrosine kinase signal transducer molecules. It is expressed throughout B-cell development (as well as in myeloid and erythroid cells) and is essential for B-cell maturation (Figure 46.1). Alterations in *BTK* result in failure of B-cell maturation beyond the pre-B stage, leading to a profound reduction in mature B cells in the blood and peripheral tissues, failure to generate plasma cells, and consequently severely reduced production of all immunoglobulin isotypes. Alterations associated with AR forms of agammaglobulinaemia similarly occur in genes that are essential for B-cell maturation and/or function. Although the majority of alterations in *BTK* in males are associated with agammaglobulinaemia and an absence of mature B cells, less severe cases have been described, with reduced, rather than absent B cells and antibody production.

Symptoms and clinical features

Most patients with XLA present in early life (<2 years of age) with recurrent sinopulmonary infections, principally with encapsulated bacteria. *Streptococcus pneumonie, Haemophilus influenzae, Streptococcus pyogenes,* and *Pseudomonas* species are the commonest infecting organisms. Infections commonly start at about 3–6 months, as actively transported transplacental (maternal) IgG protects the neonate prior to this. There is also an increased susceptibility to blood-borne enterovirus infection, leading to viral encephalitis. Due to the lack of peripheral B cells, B-cell-rich tissues such as tonsils are commonly absent or markedly reduced in size.

Diagnosis

A family history of XLA may be present. Characteristic laboratory features include:

- Profound deficiency in serum immunoglobulins IgG, IgA, and IgM.
- Markedly reduced numbers of B cells (with normal numbers of T cells and NK cells) on flow cytometric analysis of peripheral blood.
- Suspicion of XLA is strengthened by reduced or absent expression of *BTK* in peripheral blood monocytes, although normal *BTK* expression is seen in ~15% of those with alterations in the *BTK* gene.
- Genetic testing: A definitive diagnosis is made by confirmation of a alteration in *BTK* by gene sequencing.

Table 46.1 Overview of the two main subtypes of agammaglobulinaemia.

Condition	Inheritance	Alteration	Details
XLA	X-linked	*BTK* (X chromosome; Xp22.1)	Affects males. Females with heterozygous alterations act as genetic carriers
AR	AR	• *Immunoglobulin μ heavy chain* gene 14q32.33); • λ5 gene (*IGLL1*; 22q11.23); • Igα gene (*CD79A*; 19q13.2); • Igβ gene (*CD79B*, 17q23.3); • p85α subunit of PI3K (*PIK3R1*; 5q13.1); • *BLNK* gene (10q24.1).	

Clinical Genetics and Genomics at a Glance, First Edition. Edited by Neeta Lakhani, Kunal Kulkarni, Julian Barwell, Pradeep Vasudevan, and Huw Dorkins.

Management

Treatment of patients with XLA or AR agammaglobulinaemia is with (life-long) immunoglobulin replacement therapy, given either intravenously or subcutaneously. Observational studies in patients with XLA indicate that immunoglobulin replacement reduces both rates of infection (including enteroviral infections, and long-term pulmonary sequelae of infections) and hospitalisation rates. With appropriate treatment and care, most patients with XLA can now expect to survive well into adult life, with a good quality of life.

The future

Recent scientific advances make it possible to detect patients with severe defects of B-cell maturation using a blood spot test, making the prospect for neonatal screening for XLA and certain other severe T- and B-cell immunodeficiencies a reality. The test (for B cells) is based on detection of immunoglobulin kappa-deleting recombination excision circles (KRECs), which are normally formed during rearrangement of the immunoglobulin genes during B-cell development. In patients with XLA (and certain forms of SCID), KRECs are markedly reduced.

Figure 46.1 Abnormalities in B-cell development.

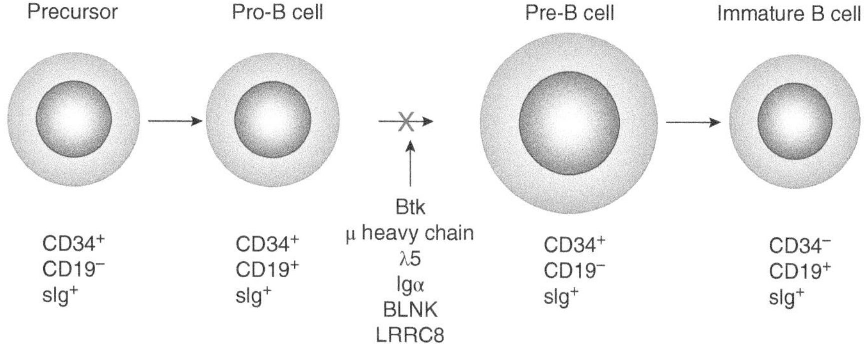

47 Wiskott-Aldrich syndrome

Background

Wiskott-Aldrich syndrome (WAS) is characterised by a combination of increased susceptibility to infections, microthrombocytopenia, and childhood eczema.

Aetiology

Estimates of the incidence of WAS-related disorders vary somewhat, but it is in the order of $1–4/10^6$ live male births. There are no obvious racial or ethnic differences.

Genetics

WAS is caused by alterations in a gene encoding a protein that links intracellular signalling pathways to actin cytoskeleton reorganisation. Three distinct clinical phenotypes are now recognized. Approximately half of patients with WAS alterations present with the classical WAS clinical phenotype, and half with X-linked thrombocytopenia (XLT). X-linked neutropenia (XLN) has only been described in a small number of families. Inheritance is x-linked, and penetrance appears complete.

The *WAS* gene encodes the WAS protein (WASp) and is located on the short arm of the X chromosome, at Xp11.23. Loss of function mutations in the *WAS* gene are responsible not only for the 'classical' Wiskott-Aldrich clinical phenotype but also for XLT (depending on the nature and site of the alteration), whilst (rare) gain of function alterations can give rise to XLN.

In addition, homozygous alterations in the *WIPF1* gene located at chromosome 2q31.1 can give rise to a clinical phenotype very similar to WAS. The *WIPF1* gene encodes a protein that stabilizes the WASp in the cell's cytoplasm).

Pathophysiology

The WAS protein is expressed only in cells of haematopoietic origin. It is a member of a family of proteins that link intracellular signalling to actin polymerization through activation of actin-related protein (Arp) 2/3. WASp is involved in several key functions of immune cells, including actin cytoskeleton reorganisation, locomotion, and formation of the immune synapse. Loss of functional WASp impacts on the function of a wide range of cells of both the innate and adaptive arms of immunity, including T cells, NK cells, granulocytes, monocyte/macrophages, and dendritic cells. Thrombocytopenia results from a combination of factors, including reduced thrombopoiesis, reduced platelet survival, increased clearance and immune mediated mechanisms. The site and type of alteration in the *WAS* gene determines the clinical phenotype and severity of disease.

Symptoms and clinical features

A WAS clinical scoring system has been developed, based on a range of clinical features including presence of thrombocytopenia, eczema, immunodeficiency, autoimmunity, and malignancy, and may be helpful in differentiating classical WAS from XLT (Figure 47.1).

- **'Classical' WAS:** Usually presents in infancy in affected males, with thrombocytopenia (often associated with bloody diarrhoea and petechial or purpuric rash), widespread eczema, and recurrent bacterial, viral, and fungal infections. Development of autoimmunity is common, including immune cytopenias, vasculitis, inflammatory bowel disease, and renal disease. There is an increased susceptibility to develop malignancies, especially EBV-associated lymphomas.
- **XLT:** Males usually present with microthrombocytopenia. Eczema and immune deficiency, if present, are usually mild. XLT patients have an increased risk of developing autoimmunity and malignancy, although this is less than in classical WAS.
- **XLN:** Presents in affected male patients as a congenital neutropenia (with associated infections), which may be associated with development of myelodysplasia and lymphocyte dysfunction.

Diagnosis

A diagnosis of WAS or XLT should be considered in any male patient presenting with congenital or early onset microthrombocytopenia and is supported by the presence of eczema, or a family history. Detection of the WAS protein can be carried out by flow cytometry, following staining of blood cells with a fluorescently labelled anti-WASp antibody, but may not detect patients with expressed WAS protein containing missense alterations. Identification of an alteration in the *WAS* gene is required for confirmation of the diagnosis.

Management

Treatment depends on the severity of disease and clinical features. Life expectancy is reduced, particularly in patients with classical WAS, with bleeding being the main cause of death. However, life-threatening infections, development of malignancies, and autoimmune manifestations all contribute to the poor prognosis. In contrast, patients with XLT have life expectancies close to those of healthy males (in developed countries, at least). Management options include:

- **Platelet transfusions:** These are given to treat bleeding episodes or to prevent blood loss during surgery.

Clinical Genetics and Genomics at a Glance, First Edition. Edited by Neeta Lakhani, Kunal Kulkarni, Julian Barwell, Pradeep Vasudevan, and Huw Dorkins.

- **Splenectomy:** May ameliorate the thrombocytopenia and bleeding tendency.
- **Prophylactic antimicrobials:** Used to prevent infections (e.g. cotrimoxazole for prevention of *P. jiroveci* pneumonia; acyclovir in patients with recurrent HSV infection).
- **Immunoglobulin replacement:** Indicated in patients with significant antibody deficiencies.
- **Immunosuppressive therapy:** May be required for treatment of autoimmune manifestations.
- **Haematopoietic stem cell transplantation (HSCT):** This is the only curative therapy available at present and is generally used in patients with higher disease severity scores (where a suitable donor is available). It is used less in patients with XLT than classical WAS, due to the more favourable long-term outcome with conservative management in these patients.

The future

As with other monogenic conditions, gene therapy offers a potential future curative therapy and has been used in a small number of patients with WAS. Improvement in clinical parameters was seen, but the treatment was associated with development of acute leukaemia in a proportion of patients (receiving retroviral-based gene therapy).

Figure 47.1 Clinical features of Wiskott-Aldrich syndrome.

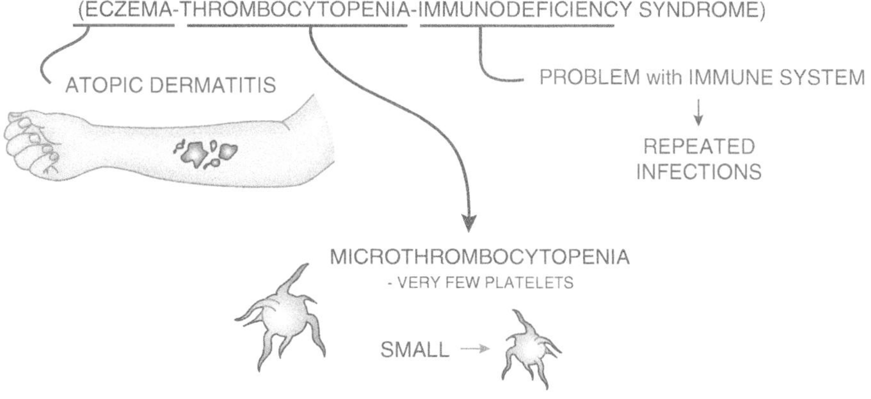

48 Hyper-immunoglobulin M syndromes

Figure 48.1 Stages of B cell development.

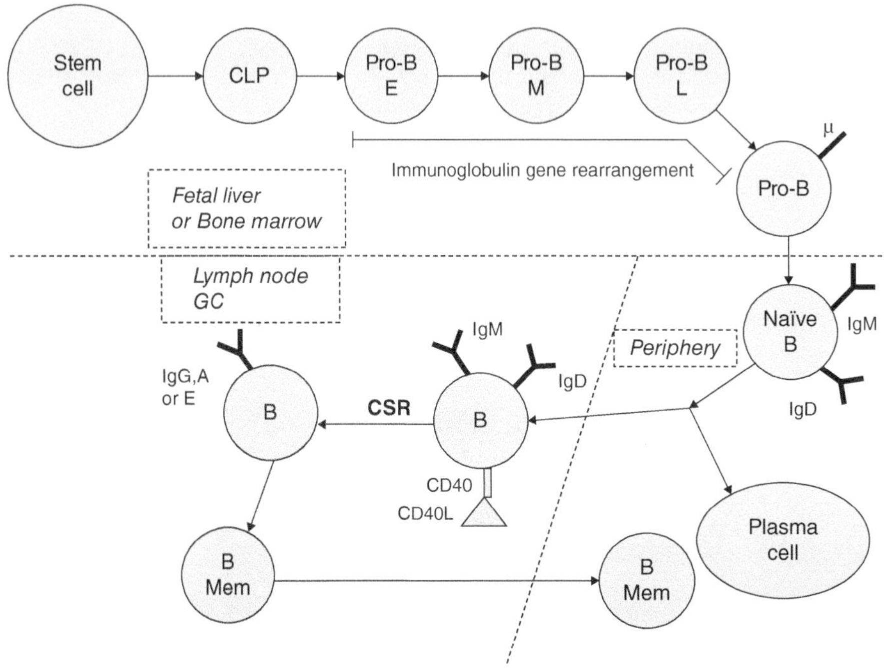

Key: CLP, Common Lymphoid Precursor; Pro B E/M/L, Precursor B cell early/mid/late; B Mem, Memory B cell; CSR, Class switch recombination.
Source: Davies EG, Thrasher AJ. Update on the hyper immunoglobulin M syndromes. British journal of haematology. 2010 Apr;149(2):167–80.

Background

The hyper-immunoglobulin M (hyper IgM) syndromes are a heterogeneous group of immunodeficiency disorders characterised by defective immunoglobulin class-switch recombination, leading to the presence of normal or increased levels of serum IgM, and markedly reduced levels of other immunoglobulin isotypes (IgG, IgA, and IgE), and associated with increased susceptibility to infections.

Aetiology

Hyper IgM syndromes are rare. The X-linked variant (HIGM1) is the commonest form of Hyper IgM syndrome, with an estimated prevalence of about 1 : 500 000 males. HIGM2 has an estimated frequency of <1 : 1 000 000, with HIGM3 and UNG deficiencies rarer still.

Genetics

To date, alterations in five genes have been identified as causing hyper IgM syndromes. Table 48.1 summarises the alterations.

Pathophysiology

Hyper IgM syndromes occur due to impaired class switch recombination of immunoglobulin production, meaning the B/plasma cells are unable to switch the class of antibody production from IgM (the 'default' immunoglobulin isotype) to other immunoglobulin isotypes, such as IgG, IgA, or IgE. The hyper IgM syndromes are therefore typified by normal or (usually) raised levels of IgM, with very low levels of IgG, IgA, and IgE. In the case of hyper IgM syndromes due to alterations in *CD40LG* and *CD40* genes, this is due to a deficient cognate receptor ligand interaction between T cells and B cells in the lymphoid follicles, which is required for class switch recombination to occur (Figure 48.1). This interaction activates the NF-*k*B signalling pathway within the B cells, hence the association of alterations in the NF-*k*B regulator, *NEMO*, with impaired immunoglobulin class switch recombination. Within B cells, NF-*k*B upregulates expression of the *AICDA* and *UNG* genes, which encode enzymes that help to mediate class switch recombination.

Symptoms and clinical features

The main clinical manifestations of hyper IgM syndromes are an increased susceptibility to infections. However, the clinical phenotypes vary, depending on the underlying genetic defect.

1 **CD40 and CD40L deficiencies:** Classified as combined immunodeficiencies, as both B-cell and T-cell functions are impaired. (Male) patients with CD40L deficiency usually present in infancy with sinopulmonary infections, predominantly with encapsulated bacteria. These patients also have an increased susceptibility to

Table 48.1 Alterations causing hyper IgM syndromes.

Condition	Inheritance	Alteration	Details
Hyper IgM syndrome type 1 (HIGM1)	XLR	*CD40LG* gene (*TNFSF5*) encoding CD40 ligand, at Xq26.3	Commonest. Female carriers of mutations in *CD40LG* are generally healthy, except in cases of extreme lyonisation
Hyper IgM syndrome type 2 (HIGM2)	AR	*AICDA* gene coding activation induced cytidine deaminase (AID), at 12p13.31	Second most common cause
Hyper IgM syndrome type 3 (HIGM3)	AR	Gene encoding CD40, at 20q13.12	
Hyper IgM syndrome type 4 (HIGM4)		Alteration not yet established	
Another AR form of hyper IgM syndrome	AR	Gene encoding uracyl N-glycosylase (UNG), at 12q24.11	
X-linked ectodermal dysplasia with immunodeficiency	X-linked	*IKBKG* gene encoding a regulator of the NF-*k*B signalling pathway (NEMO) at Xq28	Phenotype of which also involves impaired class switch recombination

opportunistic infections, such as *Pneumocystis jiroveci*, *Cryptosporidium,* and *Histoplasma*. Lymphadenopathy and hepatosplenomegaly are common, as is development of sclerosing cholangitis secondary to *Cryptosporidium* infection. There is an increased risk of malignancies, including hepatocarcinoma and lymphomas. Relatively few patients with CD40 deficiency have been described, so the clinical phenotype is less well defined.

2 **AID and UNG deficiencies:** Intrinsic B-cell defects and affect humoral immunity only. Recurrent sinopulmonary infections are the main feature, without the susceptibility to opportunistic pathogens seen in CD40L deficiency. Lymphoid hyperplasia, affecting tonsils and other secondary lymphoid tissues, is a feature of AID deficiency. Patients with AID deficiency often undergo tonsillectomy, as a consequence of the tonsillar hyperplasia.

3 **IKBKG/NEMO deficiency:** Characterised by the combination of anhydrotic ectodermal dysplasia, characteristic conical teeth, and infections in male patients (X-linked inheritance).

Diagnosis

Typically, patients with hyper IgM syndromes have normal or raised serum levels of IgM, with markedly reduced levels of the other immunoglobulin isotypes (IgG, IgA, and IgE) and with impaired antibody responses to protein and polysaccharide antigens. Circulating immunoglobulin class-switched memory B cells are absent or markedly reduced. Flow cytometry can be used to analyse expression of CD40 or CD40L on circulating B cells or activated T cells. As with other primary immunodeficiency disorders, definitive diagnosis is by identification of relevant gene alterations.

Management

1 **Immunoglobulin replacement therapy:** This is used to treat the antibody deficiency in patients with hyper IgM syndromes and reduces the incidence of sinopulmonary infection.

2 **Infection prophylaxis:** Due to the combined B- and T-cell immunodeficiency associated with CD40L and CD40 deficiencies, treatment of these patients is more complex and also involves prophylaxis against opportunistic infections such as *Pneumocystis jiroveci* (cotrimoxazole), and hygiene measures to reduce the risk of *Cryptosporidium*.

3 **Haematopoietic stem cell transplantation:** As with other combined immunodeficiencies, this offers the only current curative treatment for patients with CD40L and CD40 deficiencies.

There is a need for more current estimates of prognosis in hyper IgM syndromes. Historically, median survival in males with CD40L deficiency who had not received HSCT was poor (<25 years), but this figure does not reflect the impact of HSCT or improved management of these patients more recently. Long-term survival in AID and UNG deficiencies appears better, as use of immunoglobulin replacement and aggressive treatment of infections leads to reduced early death and prevents development of chronic lung disease as a result of recurrent infections.

The future

As indicated above, the genetic basis of HIGM4 remains to be defined. Use of HSCT is likely to continue to result in improved survival or patients with CD40L (and CD40) deficiencies. As with other monogenetic conditions, developments in gene-base therapies may offer improved curative treatments in the future.

49 Hyper-immunoglobulin E syndrome

Background

Hyper IgE syndrome (HIES) encompasses a group of clinically related phenotypes, the majority of which are now genetically defined. HIES is characterised by markedly elevated serum IgE levels, with recurrent infections, due to defects in intracellular signalling.

Epidemiology

AD HIES occurs equally in males and females, and is seen in all ethnic groups, but is best described in Caucasian populations. AR HIES with confirmed *DOCK8* alterations had been identified as in just over 100 patients worldwide (as of 2014). The true incidence is not known, but estimates range from 1 : 100 000 to 1 : 500 000. HIES associated with alterations in *Tyk2* has been reported in a single Japanese patient.

Genetics

There are AD and AR *forms* of HIES (see Figure 49.1):

- **AD:** Most common form and is well characterised. Occurs from alterations in the signal transducer and activator of transcription 3 (*STAT3*) on chromosome 17q21.2. *De novo* mutations in *STAT3* are found in up to 50% of cases. The majority are missense alterations in DNA or SH2 binding sites, and all cause loss of function.
- **AR:** Rarer, and not all cases have been genetically determined. There are known alterations in dedicator of cytokinesis 8 (*DOCK8*) on chromosome 9p24.3, cytoplasmic *TYK2* on chromosome 19p13.2, and a recently proposed variant associated with alterations in *PGM3* tyrosine kinase with a distinct clinical phenotype.

Pathophysiology

- ***STAT3* alterations:** Cause immune dysregulation. STAT3 is involved in intracellular signalling in response to pro-inflammatory cytokines activating the JAK kinases, which in turn allow homodimerisation of STAT3. STAT3 homodimers then are transported to the nucleus and increase transcription of other cytokines, both pro- and anti-inflammatory. Loss of STAT3 function most notably causes defects in signalling from IL-6 (pro-inflammatory), IL-10 (anti-inflammatory), and IL-11 (proposed to be causative of the skeletal defects). Defects in response to IL-6 lead to a lack of differentiation of Th17 T cells, which have anti-fungal actions. The immune dysregulation in AD-HIES is also associated with abnormal, often exaggerated inflammation (such as cold abscess formation).
- ***DOCK8* alterations:** Recently described, hence the immunological mechanisms are not yet fully known. The DOCK-180 family, of which DOCK8 is a member, is responsible for activating Rho GTPase by removal of GDP. There is some evidence that DOCK8 deficiency impairs cytoskeletal actin accumulation, which is important in NK cell function, accounting for some of the susceptibility to viral infection.
- ***TYK2* alterations:** Poorly characterised functionally, but may lead to impairment of the IL-12/interferon pathway. (*See Chapter 53 - Mendelian susceptibility to mycobacterial disease.*)

Symptoms and clinical features

Although there are common features to all three genetically defined forms of HIES, there are some clinical variations between the groups.

- **All forms:** Present with recurrent bacterial sinopulmonary infections, moderate to severe eczema/atopic dermatitis, and markedly **elevated total serum IgE** levels (>2000 IU/ml). The eczematous rash is classically present from birth or the first weeks of life, and an eosinophilia is normally present. Significant skin abscesses, which are typically 'cold' (pus filled but without heat or redness) are a feature of all forms, and osteomyelitis can occur. All display susceptibility to mucocutaneous candidiasis. There is an increased risk of malignancy (especially lymphoma) and of autoimmune cytopenias.
- **STAT3 deficiencies:** Present with the classical HIES picture, including coarse 'leonine' facies, a widened nose, susceptibility to fractures especially of long bones, scoliosis, and retained primary dentition. They may also have hyperintensities on brain MRI, Chiari 1 malfomations and coronary vascular malformations. They are the only group at risk of lung pneumatoceles and fungal pneumonia.
- **DOCK8-deficient patients:** Do not have the classical skeletal, dental, or facial presentation, although the great majority will present with severe, recurrent viral skin infections from HPV, HSV, molluscum, or VZV. Despite all forms having elevated IgE, this is the only form to present with asthma or food allergy.
- **HIES with Tyk2 deficiency:** Reported in a single Japanese patient, who presented with a markedly elevated serum IgE, skin abscesses, pneumonia, and BCG and Salmonella infections. Several patients with Tyk2 deficiency have been reported subsequently, who presented with atypical mycobacteriosis, but lacked the other features of HIES.

Diagnosis

All patients present with an elevated IgE, frequently above 2000 IU/ml and often above 5000 IU/ml. However, due to maturational development of immunoglobulins, this may not be apparent in early life. Neutrophil and lymphocyte cell numbers are usually normal, with a peripheral blood eosinophilia. Other immunoglobulin levels are variable, but IgG is usually normal. There is a National Institute of Health (USA) scoring system for clinical suspicion of HIES. It should be noted, however, that this was originally designed for the AD form. Testing for alterations in the known associated genes identifies subtype.

Management

Goals are prevention of infection, aggressive treatment of active infection, and management of the associated complications, as outlined in Table 49.1.

The future

Further investigation into the efficacy and optimal conditioning for stem cell transplantation may improve management. Interferon gamma is under investigation, and one patient has had treatment with omalizumab (anti-IgE monoclonal antibody), although this approach would require caution.

Clinical Genetics and Genomics at a Glance, First Edition. Edited by Neeta Lakhani, Kunal Kulkarni, Julian Barwell, Pradeep Vasudevan, and Huw Dorkins.

Figure 49.1 Molecular basis for the shared clinical and immunological phenotypes between AD (*STAT3* alteration) and AR HIES (*DOCK8* deficiency).

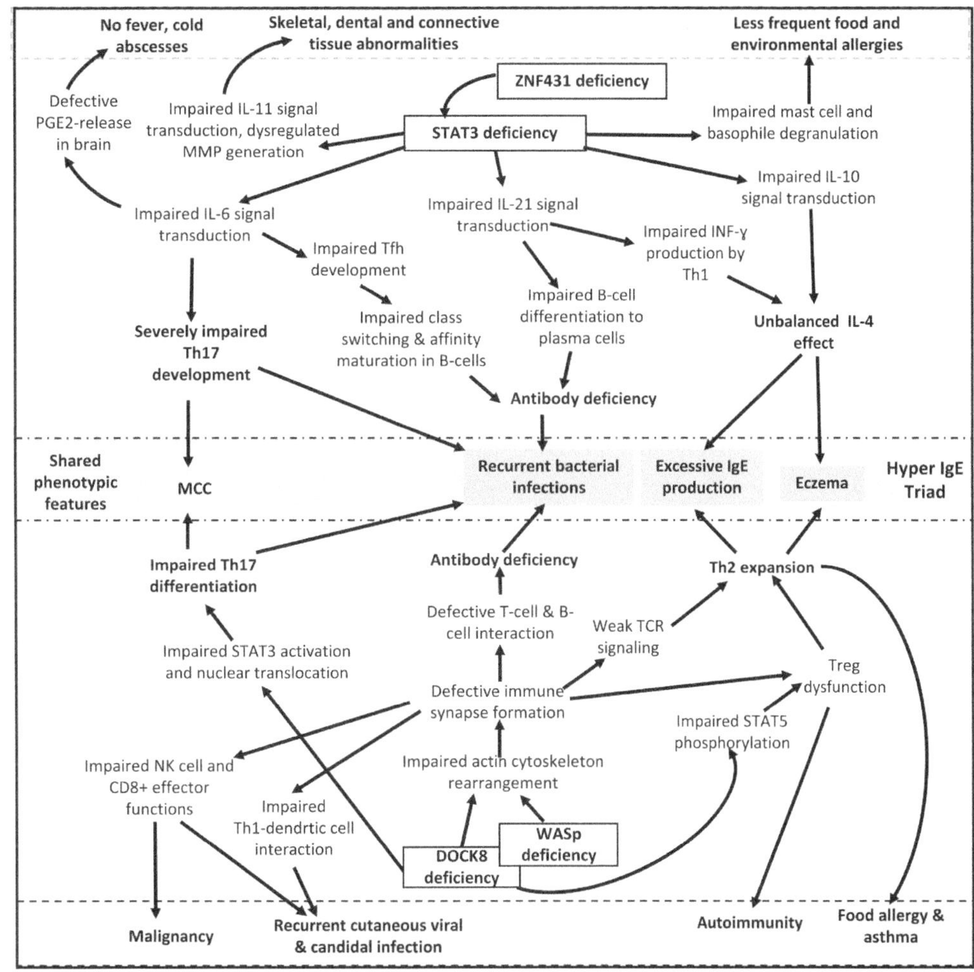

Key: MCC, mucocutaneous candidiasis; PGE2, prostaglandin E2; TCR, T-cell receptor; MMP, matrix metalloproteases; STAT3, signal transducer and activator of transcription-3

Source: Al-Shaikhly T, Ochs HD. Hyper IgE syndromes: clinical and molecular characteristics. Immunology and cell biology. 2019 Apr;97(4):368–79.

Table 49.1 Principals of management of HIES.

Issue	Details
Preventing infections	• Minimises sequelae of progressive lung damage, pneumatocele formation, and bronchiectasis. • First line is prophylactic antimicrobials that cover both skin and chest, with co-trimoxazole being a common first choice. • May also require anti-fungal prophylaxis in the form of itraconazole. • Good skin hygiene using chlorhexadine washes may help. • With structural lung damage *Pseudomonas* colonisation may occur and decolonisation may be attempted. • Immunoglobulin therapy is used in some patients, in whom there is a demonstrated impaired response to vaccination (despite a normal total serum IgG level).
Acute skin abscesses	• Treated with antibiotics and a low threshold for surgical intervention. The majority of skin infections are due to *Staphylococcus aureus*. • Patients presenting with chest symptoms should be rigorously investigated, with early, aggressive antibiotic treatment where indicated. • Microbiology testing is important, as is consideration of fungal infection as a cause.
Viral skin infections	• In DOCK8, patients should be treated with aggressive high dose anti-viral treatment, but response is often poor, and immunoglobulin replacement has little effect on viral infections in these patients.
Pneumatoceles	• If particularly troublesome, may on occasion require surgical resection.
Retained teeth	• Dental referral is often required
Scoliosis and facial features	• May require operative management.
Eczema	• Requires standard treatment but may be resistant, and there must be significant caution in the use of immunosuppression.
Haematopoietic stem-cell transplantation (HSCT)	• Occasionally used in STAT3 deficiency, with mixed success, probably due to non-haematopoietic effects of STAT3. • DOCK8 deficiency may be treated with stem cell transplantation, but it remains unclear if this is curative in the long term. • Prognosis has improved as infection rates have reduced; however, infectious lung complications remain the leading cause of death, followed by lymphoma, which is often resistant to therapy.

50 Chronic mucocutaneous candidiasis

Background

Chronic mucocutaneous candidiasis (CMC) are a heterogeneous group of disorders characterised by persistent, non-invasive candida infections of the skin, nails, and mucous membranes. Some forms are associated with the (early) development of autoimmune disease, in particular autoimmune endocrinopathies.

Aetiology

Autoimmune polyendocrinopathy, candidiasis, ectodermal dysplasia (APECED) syndrome accounts for the majority of cases of CMC in several populations (e.g. Iranian Jews, Finns, and Sardinians, where the frequency may be 1 : 9000–1 : 25 000) but is significantly less common in other populations (1 : 100 000–1 : 200 000).

Genetics

Alterations in (at least) nine genes have been associated with CMC. CMC due to alterations in *AIRE, IL17RA, IL17RC,* and *ACT1* are inherited in an AR pattern, whilst *IL17F* and *STAT1* gain of function alterations are AD.

- Alterations in several genes associated with the development or function of Th17 cells have been associated with CMC. These include alterations in the IL-17 receptor A (*IL17RA*; at chromosome 22q11) and IL-17 receptor C (*IL17RC*; at chromosome 3p25), IL-17F (*IL17F*; at chromosome 6p12), STAT1 gain of function alterations (*STAT1*; at chromosome 2q32), and ACT1 (*ACT1/TRAF3IP2*; at chromosome 6q21).
- Alterations in the autoimmune regulator (*AIRE;* chromosome 21q22.3) gene are associated with the APECED syndrome.
- Cases of CMC have also been found in patients with alterations in Dectin-1 (*CLEC7A* gene; at 12p13.2), CARD9 (*CARD9*; at 9q34.3), toll-like receptor 3 (*TLR3*; at 4q35.1), and Lyp (*PTPN22*; at 1p13.2).

Pathophysiology

- **IL-17 signalling pathway (*IL17RA, IL17RC,* and *IL17F*) defects:** Affect the development and function of Th17 cells, and their association with CMC reflects the important role that Th17 cells play in combating fungal infections.
- **Gain of function STAT1 alterations:** Similarly, these are associated with impaired development of IL-17-producing cells, whilst alterations in *ACT1* are associated with failure of fibroblasts and T cells to respond normally to members of the IL-17 cytokine family (IL-17A, F, and E).
- **AIRE deficiency:** AIRE is a transcription factor expressed in thymic medullary epithelial cells and allows the expression of a vast array of self-antigens within the thymus and plays a central role in the negative selection of potentially autoreactive T cells within the thymic tissue. Deficiency, therefore, allows T cells expressing autoreactive T-cell receptors to exit the thymus, where they expand and induce autoimmunity in peripheral tissues. The mechanism of susceptibility of AIRE-deficient patients to candidal infections is unclear but is thought to result from associated defects in adaptive and innate immunity.
- **Dectin-1 and CARD9 deficiencies:** Their relationship with CMC is explained by the roles of these molecules in immunity against fungal infections. Dectin-1 is a beta-glucan receptor expressed on innate immune cells that is involved in the detection of fungi and production of cytokines in response to them, whilst CARD9 is a downstream component of the Dectin signalling pathway. In addition, AIRE associates with components of the Dectin-1 signalling pathway, so that patients with AIRE deficiency have impaired Dectin-1 signalling in response to fungal infection.

Symptoms and clinical features

The clinical feature common to all forms of CMC is of chronic, non-invasive candidal infection of the skin, mucous membranes, and nails. This may be associated with autoimmune manifestations, including endocrinopathies and immune cytopenias. A variety of immune abnormalities may be identified, although most common is T-cell anergy to stimulation with Candida antigens. In some cases, there may be autoantibodies to IL-17. APECED usually presents with a triad of mucocutaneous candidiasis, polyendocrinopathy (including hypoparathyroidism, adrenal insufficiency, hypothyroidism, diabetes mellitus, gonadal dysfunction), and dental enamel hypoplasia.

Diagnosis

This is based on the presence of chronic skin and mucous membrane infection with Candida, with or without autoimmune features (Figure 50.1). APECED presents as distinct clinical constellation most frequently of mucocutaneous candidiasis, hypoparathyroidism, and adrenal failure. Identification of alteration(s) in a relevant gene confirms the diagnosis.

Management

Treatment is primarily symptomatic. Azole antifungals are usually effective in managing the candidal infections, for both treatment and prophylaxis (Figure 50.2). Endocrine abnormalities are managed by replacement therapy (under appropriate supervision). Severe autoimmune abnormalities are treated with standard immunosuppressive regimes, although most reports in CMC are anecdotal. Prognosis is variable, depending on age of onset and responsiveness to treatment. Most patients survive into their forties or beyond.

The future

Recent advances in the understanding of the genetics and pathophysiology of CMC have led to improved diagnosis and management, with the potential for development of novel therapies for the future.

Clinical Genetics and Genomics at a Glance, First Edition. Edited by Neeta Lakhani, Kunal Kulkarni, Julian Barwell, Pradeep Vasudevan, and Huw Dorkins.

Figure 50.1 Diagnosis of chronic mucocutaneous candidiasis.

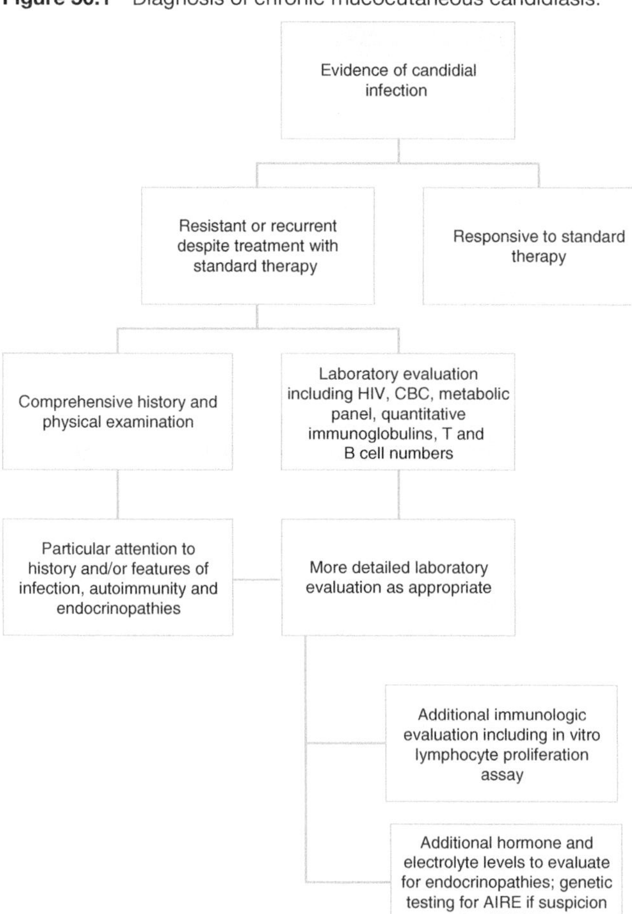

Figure 50.2 Treatment of chronic mucocutaneous candidiasis.

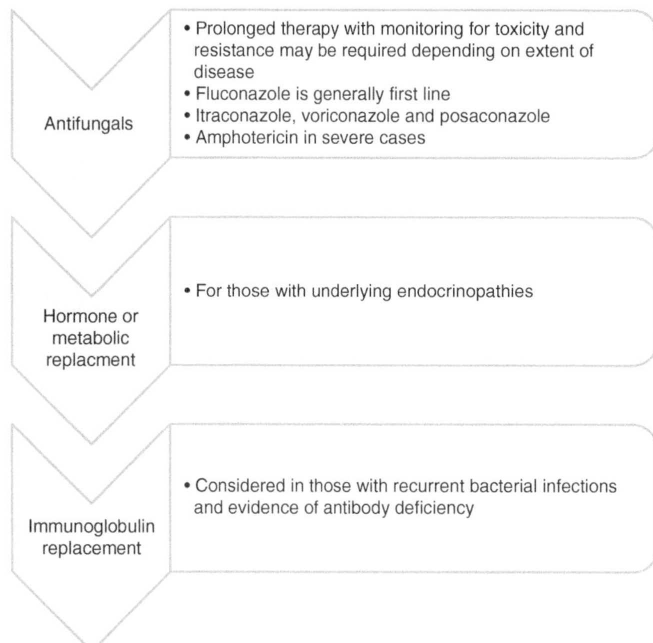

Source: Sampson, Hugh A. (2015). Allergy and Clinical Immunology (Sampson/Allergy and Clinical Immunology) || Chronic Mucocutaneous Candidiasis, 10.1002/9781118609125(), 375–381.

Genetic disorders associated with immune dysregulation and/or autoimmunity

Background

This disparate group of conditions includes the autoimmune lymphoproliferative syndromes (ALPS), immune dysregulation, polyendocrinopathy, enteropathy, X-linked syndrome (IPEX), and immune dysregulation with colitis (associated with defects of the IL-10 signalling pathway). APECED (autoimmune polyendocrinopathy, candidiasis, ectodermal dysplasia) and the X-linked lymphoproliferative diseases (XLP 1 and 2) also fall into this category but are discussed in the sections on familial mucocutaneous candidiasis and familial haemophagocytic, respectively.

Epidemiology

ALPS is rare, and there are no accurate estimates of its incidence, although cases have been reported in a range of ethnic and racial groups, with a slight predominance in males. IPEX is also rare, with an estimated incidence of around 1 : 1 500 000. Female carriers of *FOXP3* alterations do not appear to be at increased risk of developing autoimmune disease. The IPEX-like syndromes have been identified in a small number of kindreds only. IL-10 signalling pathway deficiencies are rare, and there are no accurate estimates of incidence.

Genetics

Table 51.1 highlights the genetic basis of the various disorders.

Pathophysiology

- **ALPS:** Associated with alterations in lymphoid cell apoptotic pathway genes in about two thirds, leading to dysregulated lymphocyte homeostasis. Apoptosis is important for limiting the overall size of the lymphoid compartment; defective apoptosis results in a non-malignant lymphoproliferation, with lymphadenopathy and hepatosplenomegaly, and increased lymphoma risk.
- **IPEX:** Caused by *FoxP3* alterations, a transcription factor required for the development and function of regulatory T cells (T regs), which have potent immunosuppressive activities and are important in preventing autoimmune and allergic inflammatory responses. Alterations in *FOXP3* therefore lead to a loss of development of T regs and increased autoimmune and allergic inflammation. The main autoimmune manifestations are a severe autoimmune enterocolitis, autoimmune endocrinopathy (typically diabetes or thyroid disease), and an eczematous dermatitis. Like *IPEX, CTLA4* alterations are associated with impaired function of T regs and present clinically with enteropathy, immune cytopenias, and interstitial lung disease.
- **IL-10:** This is a key anti-inflammatory cytokine, produced by a range of cell types including T regs. IL-10 plays an important role in preventing excessive inflammation leading to tissue damage in the gut. Deficiency in IL-10 or its receptor is associated with uncontrolled inflammation, leading to a severe enterocolitis.

Table 51.1 Disorders associated with immune dysregulation and/or autoimmunity.

Condition	Inheritance	Alterations
ALPS	FAS (AD) FAS Ligand (AR) Caspase-10 (AD) Caspase-8 (AR) FADD (AR) CTLA4 (AD)	Several genes associated with the apoptosis pathway: • Majority are Fas/CD95 (*TNFRSF6*; 10q23.31) germline alterations • Additional 15–20% are FAS somatic alterations • Germline alterations associated with ALPS have also been identified in the FAS ligand gene (*TNFSF6*; 1q24.3) • Others include alterations to the Caspase-10 gene (*CASP10*; 2q33.1), Caspase-8 gene (*CASP8*; 2q33.1), Fas-associated protein with death domain (FADD; 11q13.3; and CTLA4 (*CTLA4*; 2q33.2); give rise to ALPS V)
IPEX	X-linked (most cases familial, sporadic described) IPEX-like: IL2RA (AR), CTLA4 (AD), STAT3 (AD)	• Usually Loss of function alterations in the FoxP3 gene (*FOXP3*; Xp11.23) • Several 'IPEX-like' syndromes identified, with alterations in the genes encoding CD25 (*IL2RA* gene; 10p15.1), CTLA4 (see above), STAT5b (17q21.2), STAT1 (gene gain of function mutation; 2q32.2; see chronic mucocutaneous candidiasis section), STAT3 (gene gain of function mutation; 17q21.2), and LRBA (4q31.3)
IL-10 signalling pathway defects (immune dysregulation with colitis)	AR	Alterations in the interleukin (IL)-10 signalling pathway: • Loss of function in 11q23.3; or *IL10R2*; OMIM 123889; 21q22.11), or its receptor (*IL10R1*; 11q23.3; or *IL10R2*; 21q22.11)

Clinical Genetics and Genomics at a Glance, First Edition. Edited by Neeta Lakhani, Kunal Kulkarni, Julian Barwell, Pradeep Vasudevan, and Huw Dorkins.

Symptoms and clinical features

• **ALPS:** Lymphadenopathy and splenomegaly, with or without hepatomegaly, resulting from chronic lymphoproliferation. Hypersplenism features may be present. Autoimmunity is common, usually manifesting as autoimmune haemolytic anaemia and/or immune thrombocytopenia, and is seen more frequently in males than females. Other autoimmune manifestations can include glomerulonephritis, autoimmune hepatitis, immune neuropathies, but rarely involve the endocrine glands. Increased risk of developing both Hodgkin and non-Hodgkin lymphomas.

• **IPEX**: Typically present at an early age in affected male children presenting with severe chronic diarrhoea (associated with an autoimmune enteropathy), endocrinopathy (early onset type 1 diabetes and/or autoimmune thyroid disease), and an eczematous dermatitis, commonly associate with failure to thrive. Immune cytopenias, severe allergies, and exaggerated responses to infections are also common. Several IPEX-like conditions have been identified, with similar clinical features, but mutations in genes other than *FOXP3*. IPEX-like syndromes can affect females, as well as males.

• **IL-10:** Associated inflammatory bowel disease typically presents as a severe, progressive enterocolitis, often with extraintestinal manifestations, in children less than three months of age.

Diagnosis

• **ALPS:** Presence of TcR alpha/beta-positive but CD4 and CD8 double-negative T cells which, in combination with the clinical features, alert to the presence of ALPS. *in vitro* studies show impaired Fas-mediated apoptosis. Diagnostic criteria are based on clinical and laboratory criteria, including the identification of germline or somatic mutations in *FAS, FASLG*, or *CASP10*.

• **IPEX:** Clinical feature lead to sequencing and identification of mutations in the *FOXP3* gene.

• **IL-10:** Detected using *in vitro* functional studies. Diagnosis should confirmed by identification of relevant alterations.

Management

• **ALPS:** Immunosuppressive therapy (particularly targeting T cells), although the potential benefits of treating lymphoproliferation need to be offset against the potential side effects of long-term immunosuppressive therapies. Haematopoietic stem-cell transplantation (HSCT) is the only curative therapy available. Long-term prognosis is generally favourable, and lymphadenopathy often decreases with age. Patients with *FAS* alterations affecting the extracellular domains tend to have a more favourable prognosis, whilst those with homozygous or compound heterozygous *FAS* mutations have a poorer prognosis, and generally require HSCT for long-term survival.

• **IPEX:** Early and aggressive treatment of acute medical events, involving a multidisciplinary specialist team is important. Immune suppression and dietary modifications are required to control the enteropathy, and acute exacerbations may require periods of total parenteral nutrition. Hormone replacement is used to manage the endocrine manifestations. Haematopoietic stem cell transplantation has been used and offers the potential for cure in selected patients.

• **IL-10:** Enterocolitis is typically poorly responsive to standard immunosuppressive regimes. Long-term prognosis in these patients tends to be poor. HSCT offers the prospect of curative therapy for suitable patients.

The future

These conditions are rare and have only been defined in the last decade or so. Experience of their management is limited, and as more patients are identified, it is likely that treatment will improve. A broader availability of HSCT and advances in this field are also likely to lead to improved outcomes for these patients.

52 Genetic disorders associated with familial haemophagocytic lymphohistiocytosis

Background

Haemophagocytic lymphohistiocytosis (HLH) is a sudden-onset, life-threatening condition associated with excessive immune activation and multiple organ involvement. Familial FHLH (FHLH) is commonly triggered by infection in those with a genetic predisposition (and in sporadic cases). Prompt treatment is essential to prevent multi-organ failure, and mortality in untreated patients is high.

Epidemiology

The majority of cases of HLH present in (early) childhood, and account for around 1 in 3000 childhood hospital admissions, with approximately 1 in 4 of these cases representing FHLH. Syndromes associated with disorders of cytotoxic granules or granule release are rare, with a male-to-female ratio of approximately 1 : 1. Alterations in specific genes associated with FHLH are found with higher frequencies in specific ethnic groups (e.g. *PRF1* alterations in Japanese). The majority of cases of HLH (especially in older individuals) are not associated with mutations in known genes associated with FHLH. X-linked lymphoproliferative disease (XLP) is estimated to affect between one and three males per million, but this may be an underestimate as not all cases of fulminant infectious mononucleosis (FIM) are investigated for alterations in *SH2D1A* or *XIAP*.

Genetics

Both familial and sporadic forms occur, and alterations in a number of genes have been associated with FHLH. Syndromes have an AR pattern of inheritance (with the exception of Munc18-2 alterations, in which both AR and AD patterns are seen). XLP 1 and 2 are X-linked disorders, with clinically affected males, and female carriers clinically unaffected.

Alterations in a number of genes have been identified in association with FHLH:

- **Cytotoxic granules or granule release disorders:** Include perforin deficiency (*PRF1* gene alterations; 10q22.1); Munc13-4 deficiency (*UNC13D* gene alterations; 17q25.1); Syntaxin 11 deficiency (*STX11* alterations; 6q24.2), Munc18-2 deficiency (*STXBP2 alterations; 19p13.2*).
- **XLP:** Associated with alterations in two genes. *XLP1* (previously known as Duncan's syndrome) is associated with SH2 domain protein 1A (*SH2D1A*, also known as SLAM-associated protein) alterations, whilst *XLP2* is associated with alterations in the X-linked inhibitor of apoptosis (*XIAP*). Both genes are located at Xq25.
- **Other congenital immunodeficiency syndromes associated with FHLH:** Include Griscelli syndrome type 2 (*RAB27A* alterations; 15q21.3), Chediak-Higashi syndrome (*CHS1 / LYST* alterations; 1q42.3), XMEN (X-linked immunodeficiency with magnesium defect) disease (*MAGT1*; Xq21.1); Interleukin-2-inducible T cell kinase (ITK) deficiency (*ITK*; 5q33.3), CD27 deficiency (*TNFRSF7*; 12p13.31), and Hermansky-Pudlak syndrome (associated with several gene alterations).

Pathophysiology

FHLH is a condition of excessive or uncontrolled inflammation, usually triggered by an infectious episode, in a genetically susceptible individual, resulting in tissue damage to multiple organs. Uncontrolled macrophage activation in HLH leads to a cytokine storm of pro-inflammatory cytokine production (IFNγ, TNFα, IL-6, etc.), as well as haemophagocytosis (engulfment and internalisation of red cells, platelets, or white blood cells by macrophages) (Figure 52.1). The predisposing genetic causes can be split into two main groups: those alterations associated with defects of cytotoxic granules or granule release, leading to impaired function of natural killer (NK) cells and cytotoxic T cells (*PRF1; Munc13-4, Munc18-2, STX11*); and those associated with a failure to handle EBV (or other viral) infections (XLP1, XLP2, XMEN, ITK, and CD27 deficiencies).

Symptoms and clinical features

The initial presentation of FHLH is usually of a young child with fever and evidence of multiple organ involvement. Hepatomegaly and splenomegaly (~90%) and cytopenias (especially anaemia and/or thrombocytopenia; 80%) are very common, with lymphadenopathy, rash, or neurological symptoms each seen in 33% of cases. An infectious trigger is common, in particular EBV infection in the case of XLP1/2, XMEN, ITK, and CD27 deficiencies. If untreated, the condition leads to progressive multi-organ failure and death.

In the X-linked lymphoproliferative syndromes, there is significant overlap between HLH and FIM (although HLH may be triggered by other virus infections, as well as EBV). Collectively, HLH and FIM account for approximately 50% of clinical presentations of XLP, with approximately one third of patients presenting with lymphoma, and about 20% with dysgammaglobulinaemia (most commonly reduced serum IgG with normal or raised IgA and IgM).

Clinical Genetics and Genomics at a Glance, First Edition. Edited by Neeta Lakhani, Kunal Kulkarni, Julian Barwell, Pradeep Vasudevan, and Huw Dorkins.

Diagnosis

The HLH-2004 diagnostic criteria require either a molecular diagnosis consistent with HLH (i.e. relevant gene alteration)or at least 5 of the 8 following clinical findings:

- Fever > 38.5 °C
- Splenomegaly
- Cytopenia (two lineages affected)
- Raised ferritin (>500 ng/ml)
- Raised serum triglycerides and/or low fibrinogen
- Raised soluble CD25
- Evidence of haemophagocytosis in tissue biopsy
- Low or absent NK activity

Table 52.1 provides details on some specific laboratory tests.

Table 52.1 Specific laboratory markers.

Specific laboratory markers include:
• **Serum ferritin:** Markedly elevated (usually >1000 ng/ml). May be useful diagnostically.
• **Serum triglyceride and liver enzyme levels:** Elevated.
• **Coagulation abnormalities:** Common.
• **Soluble IL-2 receptor alpha (CD25):** Typically elevated.
• **Bone marrow examination:** May show evidence of haemophagocytosis, although its absence (especially in the earlier stages of disease) does not exclude HLH.
• **Flow cytometry:** Natural killer (NK) cell function is typically low or absent on **CD107alpha granule release assay**. Also used to detect expression of perforin, granzyme B, SAP, and XIAP proteins in white blood cells.
• **Genetic testing:** Identification of candidate causative genetic alterations is confirmatory.

Figure 52.1 Cytotoxic lymphocyte granule-mediated cytotoxicity pathway.

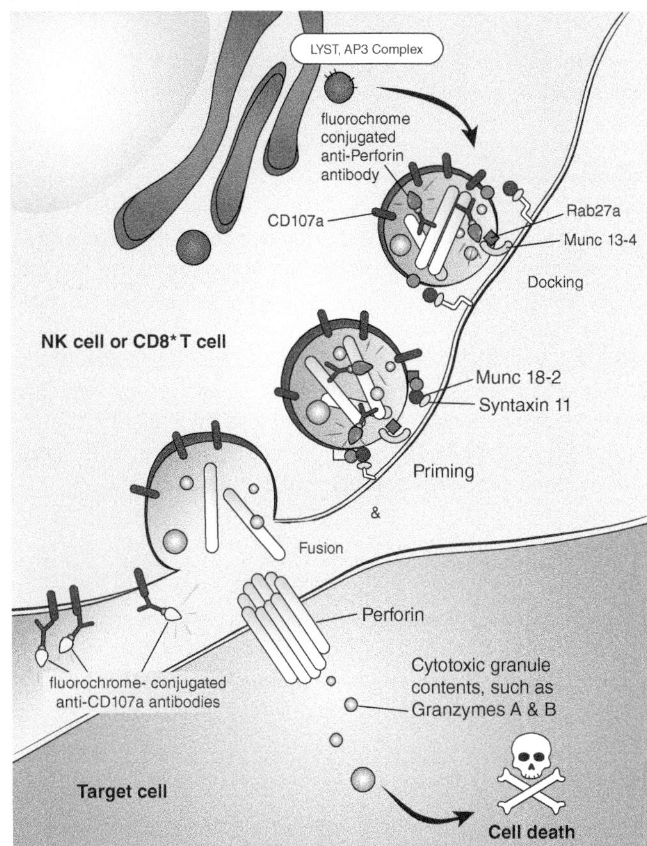

Source: Marsh RA, Haddad E. How i treat primary haemophagocytic lymphohistiocytosis. British journal of haematology. 2018 Jul;182(2):185–99.

Management

The goals of treatment are to suppress the aberrant inflammatory response. The HLH 2004 treatment regime involves a combination of dexamethasone, cyclosporine A, and etoposide, with intrathecal methotrexate and steroids for those with CNS involvement (although other treatment regimens are also available, and many centres continue to use the HLH 94 regimen, which does not include cyclosporin A). Subsequent haematopoietic stem cell transplantation (HSCT) is recommended for those with familial disease or a molecular diagnosis. Mortality without treatment is extremely high, particularly in those with an inherited alteration in a known HLH gene (median survival around two months). Prognosis has improved dramatically since the introduction of HLH-specific treatment regimens and HSCT. Following HLH 94, three-year survival in those undergoing HSCT was 64%. With improved, reduced intensity regimens prior to HSCT, three-year survival following FHLH has improved to >90%, with normal or near-normal quality of life for those surviving.

The future

Treatment has improved dramatically over the past two decades. However, the optimum therapeutic regime has yet to be defined, and new targets for therapy and novel immunosuppressive agents are likely to continue to lead to improvements in treatment. HSCT offers the potential for curative therapy, and as regimens improve, early genetic diagnosis may offer the prospect of curative treatment in genetically susceptible individuals prior to the onset of HLH.

53 Mendelian susceptibility to mycobacterial disease

Background

Mycobacterium tuberculosis is the archetypal pathogenic mycobacterial infection in humans, and infection is endemic in many parts of the world. Of interest are the individuals who get recurrent atypical mycobacterial infections with mycobacteria that would not normally be pathogenic in healthy individuals. These patients also have susceptibility to other infections. Where susceptibility is genetically determined, these cases are referred to as Mendelian susceptibility to mycobacterial disease (MSMD). Note that the majority of non-tuberculous mycobacterial (NTM) infections occur in individuals with structural lung disease, as opposed to immunodeficiency.

Aetiology

These are rare, with <100 cases of each genetic disorder described in the literature. Prevalence may rise with greater awareness of the phenotypes. MSMD may be caused by alterations in a number of genes. Assessment of these conditions may be difficult, as this often requires complex functional assays to assess cytokine release profiles.

Genetics

Table 53.1 highights the genetic basis of the various MSMDs.

Table 53.1 Inheritance and alterations associated with the various MSMDs.

Condition	Inheritance	Alteration
IL-12B deficiency	AR	*IL-12B*, 5q33.3
IL12 receptor B1 subunit deficiency	AR (poor penetrance)	*IL12RRB1*, 19p13.11. Homozygous and compound heterozygous alterations. Mostly associated with an absence of protein. On occasion, non-functional protein is detected
Interferon gamma (IFNγ) receptor 1 defects	AD (less severe) and AR (more severe)	*IFNGR1*, 6q23.3
IFNγR2 deficiencies	AR	*IFNGR2*, 21q22.11 – homozygous and compound heterozygous alterations. Most have absent protein. One report of a partially functional protein and mild phenotype. Interferon gamma antibodies that neutralise IFNγ have been detected in some patients with MSMD, although there are no known specific genetic defect leading to formation of these antibodies)
GATA-2 deficiency (monocyte deficiency with mycobacterial disease, MonoMAC)	AD	*GATA2*, 3q21.3. Haploinsufficiency. Phenotype distinct from the defects of the direct IL-12: IFNγ pathway
STAT1 gene alterations	AD and AR	*STAT1*, 2q32.2. Distinct alterations from those causing chronic mucocutaneous candidiasis. Each have distinct phenotypes: AR (defects in IFNα and β pathways as well as IFNγ); AD (IFNγ only). AR has a broader spectrum of pathogens. AD has low penetrance and a mild phenotype

Pathophysiology

Mycobacteria are intracellular pathogens and can be fast or slow growing (Figure 53.1). The key requirement for their killing is a strong response from macrophages; however, there is a complex interaction between T cells driving macrophage recruitment and activation. In some instances, the mycobacteria cannot be cleared and will reside within phagocytic cells, forming the classical granulomata seen in TB infection. However, why some patients exposed to TB develop infection, why some clear the bacteria, and why others end up with latent TB remains complex. The majority of MSMD resides around the T cell:macrophage activation axis, which is reliant on interferon γ and IL-12 and their intracellular signalling pathways. IL-12 is produced by activated macrophages, whereupon it will interact with its receptor on CD4 T cells and some NK cells to activate them and drive them down the Th1 differentiation route. Th1 CD4 cells then produce IFN-γ, which is made up of multiple subunits and acts on the IFN-γ receptor on macrophages, causing phosphorylation of STAT-1 and upregulation of pro-phagocytotic and inflammatory transcription factors. Defects anywhere in this pathway can give rise to increased susceptibility to intracellular pathogens as can defects in macrophage function. GATA-2 is a transcription factor involved in erythropoiesis and proliferation and differentiation of haematopoietic cells from an early stage. It is associated in particular with low numbers of monocytes and NK cells.

Symptoms and clinical features

Although the predominant reported infections are with atypical mycobacteria (most commonly pulmonary, but extra pulmonary sites can be involved), other intracellular pathogens are seen.

Clinical Genetics and Genomics at a Glance, First Edition. Edited by Neeta Lakhani, Kunal Kulkarni, Julian Barwell, Pradeep Vasudevan, and Huw Dorkins.

Figure 53.1 Mycobacterium Tuberculosis structure.

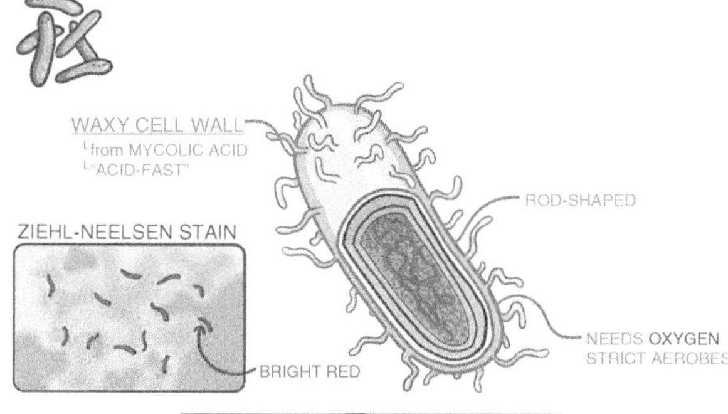

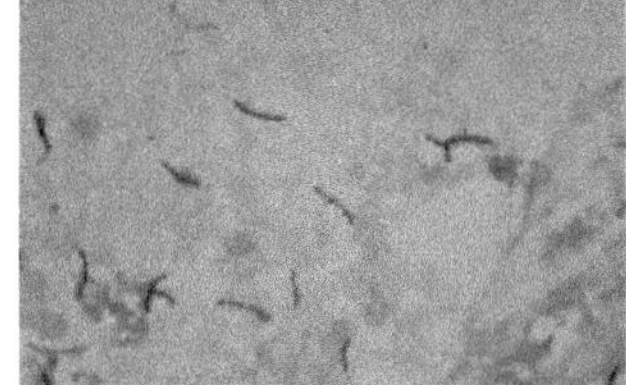

AFB on Ziehl-Neelsen stain

Source: Dr. George P. Kubica / U.S. Department of Health & Human Services (CDC) / Public Domain.

These include Salmonella and, in some cases, fungal infections. Classically, those individuals, immunised with BCG will get 'BCG-itis', which can be localised or disseminated, and culture will produce the M bovis strain of that batch of BCG. Patients are also more at risk of *Mycobacterium tuberculosis* and suffer a more severe infection from it. Other infections reported in MSMD include Listeria, Nocardia, HHV8, CMV, and other viral infections. There are reported tumours, including B-cell lymphomas; however, it is unclear if these relate directly to the immunodeficiency or result from repeated viral infections.

GATA2 deficiency presents with a similar spectrum of infections, although viral infections tend to predominate. There is a notable lack of peripheral blood monocytes and of NK cells. They often present with myelodysplasia, which has a hypoplastic appearance on bone marrow examination, and can progress to AML more frequently than other MDS.

Diagnosis

Investigation of patients with clinical patterns of MSMD is complex.

- **Flow cytometry:** The absence of IFNγ or IL-12 receptors may be detected, although this would not exclude defects in other pathways.
- **Functional cytokine stimulation assays:** Are performed to see if collected leucocytes can recognise and produce the relevant cytokines. If a defect in a pathway is identified, then genetic testing may be undertaken to confirm this.
- **GATA-2 deficiency:** Investigated based on the clinical picture, low numbers of monocytes and NK cells, and a hypocellular bone marrow biopsy. If these raise suspicion of the defect, then genetic testing is undertaken.

Management

High-dose interferon γ has been used in patients with defects in the interferon receptor or IL-12 receptor pathways, alongside standard anti-mycobacterial antibiotics. The results have been variable, and most patients will still get recurrent infection. High-dose interferon γ is often given when the patient is acutely unwell to try to aid stimulation of the immune system. Stem-cell transplants have generally had poor results, with significant graft versus host disease. There is no specific therapy for GATA-2 deficiency other than treatment of infections, and most will progress to haematological malignancy.

The future

Gene therapy may be a potential option for MSMD; however, given the rarity of each individual mutation, no current clinical trials are in progress.

54 Chronic granulomatous disease

Background

Chronic granulomatous disease (CGD) represents a group of genetically defined disorders, characterised by an inability to produce the oxygen radicals that are involved in intracellular killing of phagocytosed micro-organisms. CGD is characterised by life-threatening infections with fungi and certain types of bacteria and by granuloma formation.

Epidemiology

CGD affects an estimated 1 : 200 000 individuals. Males are affected more than females (X-linked variant is most prevalent and can form part of a contiguous gene deletion syndrome). Rates of X-linked CGD appear similar across racial and ethnic groups, although in cultures with high levels of consanguinity, AR variants may predominate.

Genetics

To date, alterations in six genes have been identified as causing CGD (Table 54.1).

Pathophysiology

Phagocytic cells use nicotinamide adenine dinucleotide phosphate (NADPH) oxidase to generate oxygen radicals, which are involved in the killing of internalized micro-organisms. The genes associated with CGD encode proteins that make up a cytochrome complex, which catalyses the production of superoxide, by transfer of an electron from NADPH to oxygen. Alterations in any one of these genes disrupts the formation of the NADPH oxidase complex, resulting in defective superoxide formation and impaired microbial killing by phagocytic cells. In addition to impaired microbial killing, the defects lead to an enhanced inflammatory response, which results in patients with CGD being prone to the formation of tissue granulomata and other inflammatory complications (Figure 54.1).

Symptoms and clinical features

Patients with chronic granulomatous disease usually present in early life with severe and/or recurrent, often life-threatening bacterial and fungal infections. The most common types of infections are pneumonias, abscesses, suppurative adenitis, osteomyelitis, and more superficial skin infections. Organisms causing infections in patients with CGD are mainly catalase producing, and (in the USA) the great majority of severe infections have been attributed to five types of micro-organisms: *Aspergillus* species, *Staphylococcus aureus, Burkholderia cepacia* complex, *Serratia marcescens,* and *Nocardia* species. Fungal infections, particularly of the respiratory tract, are particularly common and remain a major cause of mortality in patients with CGD.

Other common clinical features include poor growth, abnormal wound healing, diarrhoea, hepatic and genitourinary symptoms. As indicated above, enhanced inflammation and formation of tissue granulomata is common and can give rise to strictures, obstruction, and fistula formation in the gastrointestinal and urogenital tracts. Granulomatous lesions seen on tissue histology can also give rise to misdiagnosis of conditions, such as Crohn's disease or mycobacterial infections.

Table 54.1 Alterations causing CGD.

Alteration	Inheritance	Details
***CYBB encoding* gp91 phox** (cytochrome b(-245) beta subunit), Xp21.1	X-linked	2/3 cases (USA/Europe). 1/3 *CYBB* alterations arise *de novo*, with 2/3 inherited. Females with *CYBB* mutations are usually (asymptomatic) carriers, although some may show an attenuated form (depending on degree of WBC lyonisation)
CYBA encoding **p22 phox** (cytochrome b(-245) alpha subunit), 16q24	AR	Approximately 5% of cases
NCF1 (neutrophil cytosolic factor 1; encoding **p47 phox**, 7q11.23	AR	Approximately 25% of cases of CGD
NCF2 (neutrophil cytosolic factor 2; encoding **p67 phox**, 1q25.	AR	Approximately 5% of cases of CGD.
NCF4 (neutrophil cytosolic factor 4; OMIM*601488), encoding **p40 phox**, 22ca13.1	AR	Very rare variant of CGD
Alteration = *CYBC1* Inheritance = AR Details = Very rare (few individuals only)		

Clinical Genetics and Genomics at a Glance, First Edition. Edited by Neeta Lakhani, Kunal Kulkarni, Julian Barwell, Pradeep Vasudevan, and Huw Dorkins.

Diagnosis

This is based on identification of the defective neutrophil oxidative burst (reflecting the defect in NADPH oxidase activity). Two screening tests are commonly used:

- **Dihydrorhodamine 123:** This non-fluorescent dye is taken up by phagocytic cells. On activation of the cells, the dye is oxidised to produce a green fluorescent colour by the NADPH oxidase complex, which is generally detected using flow cytometric analysis. Patients with CGD either fail to oxidise the colour change in DHR or show a significantly reduced colour change. The DHR test can also be used to identify female carriers of X-linked CGD, whose cells produce a biphasic pattern of response, depending on whether the inactivated X chromosome was normal or contained the mutation.
- **Nitroblue tetrazolium:** In this slide-based test, superoxide produced by normal phagocytic cells reduces the (yellow) NBT to a dark blue formazan precipitate within the cells. CGD patients' phagocytic cells fail to reduce the dye. As with the DHR test, the NBT test can also identify female carriers of X-linked CGD.

Following an abnormal DHR or NBT test suggestive of CGD, confirmatory tests should be performed, including immunoblotting for the relevant proteins of the NADPH oxidase complex and sequencing of the relevant genes to identify mutations.

Management

Treatment of chronic granulomatous disease can be categorized into three categories: treatment of infectious complications, treatment of inflammatory complications, and curative therapies.

- **Infectious complications:** Antimicrobial prophylaxis, and early diagnosis and aggressive treatment of infections, commonly with a combination of cotrimoxazole (antibacterial) and itraconazole (antifungal). Prophylactic interferon-gamma may sometimes be used.
- **Acute inflammatory complications:** Steroids, alongside azathioprine used in longer-term, glucocorticoid-sparing regimens for chronic inflammation. Sulfasalazine and its derivatives are usually effective for treating the inflammatory bowel disease associated with CGD.
- **Haematopoietic stem cell transplantation** (HSCT) is the only current curative therapy. However, many can be managed effectively without undergoing HSCT, and so the decision to undergo HSCT is taken on a case-by-case basis following individual risk / benefit analysis.
- **Gene therapy:** Trialled in small numbers.

The future

Average survival is improving, and most will now survive beyond 40 years, with better survival in the AR than X-linked variants. Quality of life has also improved significantly since the advent of effective antimicrobial prophylaxis. Early diagnosis, improved patient management, and emerging gene therapy approaches may offer definitive treatment in the future (at least for those without suitable HSCT donors), although HSCT remains the main curative therapy for the foreseeable future.

Figure 54.1 Phagosome formation and oxidative killing of microbes by phagocytic cells.

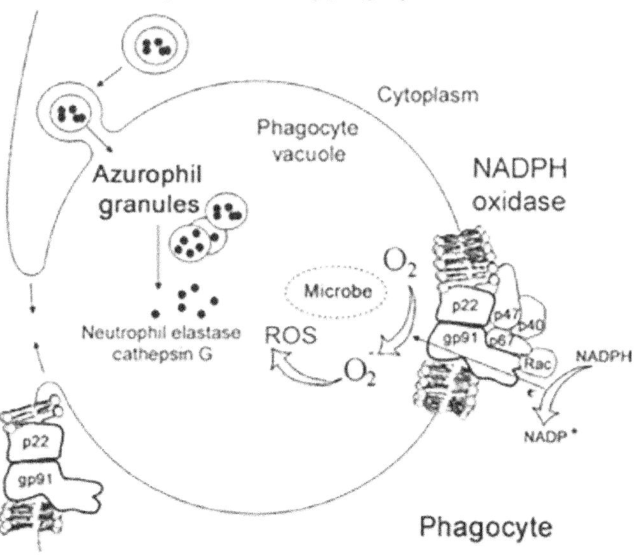

Source: Seger RA. Modern management of chronic granulomatous disease. British journal of haematology. 2008 Feb;140(3):255–66.

55 Defects in leukocyte migration

Background

Defects in leukocyte migration have been described, giving specific clinical phenotypes and classically affecting multiple cell lineages. They cause problems in the ability of myeloid and lymphoid cell attachment to the vascular endothelium and/or egress into the peripheral tissues. This group of conditions are called the leucocyte adhesion deficiencies (LAD). Depending on the specific defect, there may be problems at different points of leucocyte migration (Figure 55.1).

Epidemiology

All three forms of LAD are rare. LAD-1 has approximately 300 cases described worldwide, with LAD-2 having about 10 known cases, and LAD-3 having approximately 25 known cases (almost all of which are of Middle Eastern origin).

Genetics

- **LAD1** is caused by an alteration in **β-2-integrin**, *ITGB2* gene (21q22.3). It is inherited in an AR manner with variable penetration, and carriers of the alteration show half normal levels of the affected molecules.
- **LAD2** is caused by an alteration in a **GDP–fucose transporter FUCT-1**, *SLC35C1* gene (11p11.2). It is inherited in an AR fashion. It has both homozygous and compound heterozygous mutations, and leads to impaired fucose metabolism.
- **LAD3** is an AR alteration in **Kindlin 3**, *KINDLIN3* gene (11q31.1).

Pathophysiology

Leucocyte migration to the site of infection is mediated by chemotaxis (the signals to attract leucocytes to the infection) and then the movement of leucocytes from the blood stream into peripheral tissue. Movement across the vascular endothelium is reliant upon a number of processes. Firstly, the cell is slowed as it undergoes 'rolling' along the endothelium, mediated by weak adhesion molecules such as selectins on the endothelium. Then comes triggering by chemokines from the site of infection, which prime the leucocyte to upregulate and display adhesion molecules. Then comes adhesion, mediated by ICAMs on the endothelium and integrins on the leucocyte forming a strong bond. Finally diapedesis occurs where the leucocyte moves through the gap junctions between the endothelial cells.

β-2-Integrin is a key component of multiple integrin complexes, including LAD-1. Defects in LAD-1 lead to failure of adhesion of leukocytes to the endothelium, and an inability to undergo the adherence stage of migration. LAD-2 lacks the ability to form selectins, which rely on the sialyl Lewis-x as they require fucosylation. It is the lack of selectins, which leads to an inability to undergo rolling, leading to defective leukocyte adhesion to endothelium. However, the lack of ability to fucosylate goes further than the immune system and affects other proteins as well, giving a unique phenotype. Kindlin 3 (LAD-3) is required for activation of the β integrin family, and defects again lead to a lack of adhesion.

Although the classical reason for leucocyte migration to peripheral tissues is to enable defence against pathogens, they are also required for removal of apoptotic cell remnants and necrotic cells. An inability to get neutrophils and macrophages to the site of cell death leads to clinical effects, which are separate from the increased susceptibility to infection. These include abnormal wound healing and aberrant scar formation.

Symptoms and clinical features

- **Increased propensity to infection:** All forms. In LAD-1 and LAD-3, this is the most common bacterial or fungal skin and mucosal infection, notably without pus formation due to the lack of neutrophil migration. As patients get older, they develop periodontitis and gingivitis, leading to tooth loss if untreated. The severity of LAD-1 is variable depending on the degree of penetrance. LAD-2 tends to have milder infections, most commonly of the sinopulmonary tract and middle ear. They can get infective periodontitis and can develop cellulitis.
- **Delayed wound healing:** LAD-1 and LAD-3. Classically described as delayed separation or healing of the umbilical cord, taking more than 10 days. Other wounds and surgical incisions may also be slow to heal, and vaccination sites may scar.
- **LAD-2:** Slightly different phenotype, involving learning difficulties, growth deficiency, hypotonia, and classical facies due to defects in fucosylation of proteins other than sialyl Lewis-x. Also have a classical blood type called 'Bombay' or 'hh' blood group.
- **LAD-3:** Bleeding diathesis that can be life threatening, likely due to defects in platelet adhesion. Easy bleeding from wounds, epistaxis and subcutaneous tissues.

Diagnosis

Some forms of LAD can be detected by flow cytometry for the cell surface molecules; milder phenotypes may require PMA stimulation of granulocytes. There is usually a peripheral blood neutrophilia due to the lack of migration. Genetic testing is possible if LAD is suspected or variant phenotype considered.

Management

All forms require primary treatment with prompt recognition of infection and aggressive anti-microbial therapy. LAD-1 is often treated with antibiotic prophylaxis, whereas LAD-2 may not require this due to the milder severity of infection. LAD-1 and LAD-3 can be treated with stem-cell transplant if severe; however, due to the fact that non-haematopoietic cells are affected in LAD-2, stem cell transplant is not normally indicated.

Clinical Genetics and Genomics at a Glance, First Edition. Edited by Neeta Lakhani, Kunal Kulkarni, Julian Barwell, Pradeep Vasudevan, and Huw Dorkins.

The future

LAD-2 has been treated with high-dose oral fucose. There is a variable response to this, and there is a concern about risk of development of auto-antibodies to the fucosylated proteins. There is investigation into gene therapy, especially for LAD-1. Anti-CD18 antibodies have been used in non-LAD stem-cell transplants to reduce GvHD due to the very low levels of GvHD seen in transplanted LAD patients, showing how information from one disease can inform on treatment for other conditions.

Figure 55.1 Leucocyte migration.

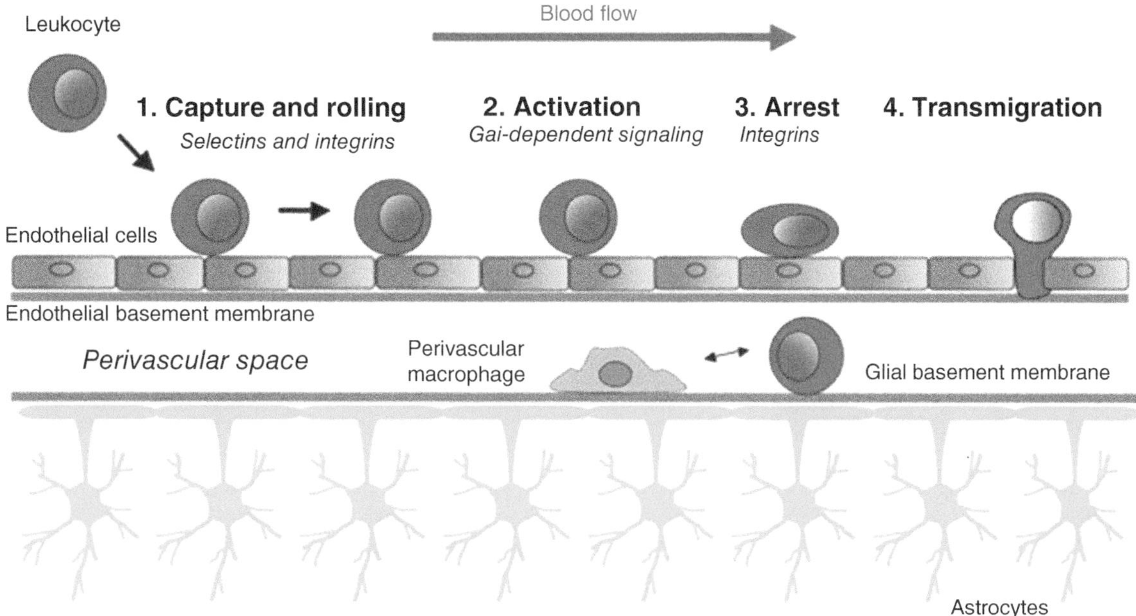

56 Defects of toll-like receptors and their signalling pathways

Background

Toll-like receptors (TLRs) were named due to their similarity to already identified receptors in Drosophila. They are relatively conserved across species and are a major component of the innate immune system. They recognise 'molecular patterns' found on pathogens or from necrotic cells, but they do not have the same degree of specificity that antibodies do and do not produce a memory response. They have important roles in viral, bacterial, and fungal immunity.

Aetiology

These are all exceptionally rare defects, with fewer than 1 : 1 000 000 million population cases.

Genetics

Table 56.1 summarises the genetic basis of TLR defects.

Pathophysiology

Defects of the innate immune system, which limit the ability to recognise or respond to generic molecules seen on different bacteria or from necrotic/apoptotic cells. Defects at different points have different impacts, hence the different phenotypes. TLRs recognise conserved microbial molecules and activate a pro-inflammatory cascade *via* NFκB (transcription molecule) (Figure 56.1). Majority of TLRs are expressed on the cell surface, recognising extracellular ligands; however, TLRs 3/7/8/9 are intra-cellular (on endosomes) to enable recognition of intracellular

Table 56.1 Genetic basis of TLR defects.

	Inheritance	Alteration	Details
Myd88 deficiency	AR	*MYD88,* 3p22.2. Homozygous/ compound heterozygous	Second messengers in TLR path (for all except TLR3). Bound to IRAK4 and IRAK1
IRAK4 deficiency	AR	*IRAK4,* 12q12. Homozygous/ compound heterozygous	Second messengers in TLR path. Forms scaffold with Myd88 to recruit and activate NEMO
TLR3 deficiency	Complex, AR and AD	*TLR3,* 4q35.1. AR = total vs AD = partial deficiency	Only described defect of specific TLR (recognises viral dsRNA). Most viruses detected by other mechanisms, but HSV-1 specific to TLR3 (encephalitis risk)
NEMO (IκB kinase complex) deficiency	X-linked	*IKBKG,* Xq28. Also v. rare defects in IκBα, (interacts with NEMO), same clinical pattern (AD inheritance)	Also called X-linked ectodermal dysplasia, anhydrotic with immune deficiency (EDA-ID). Activates NFκB, enabling its movement to nucleus to act as transcription factor and upregulate TNF-α, IL-1β, and IL-6
WHIM syndrome	AD	Gain of function alteration of *CXCR4,* 2q22.1	Co-receptor used by HIV to gain cellular entry. Defect = alterations in myeloid cell development/maturation, so neutrophils retained in marrow and not released into blood (myelokathexis). Unclear why mutations cause B-cell lymphopenias or how they relate specifically to HPV
STAT2 deficiency	AR	*STAT2,* 12q13.3	Signal transduction molecule for production of interferon α and β, (cytotoxic responses to intracellular viral infections)

Figure 56.1 Defects in TLR pathways.

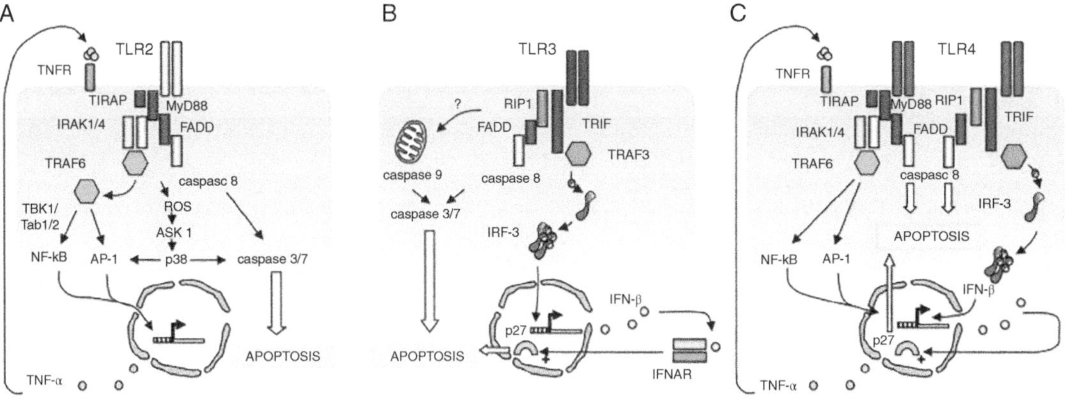

Source: Salaun, B., Romero, P. and Lebecque, S., 2007. Toll-like receptors' two-edged sword: when immunity meets apoptosis. European journal of immunology, 37(12), pp.3311–3318.

Clinical Genetics and Genomics at a Glance, First Edition. Edited by Neeta Lakhani, Kunal Kulkarni, Julian Barwell, Pradeep Vasudevan, and Huw Dorkins.

pathogens. Loss of Myd88, IRAK-4, or NEMO causes significant disruption to TLR signalling, but due to multiple redundancies in the innate immune system, infectious susceptibility is limited to organisms such as pneumococcus, Staphylococcus, and Shigella. STAT2 and CXCR4 alterations are included here due to roles of these molecules in innate immune signalling.

Symptoms and clinical features

- **Myd88 and IRAK4 deficiencies:** Recurrent childhood sinopulmonary infections, especially with encapsulated organisms (especially pneumococcus) and Shigella. Severity of presentation often reduces with age, as adaptive immune system matures. May be associated with impaired antibody production to polysaccharide antigens.
- **NEMO defects:** Anhidrotic ectodermal dysplasia in some patients, and susceptibility to multiple types of infection, including bacteria, viruses, fungi, and mycobacteria. Can have a spectrum of antibody defects from hypogammaglobulinaemia to specific deficiencies. Some have colitis.
- **TLR3 deficiency:** Almost exclusively early onset, severe HSV-1 encephalitis, which is recurrent.
- **STAT2 deficiency:** Severe/frequent viral infections. Notably, post-live viral vaccination (e.g. MMR).
- **WHIM syndrome:** Presents in childhood. Characterised by recurrent severe infections, both those expected from neutropenia and those due to antibody deficiency. Recurrent, severe viral warts and a risk of cervical carcinoma in girls are a major feature, along with granulocytopenia, lymphopenia, and hypogammaglobulinaemia. Of note, the neutropenia can be overcome during severe infection and therefore may not present acutely with absolute neutropenia (but neutrophil count may be out of keeping with severity of infection).

Diagnosis

Diagnosis of the innate immune defects is complex, as there is rarely a simple test.

- Most initially rely on ***cytokine release assays*** – tests of various activation and inhibition compounds' abilities to stimulate leucocytes. Complex to perform and interpret, and only done in specialised laboratories, therefore clinical assessment guides investigation.
- **Myd88 and IRAK4 deficiencies:** Normally identified through observing defects in response to IL-6 and TNF-α, before undergoing genetic analysis and/or Western blotting.
- **NEMO deficiency:** Usually has a clear clinical picture indicating direct genetic testing. Tend to have impaired IL-10 production. Diagnostic delays in subgroup with subtle ectodermal dysplasia.
- **TLR3 defects:** Require primary human fibroblasts (usually cultured from skin biopsies) to test the TLR-3 pathway response, making it a complex process. If impaired TLR3 pathway responses seen, then genetic testing can be done by whole exome sequencing.
- **STAT2 deficiency:** Gives impaired release of IFNα and IFNβ on stimulation of leukocytes.
- **WHIM syndrome:** Is primarily investigated with the correct set of clinical symptoms in conjunction with a neutropenia (during convalescence). Bone marrow biopsy usually show high neutrophil numbers retained in the bone marrow, differentiating it from other neutropenia syndromes. Genotyping of *CXCR4* can then be undertaken.
- Note that as the various pro-inflammatory cytokines are important in forming the acute phase response, inflammatory markers (e.g. CRP) are often normal even during severe infection.

Management

All immunodeficiencies: prompt identification and aggressive management of acute infections is key.

- **Myd88 and IRAK4:** Usually prophylactic antibiotics. If an identified antibody deficiency, then immunoglobulin replacement therapy may be indicated, especially in younger patients.
- **NEMO:** Antibiotic prophylaxis. Most require immunoglobulin replacement. Some have required anti-viral prophylaxis to reduce the risk of herpes virus infection, and stem-cell transplantation has been successfully used. Prognosis depends on severity of the phenotype and the number of infections; with adequate treatment, most have a near normal lifespan.
- **TLR3:** Little evidence base for treatment. Current recommendation is close follow-up for relapse of HSV encephalitis, and if it occurs then early aggressive anti-viral therapy should be used.
- **STAT2:** Due to the rarity of the disease, there is no specific known treatment.
- **WHIM:** Aggressive therapy for acute infections, usually including administration of G-CSF or GM-CSF to promote neutrophil differentiation. Prophylactic antibiotics used. If evidence of an antibody deficiency, then immunoglobulin replacement is indicated.

The future

TLR3 deficiency patients with recurrent HSV encephalitis may benefit from IFN-α2β administration during acute infections based on evidence from *in vitro* studies. It is currently unclear if anti-viral prophylaxis is useful or not. WHIM syndrome has investigational treatment of Plerixafor, an inhibitor of CXCR4 previously used in chemotherapy and stem-cell transplant conditioning regimens, and there is consideration of stem-cell transplantation. However, there have been technical issues with this, and so gene therapy is being investigated.

Autoinflammatory diseases and periodic fever syndromes

Background

Autoinflammatory (AI) diseases are characterised by abnormal systemic inflammation. They are distinct from autoimmune diseases as the predominant defect is in innate rather than adaptive immunity. Both present with inflammation, and the associated symptoms can have organ-specific effects, but AI diseases are not associated with pathogenic autoantibodies. Several AI diseases were initially described in specific geographical or ethnic populations (hence the nomenclature), although most have since been identified in other groups. There are multiple identified periodic fever syndromes and AI diseases. The four commonest, with clear monogenic links, are described here (see http://www.autoinflammatory.org/ for others). In addition, juvenile idiopathic arthritis and adult onset Still's disease are now usually classified as AI diseases.

Epidemiology

Familial Mediterranean fever (FMF) is the commonest inherited AI syndrome, with carrier mutations seen in up to 1 : 5 of the population in high-risk areas, with clinical cases more common in Turkish, Armenian, Italian, and Sephardic Jewish populations. Of the cryopyrin associated periodic fever syndrome (CAPS) group, familial cold autoinflammatory syndrome (FCAS), and Muckle–Wells syndrome (MWS) cases each occur in around 1 : 1 000 000, often clustering in large family groups affecting any ethnicity. Neonatal onset multisystemic autoinflammatory disease (NOMID/CINCA) also occurs in around 1 : 1 000 000, but, as it is mostly caused by spontaneous mutations, there is not the same family clustering. TNF-receptor associated periodic syndrome/familial Hibernian fever (TRAPS) has an estimated prevalence of >1 : 1 000 000, with >1000 cases worldwide, making it the second commonest monogenic AI syndrome. Mevalonic kinase defects, such as mevalonic aciduria (MA), are very rare, with hyper IgD syndrome (HIDS) accounting for most cases, totalling >300 worldwide (with another <100 other mevalonic kinase defect patients identified). They are mostly described in Dutch and European populations (possibly due to the availability of testing).

Genetics

Table 57.1 summarises the inheritance and alterations associated with autoimmune diseases.

Table 57.1 Genetic basis of autoinflammatory diseases.

Defect	Inheritance	Alteration
FMF	AR	Pyrin (*MEFV*) gene, chromosome 16p13.3. Most are missense
CAPS (FCAS, MWS, NOMID)	AD	NLRP3 protein (cryopyrin). *NLRP3* gene, chromosome 1q44
HIDS and MA	AR	Each have distinct alterations. MA = complete mevalonate kinase deficiency. Mevalonate kinase gene (*MVK*), chromosome 12q24.11
TRAPS	AD	55kD TNF receptor. *TNFRSF1A gene,* chromosome 12p13.31

Pathophysiology

The key concept is disruption of the 'inflammasome' – pathways that enable production of inflammatory IL-1. Several are described. These can respond to different stimuli but converge on the common pathway of IL-1β production. All inflammasome complexes contain the protein pyrin; this is altered in FMF, causing overactivation of some pathways leading to increased IL-1β production. The best described individual inflammasome is NLRP-3, which is specifically altered in CAPS. This may account for the different phenotype from other AI syndromes. In HIDS, the defect is in the mevalonic kinase enzyme, part of a metabolic pathway that results in activation of PI3 kinase, Rac1, and protein kinase B. These enzymes are then involved in the post-inflammasome activation of IL-1β from pro-IL-1β. The TRAPS alteration is in the 55kD TNF receptor; this causes overstimulation, resulting in upregulation of transcription factors that increase production of pro-IL-1β. Other signals involved in activation of inflammasomes include pathogen-associated molecular patterns (PAMPs) and danger-associated molecular patterns (DAMPs), which may act directly via formation of reactive oxygen species, or by signalling through toll-like receptors (TLRs).

Symptoms and clinical features

- **FMF:** Symptoms classically last 12–72 hours. Frequency of attacks is variable. Normally presents in early life (before 20 years). Commonly present with arthralgia and serositis (abdominal or chest pain), an erythematous rash that mimics erysipelas, fever, and elevated ESR, CRP and possible leucocytosis. Eye involvement and splenomegaly rare. No auditory involvement (Figure 57.1).
- **CAPS:** FCAS presents with a near daily rash, and flares of cold induced urticaria, fever, and headaches during flares, with associated arthralgia and conjunctivitis. Serositis, splenomegaly and vasculitis are not features. Symptoms last 12–24 hours, with flares induced within 1–3 hours of encountering cold. MWD presents with random flares lasting 2–3 days, presenting in infancy with a near daily uriticarial rash (increases with flares) and arthralgia. Conjunctivitis during flares, without serositis. Abdominal pain may be a feature. Progressive sensorineural hearing loss (SNHL) moving into adolescence. NOMID presents from birth with an urticarial rash that increases with flares, chronic aseptic meningitis (with high CSF pressures and papilloedema), uveitis, iritis, or conjunctivitis. May have hepatosplenomegaly and lymphadenopathy,

Clinical Genetics and Genomics at a Glance, First Edition. Edited by Neeta Lakhani, Kunal Kulkarni, Julian Barwell, Pradeep Vasudevan, and Huw Dorkins.

pericardial effusions, and SNHL from childhood. Significant joint arthralgia, with deformities, contractures, and bony overgrowth. Continuous symptoms, chronically elevated inflammatory markers (Figure 57.2).

- **TRAPS:** Flares last from days to weeks, occurring approximately every three weeks, with most having flares before age of 20. Commonly a painful, migratory rash, with high fevers and headaches. Conjunctivitis, periorbital oedema, serositis (including pleurisy and peritonitic pain), and potential splenomegaly during attacks. Arthralgia during attacks. Can develop finger clubbing and a lymphocytic vasculitis. A predominant feature is localised myalgia (vague in some) (Figure 57.3).
- **HIDS & MA:** Present differently. HIDS has attacks lasting 2–7 days, every 2–12 weeks, whereas MA has attacks lasting 4–5 days, every 3–4 weeks. Both have a diffuse maculopapular rash with headaches, fevers, lymphadenopathy, abdominal pain, and diarrhoea, although neither have classical serositis. No eye involvement in HIDS, but MA has uveitis, cataracts, and tapetoretinal degeneration. MA has significant neurological involvement, with microcephaly, learning difficulties, and cerebellar ataxia, with epilepsy developing over time. HIDS can develop cutaneous vasculitis (not in MA). In HIDS, vaccination is a common trigger of attacks.

Diagnosis

The first step in diagnosis is to establish the pattern of flares. This is done clinically, but temperature and CRP charting is important, as true autoinflammatory diseases show a rise in inflammatory markers during attacks. Once the pattern is established, then diagnosis is usually based on sequencing the gene(s) of the most likely syndromes. It is notable, however, that a significant percentage of FMF patients (as well as some patients with other autoinflammatory diseases) do not have identified mutations and are diagnosed clinically. In some countries where genotyping is not easily available, a clinical response to colchicine is used diagnostically for FMF. HIDS-type syndromes can be identified by checking IgD levels, although in some cases these are normal. However, during flares, elevated urinary mevalonic acid is seen in all mevalonic kinase autoinflammatory diseases.

Management

Aims of treatment are to reduce symptoms (allowing patients to undertake activities of daily living) and secondly to prevent secondary amyloidosis. Prior to effective treatment, the rates of systemic amyloidosis in FMF was >50%. It is also seen in MWD, FCAS, and TRAPS, although less frequently than in FMF. HIDS does not have systemic amyloidosis as a complication. Monitoring for proteinuria as a marker of the presence of amyloidosis is important. FMF is treatable with colchicine, which reduces flares and significantly decreases rates of amyloidosis in most. Monoclonal antibodies to IL-1 (e.g. Anakinra, a daily subcutaneous injection) have become the mainstay in colchicine-resistant cases and other types of AI disorders. Newer forms are available, e.g. canakinumab, a 3-monthly injection. Rilonacept, a IL-1 fusion protein combined with in IgG Fc portion, has also been used as anti-IL-1 therapy. Anti-TNF therapy is commonly used in TRAPS, as the mutated protein is a TNF receptor.

The future

As the role of the inflammasome has been better understood, newer therapies which directly target the inflammasome or its activators are being considered. These include purine receptor inhibitors, potassium channel inhibitors, and drugs which affect uric acid. Caspase 1 inhibitors are in trials, but these have so far been limited by side effects.

Figure 57.1 Erysipelas-like erythema during an attack of FMF.

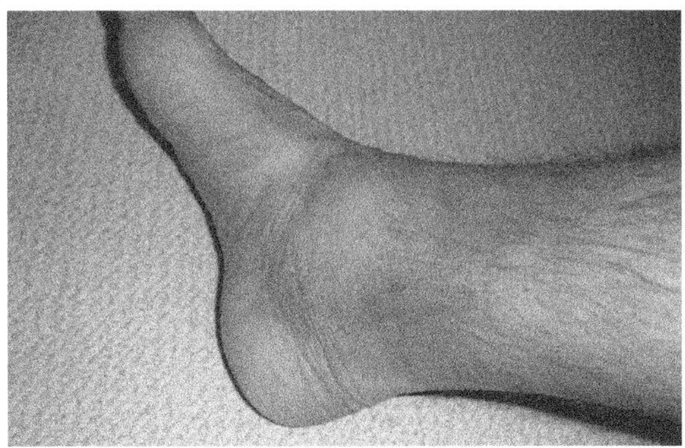

Source: Lachmann (2011) / Oxford University Press.

Figure 57.3 Typical rash accompanying an attack of TRAPS.

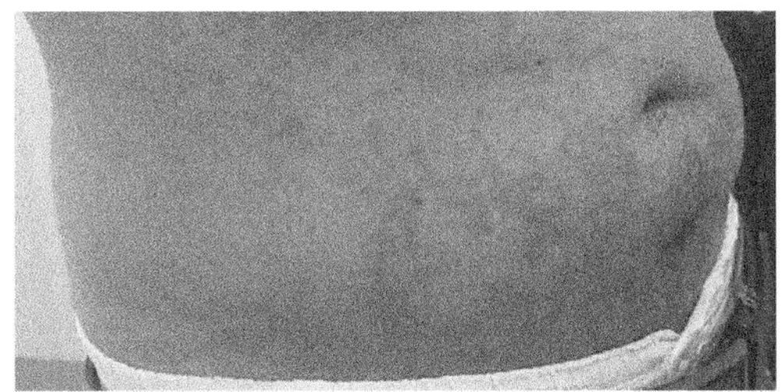

Source: Lachmann (2011) / Oxford University Press.

Figure 57.2 Classical diffuse urticarial rash of CAPS.

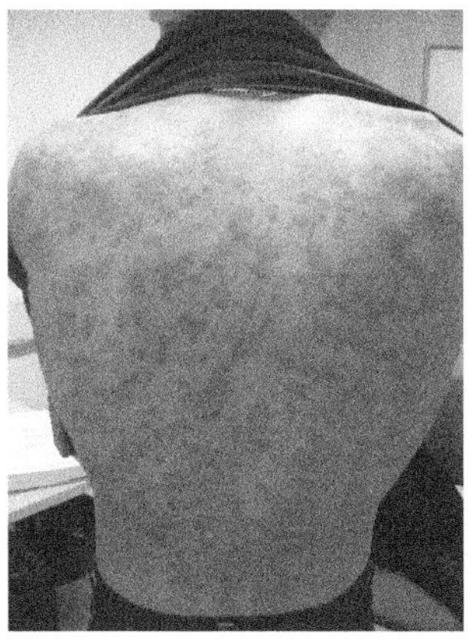

Source: Lachmann (2011) / Oxford University Press.

58 Complement deficiencies

Background

The complement system is an amplification cascade of multiple soluble proteins involved in the innate immune system, and with some impact on the adaptive system (Figure 58.1). There are three main activation pathways, classical, alternative, and lectin binding. The major end points of complement activation are opsonisation for improved phagocytosis, anaphylatoxin formation for enhancement of inflammation, and the formation of the membrane attack complex (MAC) for direct killing of cells. The cascade has multiple amplification and regulatory proteins involved within it, and there are described defects of all the proteins. Defects in complement regulation not only cause classical immunodeficiency predisposing to infection but also inflammatory complications and issues relating to complement deposition. The impact of defects of the lectin binding pathway is unclear. Mannose binding lectin deficiency is no longer considered as an immunodeficiency if found in isolation in adults, and children would generally outgrow the effects of a deficiency over time, whilst MASP-2 deficiency has been identified in a small number of individuals with increased respiratory infections, as well as in a number of healthy individuals.

Aetiology

Pathogenic defects are all rare. There are <100 known cases of C1 complex deficiency, and only 30 described cases of complete C4 deficiency. There are at least four alleles of C4, and partial deficiencies stemming from defective alleles are relatively common, but not disease causing, except for increased rates of SLE from having only one working allele. 1 : 10 000 individuals have homozygous deletions of C2, but only 10–30% develop disease. C9 deficiency was identified in 1 : 1000 Japanese blood donors, but rates are much lower in other populations. Atypical HUS occurs in 1 : 2 000 000, with 30% due to factor H alteration, 5–10% Factor I alteration, and 5% due to C3 alteration. HAE occurs in 1 : 50 000 (ethnic variations).

Genetics

Table 58.1 summarises the inheritance and alterations associated with various complement deficiencies.

Pathophysiology

- **MAC deficiencies:** Most straightforward. The MAC is made of C5, C6, C7, C8 complexes binding to multimers of C9 to form a circular ring, which penetrates the cell membrane causing **direct lysis.** On 'self' cells, there are molecules such as CD46, CD55, and CD59, which prevent MAC binding, thus preventing self-lysis. A defect in any of the complement components of the MAC will prevent the formation of the complex or inhibit the ability of the complex to penetrate the cell membrane, and therefore complement-mediated lysis cannot occur. This is most relevant in immunity to encapsulated bacteria such as *Neisseria* species, where the MAC is of particular significance in bacterial killing. Properdin is a key stabiliser of the C3 convertase of the alternative pathway and is therefore required for the activation of C3, a key component in the killing of *Neisseria* (especially *N. meningitides* serogroups Y and W135).
- **Early classical and lectin pathway deficiencies:** In C1, C2, and C4 forms, cause a lack of response to microbial oligosaccharides and pathogen-associated recognition molecules (including recognition of antigen bound IgM). In turn, this reduces activation of anaphylatoxins and failure to form the MAC by these pathways. However, the alternative pathway of autolysis of C3 remains intact. This leaves patients at some risk of pyogenic infections. However, the most notable effect is the development of autoimmune manifestations due to the importance of complement in targeting apoptotic and necrotic cells for lysis and clearance by phagocytes.
- **C3 deficiency:** Leaves patients predisposed to (mainly pyogenic) infections, due to failure to form the MAC, and inability to activate C3a anaphylatoxin. The commoner gain of function mutations in C3, or loss of function mutations in Factor H or Factor I, lead to a sustained activation of the alternative pathway and consumption of C3. However, the activated C3 must be deposited somewhere, and the primary target is the kidney, resulting in either aHUS or membranoproliferative glomerulonephritis type II (MPGN II). Gain of function mutations in Factor B also lead to aHUS, but without evidence of increased rates of infection.
- **C1 Inhibitor (C1Inh) defects:** Cause HAE due to C1Inh's effects on the bradykinin pathway. C1Inh is key to the negative regulation of the classical pathway but is also involved at several

Table 58.1 Genetic basis of complement deficiencies.

Deficiency	Inheritance	Alteration
Classical pathway	AR	Any of the components of C1qA, C1qB, C1qC, C1r, C1s, C4A/C4B, or C2
C1 inhibitor/hereditary angioedema (HAE)	AD	*HAE type 1:* protein deficiency. *HAE type 2:* reduced function but normal levels of C1 inhibitor protein. *Both:* alterations in SERPING1 gene, on chromosome 11
C3	AR. Also C3 gain of function (AD)	*AD:* consumption of C3 and, due to dysregulated inflammation, can cause atypical haemolytic uraemic syndrome (aHUS)
Properdin	X-linked	*CFP,* Xp11.23
Factor H/I	AR	H (CFH), I(CFI), B (CFB). All: dysregulated complement activation,
Factor B	AD	leading to aHU
Membrane attack components	AR	C5, C6, C6, C8, C9

Clinical Genetics and Genomics at a Glance, First Edition. Edited by Neeta Lakhani, Kunal Kulkarni, Julian Barwell, Pradeep Vasudevan, and Huw Dorkins.

points in the later stages of the coagulation cascade, involving formation of bradykinin. In HAE, there is increased bradykinin, but normal histamine (hence oedema and pain, but no rash or significant itch). No increased infection rates as anti-microbial aspects of the complement system are largely intact.

Symptoms and clinical features

- **MAC and properdin deficiency:** Present with *Neisserial* infections, mostly meningitis/encephalitis, but also fulminant septicaemia. There is not usually a history of recurrent chest or sinus infection. The rate of meningococcal disease is 7000–10 000 times greater than the healthy population. The initial infection may be less clinically severe than in the healthy population, due to a reduction in immune response-mediated inflammation. These patients are normally capable of making good antibody responses to vaccinations, including to *N. meningitidis*. Any patient with a second episode of bacterial meningitis or meningitis with a family history of meningitis should be investigated for a complement deficiency.
- **Early classical complement defects:** May present with recurrent sino-pulmonary infections from an early age. These are normally due to common organisms, such as pneumococcus and haemophilus, although increased rates of *Neisseria* are also seen. However, the most frequent presentation is with early onset severe autoimmune disease, most frequently systemic lupus erythematosus (SLE), with a higher frequency of anti-Ro antibodies. Depending on the complement protein affected, the frequency of SLE ranges from 10% in C2 deficiency to 100% in C1q deficiency. Cutaneous and discoid lupus can also be seen, and undifferentiated connective tissue disease has been reported in C2 deficiency.
- **Defects of C3, Factor H/I:** Can present with recurrent skin, sino-pulmonary, and ear infections (most commonly pneumococcal, meningococcal, and haemophilus), and progressive renal failure from MPGN, or from acute haemolysis and renal failure in aHUS. Factor I-deficient patients develop more infections than Factor H-deficient patients; however, they do not develop MPGN II. Not all patients develop aHUS, and the triggering and modulatory factors remain unclear.
- **Hereditary angioedema:** Classically presents with episodes of angioedema without an urticarial rash. Externally, these can affect any part of the body including limbs, trunk, face, and genitals. Often have recurrent abdominal pain, with or without diarrhoea, secondary to intestinal oedema. Patients often undergo multiple investigations before HAE is considered. Laryngeal oedema is the most serious and life-threatening presentation and can present with stridor, wheeze, and respiratory distress. Attacks are made worse by use of oestrogen therapies or ACE inhibitors, and triggers include stress, trauma, and infection. Classically, onset is in the teens or early 20s.

Diagnosis

- **Assessment of complement functional activity** is the initial test of classical and alternative pathways, using CH100 and AP100 tests. Determines whether defect is isolated to one pathway or (if both CH100 and AP100 are low) suggests a defect in C3 or the terminal pathway (MAC).
- **Individual component levels** can then be measured, or **genetic testing** of the relevant components. Exception to this is in properdin deficiency, where AP100 may be normal, and **direct measurement of properdin** may be indicated.
- **HAE** is diagnosed by **direct testing for C1 inhibitor level and function.** C4 levels are almost always low during attacks, but can be rarely normal in between. **Genotyping** is now available (useful in diagnosing children of affected parents), as **C1inh and C1inh function** cannot be accurately tested until at least the age of five years.

Management

- **Antibiotics:** In all forms of complement deficiency (apart from HAE) prompt aggressive treatment of infections with prolonged courses of appropriate antibiotics is essential. Penicillin or erythromycin prophylaxis is used for those patients with clear susceptibility to meningococcus, especially terminal complex defects and properdin deficiency. Other prophylactic antibiotics may be used for those patients with recurrent chest, sinus, or skin infections.
- **Vaccines:** There is no role for immunoglobulin replacement therapy. As the majority of patients can mount a normal antibody response, vaccination with pneumococcal, *Haemophilus influenzae* type B, and all available meningococcal vaccines is recommended. Immunologists can measure vaccination response and maintenance of response, with boosters as needed.
- **Immunosuppressive therapies:** Used for the autoimmune manifestations of the classical pathway defects; however, note that this adds to their risk of infection.
- **aHUS:** Eculizumab (C5 inhibitory monoclonal antibody) has revolutionised treatment. Preserves renal function and delays transplant (one of the costliest drugs approved by UK NICE).
- **HAE management:** Involves prophylactic and acute therapy (treat attacks early). Watchful waiting possible for those with low attack burden. Standard adjustments needed (e.g. avoid combined contraceptive pill, oestrogen therapies, and ACE inhibitors). Prophylaxis using attenuated androgens (danazol, stanozolol, and oxandrolone) has good evidence. Prophylactic tranexamic acid has been used but weak evidence. Severely affected patients may have prophylactic infusions of purified human C1 inhibitor. Emergency management can be at home (e.g. severe abdominal or peripheral attacks). Use IV human C1 inhibitor or a bradykinin inhibitor (Icatibant) for acute angioedema. A new kallikrein inhibitor (Ecallantide) is available. Review laryngeal attacks in hospital. Prophylactic C1 inhibitor prior to procedures (e.g. dental, endoscopy, surgery).

The future

There is much in development, including potential subcutaneous C1inh for ease of administration in home prophylactic therapy, and prophylactic/emergency oral inhibitory therapies. Due to wide clinical heterogeneity, there is little in the pipeline for the immunodeficiency-associated complement disorders. aHUS treatment is evolving, with interest in monoclonal antibodies (e.g. Eculizumab).

Figure 58.1 Complement pathways.

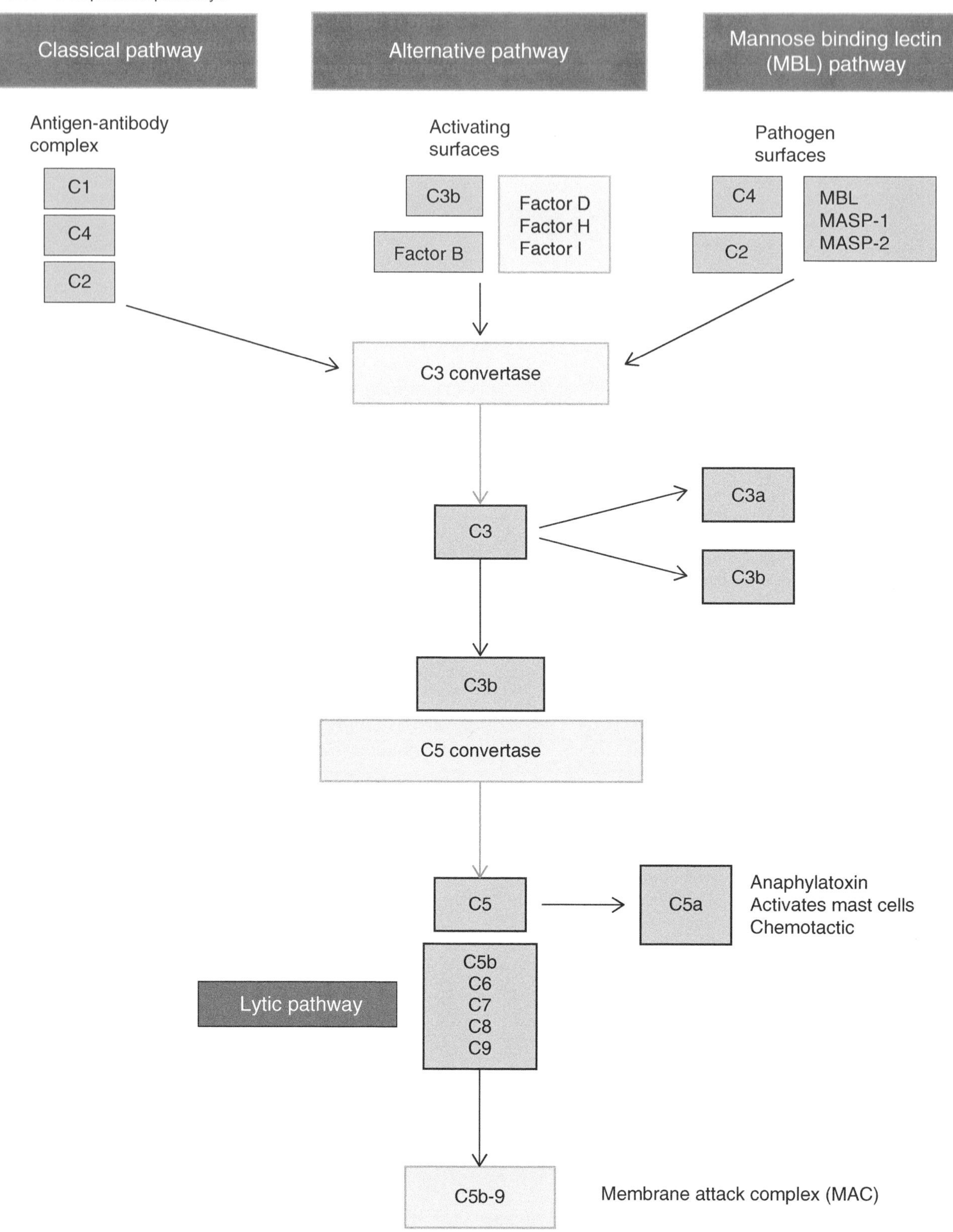

Neurology

Chapters

59 Spinal muscular atrophy

Background

Spinal muscular atrophy (SMA) is a neuromuscular disorder characterised by progressive muscle weakness and atrophy. It results in progressive degeneration and ultimately irreversible loss of the anterior horn cells of the spinal cord. Prior to genetic testing, SMA was categorised into classical subtypes (Table 59.1). It is now known that SMA is a continuum, with no clear discrimination between the different subtypes, although these classic definitions may still be encountered in clinical practice.

Epidemiology

SMA is a relatively rare condition and the exact prevalence is unknown. The estimated incidence of SMA is around 4–10 per 100 000 live births, with a prevalence of 1–2 per 10 000. The carrier rate is estimated to be between 1 in 50 and 90.

Genetics

SMA is inherited in an AR manner and is associated with alterations (deletions and small intragenic alterations) in the survival motor neurone gene (*SMN1*), located on chromosome 5q13; 94% of individuals with SMA have a homozygous deletion of exon 7 of the *SMN1* gene. The remaining 6% with SMA have a deletion in one *SMN1* copy and an intragenic alteration in the other copy. There are individual case reports of homozygous *SMN1* deletions in unaffected individuals.

It is not uncommon to have two copies of *SMN1* on one chromosome; around 7% of individuals who do not have SMA or a family history of SMA have been found to have three or four copies of the *SMN1* gene. This can cause concerns when delineating inheritance and the concept of a silent carrier is well documented.

One factor possibly accounting for the variable phenotype of SMA is copy number of the *SMN2* gene, also located on chromosome 5. The *SMN1* and *SMN2* genes are almost identical, and loss of the *SMN1* gene may be partially compensated by protein synthesis from *SMN2*. On average, individuals with a milder phenotype have more copies of the *SMN2* gene than those with type I or type II SMA.

Pathophysiology

SMA is caused by progressive degeneration and irreversible loss of the anterior horn cells of the spinal cord and brain stem nuclei. Loss of these cells leads to progressive proximal muscle weakness (lower motor neurone disease) (Figure 59.1). Enhanced neuronal death is detected as early as 12 weeks gestation in individuals with SMA type I.

Symptoms and clinical features

The primary symptom of SMA is progressive proximal muscle weakness and loss of movement secondary to muscle wasting. There may be a history of motor difficulties or motor regression. The age of onset of symptoms can range from birth to adulthood and severity of symptoms can vary (see Table 59.1). Findings on examination may include proximal muscle weakness (greater than distal muscle weakness), hypotonia, hyporeflexia or areflexia, tremors of the hand, and tongue fasciculations

Table 59.1 Clinical classification of SMA subtypes.

Subtype	Severity	Age of onset	Life span	Developmental milestones
Type 0 SMA	Severe	Prenatal. Reduced fetal movements may be noted antenatally	<6 mo	Motors milestones are not achieved. Other features may include arthrogryposis multiplex congenital, severe neonatal hypotonia, and respiratory failure at birth
Type I SMA (Werdnig–Hoffmann)	Severe	<6 mo Often, in the first few months of life	Median survival is 8–10 mo Mortality due to respiratory failure often occurs by the 2 yr of age	Symptoms of severe muscle weakness and hypotonia present in the first few months of life; most infants are never able to sit up or walk
Type II SMA (Intermediate form; Dubowitz disease)	Intermediate	6–18 mo	70% of individuals survive into adult life	Infants are usually able to sit independently but unable to walk independently
Type III SMA Kugelberg–Welander)	Mild	>18 mo	Normal	Infants are initially able to walk independently but may have difficulty with stairs and running
Type IV	Mild	>30 yr	Normal	May present with fatigue and proximal muscle weakness. Loss of ambulation may occur after the fifth decade

Clinical Genetics and Genomics at a Glance, First Edition. Edited by Neeta Lakhani, Kunal Kulkarni, Julian Barwell, Pradeep Vasudevan, and Huw Dorkins.

Diagnosis

- Electromyography (EMG) is a diagnostic technique that measures the electrical activity and muscle response to nerve stimulation. Prior to genetic testing, this was used as a diagnostic method for SMA, typically showing evidence of neuronal/axonal loss.
- If clinically suspected, the diagnosis of SMA can be confirmed via molecular genetic testing; this involves *SMN1* and *SMN2* dosage and alteration analysis. The copy number of *SMN2* may affect the clinical phenotype.

Management

Targeted treatments are now emerging for the management of SMA. The disease-modifying agent Nusinersan is an anti-sense oligonucleotide that alters splicing to increase the amount of SMN2 protein. Studies suggest this can help achieve motor milestones and prolong survival in SMA type I and encourage progression of motor milestones in SMA type II.

Multidisciplinary team involvement is also important in the management of complications of SMA. This may include physiotherapy; gastrostomy placement for nutrition or dysphagia; consideration of tracheostomy or non-invasive ventilation; and management of joint contractures.

The future

A new therapy called Zolgensma® (onasemnogene abeparvovec-xioi) has been licenced for use; this an adeno-associated virus vector-based gene therapy that provides a new copy of the gene that makes the SMN protein. The long-term side effects and phenotypic consequences of new treatments are yet to be determined.

Figure 59.1 Genetic and cellular defects underlying motor system dysfunction in SMA. SMA is the result of homozygous deletion or mutation of the SMN1 gene with retention of the nearly identical SMN2 gene. Most transcripts from SMN2 lack exon 7 due to alternative splicing and produce an unstable truncated form of the protein (SMNΔ7), leading to a setting of ubiquitous SMN deficiency in SMA.

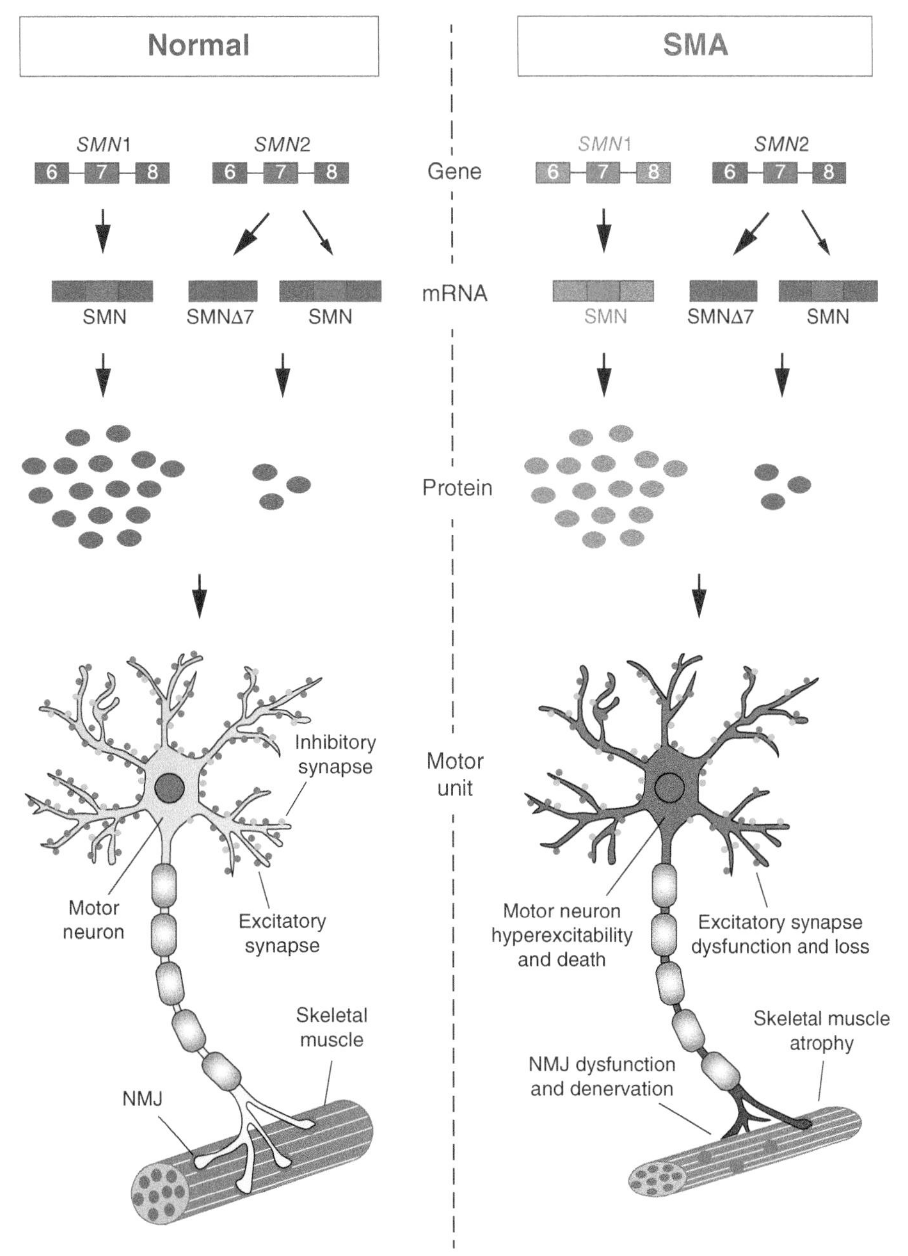

Source: https://europepmc.org/article/med/27472505

60 Motor neurone disease/Amyotrophic lateral sclerosis

Background

Motor neurone disease (MND), also known as amyotrophic lateral sclerosis (ALS), is a progressive neurodegenerative condition. It can affect motor neurones, both upper and lower, resulting in muscle wasting, paralysis, and death.

Epidemiology

Incidence is approximately 2 per 100 000 per year, with a prevalence of around 5 cases per 100 000. In 15% of patients, the MND may be accompanied by degeneration of neurones in temporal and prefrontal cortex, giving rise to frontotemporal dementia (FTD).

Genetics

- The majority of MND is sporadic, but approximately 10% of cases are familial. Most familial MND is transmitted as an AD trait, but there can be incomplete penetrance. In addition, oligogenic effects are recognised – i.e. interactions between variants in different MND susceptibility genes resulting in disease.
- The most important genes in which variants can cause MND are *C9ORF72, SOD1, TARDBP, FUS,* and *OPTN*. Of these, *C9ORF72* accounts for almost 40–50% of familial MND, while *SOD1* variants account for another 20–25%. The other genes listed above each contributes <5%. Variants in over 30 other genes have been associated with familial MND, although these account for a small proportion of patients with this disorder.
- Variants in four of the five major susceptibility genes above can give rise to FTD either in isolation or with MND; the exception is *SOD1*.

Pathophysiology

Protein misfolding, aggregation, ubiquitination, and deposition cause cell death of motor neurones. Missense alterations in *SOD1* for example may cause a spreading MND possibly through inducing misfolding of the normal SOD1 protein. Other classes of genes associated with MND (e.g. *C9ORF72, FUS*) are thought to interact with trafficking of RNA, while yet others may modify the cytoskeleton of the neuron. A final common pathway is inflammation and motor neurone death (Figure 60.1).

C9ORF72 contains a hexanucleotide repeat GGGGCC, which is expanded in MND and/or FTD. Healthy individuals carry alleles of this gene with 2–23 repeats, while MND or FTD patients have one allele with 700–1600 repeats. The repeat sequence is not translated into a protein product. The mechanism of action of the expanded repeat in causing neurodegeneration is not yet understood. Consequently, next generation sequencing would not identify *C9ORF72* expansions.

Symptoms

Sporadic and familial forms of MND have similar presenting symptoms. Patients may complain of cramps or muscle weakness affecting just one side initially. There can be wasting of the small muscles of the hand or a unilateral foot drop. As the disease progresses, there is more generalised muscle weakness, wasting of the tongue, dysarthria, and difficulty with swallowing.

The symptoms of FTD include personality changes, impulsive behaviour, apathy, inertia, and loss of interpersonal skills.

Clinical features

Although progressive muscle wasting and weakness are key features of the disease, there is variation in the extent of upper motor neurone (UMN) and lower motor neurone (LMN) involvement. UMN features are increased muscle tone, hyperreflexia, and extensor plantar responses. LMN involvement gives rise to fasciculation, muscle wasting and weakness, and reduced reflexes.

In some patients, LMN features are the only feature (progressive muscular atrophy), while more rarely in others, a pure UMN picture is seen giving rise to a pseudobulbar palsy and progressive tetraparesis (primary lateral sclerosis). In most patients, there is a mixture of UMN and LMN features.

The mean age of onset of sporadic MND is 56, while that for familial MND is 10 years earlier.

Diagnosis

MND is a clinical diagnosis. Investigations that support the diagnosis include the following:

- Electrophysiological testing can support the diagnosis by demonstrating diffuse fibrillation and fasciculation on EMG.
- Imaging of the spinal cord may be needed to exclude cord or nerve root compression.
- Genetic testing has not been undertaken in sporadic cases in the past; this may now change. Testing is appropriate in the context of a family history of the disease and/or of FTD. An earlier age of onset of symptoms may suggest an underlying genetic cause, particularly *SOD1*.

Management

MND is a relentlessly progressive disorder in the majority of cases. Psychological and social support for the patient and family are important. In later stages of the disease, patients may have a gastrostomy to permit feeding.

Median survival from the onset of symptoms is approximately 30 months, but a significant minority of patients (5–10%) survive

Clinical Genetics and Genomics at a Glance, First Edition. Edited by Neeta Lakhani, Kunal Kulkarni, Julian Barwell, Pradeep Vasudevan, and Huw Dorkins.

Figure 60.1 Motor neurone degeneration in MND can be brought about by mutant SOD1 through a variety of mechanisms. These operate in the motor neurone itself but other closely associated cells such as astrocytes, microglia and glutamatergic neurones are also implicated in the disease process.

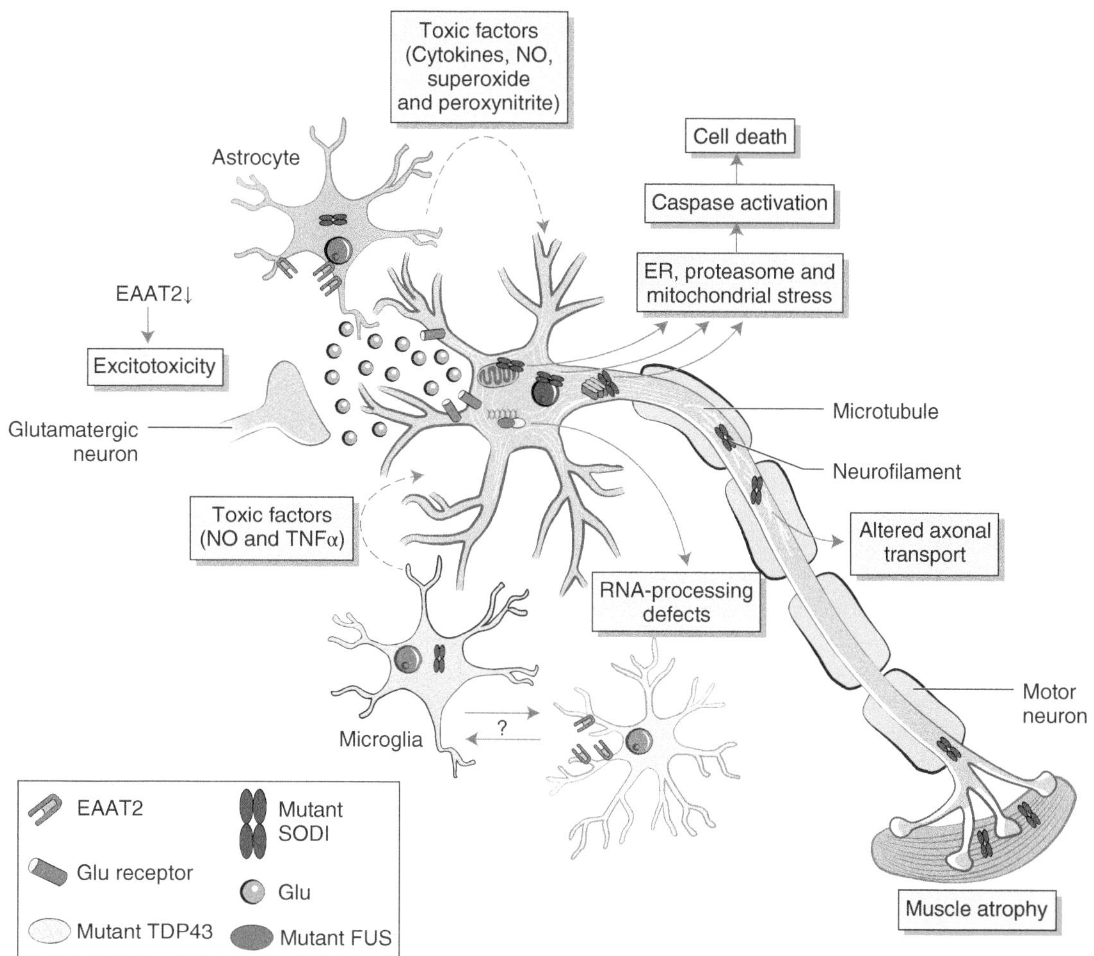

Source: https://www.nature.com/articles/nrg2680

for much longer (>10 years). Treatment with Riluzole has a small effect on life expectancy, increasing it by around three months.

The future

SOD1 was the first gene found to have a causative role in MND. Current approaches are focussing on *SOD1* knockdown in patients with intrathecal antisense oligonucleotides. In the more distant future, virally delivered RNA interference therapies targeting *SOD1* may become practicable. *C9ORF72* is a focus of intensive research at present, but insufficient is currently known about the function of the gene and its product to enable the development of novel therapies.

Genetic testing in neurodegenerative diseases

A common problem in much familial neurodegenerative disease – HD, PD, dementia, and MND is the scope for genetic testing of unaffected relatives when a pathogenic gene variant has been identified in a symptomatic individual. When few if any interventions have been available to treat the disease or to slow its progression, uptake of presymptomatic testing has been limited.

Some individuals at risk of a familial neurodegenerative disease do choose to establish their genetic status. Carefully designed protocols for genetic testing in these circumstances have been developed. These involve a series of appointments prior to undertaking the genetic test. These permit careful consideration of the implications for that individual of learning their genetic status, in areas such as such employment, insurance, career plans, reproductive decisions (including prenatal diagnosis), and relationships with their partner and other family members.

Presymptomatic testing is best managed in a centre with experience of such work, for example a clinical genetics service or a specialised neurogenetics clinic, which offers such a service on a regular basis. It seems likely that demand for presymptomatic testing will increase with the advent of clinical trials of potentially effective therapies for which knowledge of an individual's genetic status may be a prerequisite.

61 Fragile X syndrome

Background

Fragile X syndrome (FXS) is a disorder of triple-repeat-expansion and is the most common genetic cause of learning disability in males and a significant cause of learning disability in females.

Epidemiology

Approximately 1 in 4000 males and 1 in 8000 females carry a full alteration for FXS. It is known to affect people from all ethnic groups and races.

Genetics

FXS is caused be alterations in the *FMR1* gene, located on the X chromosome (Xq27.3). It is inherited in an X-linked manner. Males with alterations in the *FMR1* gene are usually affected by FXS as they only have one X chromosome and therefore only one copy of the *FMR1* gene. As females have two X chromosomes and therefore two copies of the *FMR1* gene, the unaffected copy of the gene can reduce the effects of the disease-causing copy; they may still be affected but are usually affected to a lesser extent than males.

The *FMR1* gene contains a triplet-repeat region (CGG). It is the number of triplet-repeats that determines the function of the gene (Table 61.1). Alleles outside of the normal triplet-repeat range are unstable in meiosis and at risk of expanding (increasing the number of triplet-repeats in the CGG region). The risk of *FMR1* allele expansion increases with size; the greater the number of CGG copies, the more likely these will increase in size.

Occasionally, FXS can be seen in individuals with partial or complete loss of the *FMR1* gene.

Table 61.1 Full, permutation, intermediate, and normal allele sizes.

Number of CGG triplet-repeats	Category
<45	Normal range Alleles in this size range usually remain stable when passed on from one generation to the next
45–58	Intermediate allele This is known as a 'grey zone' and does not lead to symptoms of FXS. There is a minor instability in this range
59–200	Pre-mutation carriers Pre-mutation carrier females and normal-transmitting males have 59–200 triplet-repeats (these are unmethylated) Individuals who are pre-mutation carriers are at risk of having children or grandchildren with FXS It is estimated that approximately 0.5% of the population are pre-mutation carriers
>200	Affected individuals and full alteration carriers females *FMR1* gene is methylated (silenced)

Pathophysiology

The *FMR1* gene is responsible for the production of a protein called FMRP. This protein is thought to be involved in development and maintenance of neuronal synaptic connections. Where more than 200 CGG triplet-repeats are present in the *FMR1* gene (full mutation allele), an abnormal chemical change called methylation (silencing) occurs. This inactivates the *FMR1* gene and causes absent or low levels of the FMRP leading to symptoms of FXS. Lower levels of FMRP in males and females correlate with the degree of cognitive impairment.

Symptoms and clinical features

Full alteration alleles can cause:

- Developmental delay such as mild motor delay and hypotonia.
- Speech and language difficulties, ranging from no speech to mild communication difficulties. Individuals may exhibit repetition, echolalia and use incomplete sentences.
- Learning difficulties.
- Behavioural difficulties such as hyperactivity, concentration issues, and impulsiveness.
- Autistic spectrum disorder.
- Difficulty with social interaction (shy and anxious in group situations).
- May have particular features such as macrocephaly, a long face, protruding ears and prominent forehead and chin (Figure 61.1).

Females with full alterations tend to have milder features than males; this is because they have a second working copy of the *FMR1* gene on their other X chromosome. They may still have mild learning difficulties (usually less severe than affected males).

Pre-mutation carriers

Individuals who are pre-mutation carriers may occasionally have learning difficulties; however, usually do not have any symptoms associated with FXS. Pre-mutation carriers are at risk of FMR1-related disorders including:

- Fragile X tremor-ataxia syndrome (FXTAS); this causes a late-onset progressive cerebellar ataxia, intention tremor, and cognitive impairment. The average age of onset is between 60 and 65 years.

Clinical Genetics and Genomics at a Glance, First Edition. Edited by Neeta Lakhani, Kunal Kulkarni, Julian Barwell, Pradeep Vasudevan, and Huw Dorkins.

- Pre-mature ovarian insufficiency (FXPOI); this is defined as hypogonadotropic hypogonadism before the age of 40 years and has been noted in approximately 20% of female pre-mutation carriers.

Intermediate alleles

Individuals with intermediate alleles do not tend to have any symptoms of FXS or FMR1-related disorders.

Diagnosis

FXS can be diagnosed via molecular genetic testing of the *FMR1* gene to detect the number of CGG triplet-repeats and abnormal methylation of the gene.

Management

Management of FXS is usually symptom based and focuses of supportive multi-disciplinary management. Individuals may benefit from:

- Speech and language therapy for speech difficulties
- Occupational therapy input for gross motor delay
- Educational support for learning difficulties
- Community paediatric support
- Behavioural intervention

Females with FXPOI should be referred for reproductive endocrinology for further management and counselling for reproductive options.

The future

While a 'cure' has proved challenging, for example with FMRP replacement, more targeted treatments that control activity and alleviate symptoms are the subject of ongoing studies.

Figure 61.1 Clinical features of Fragile X Syndrome.

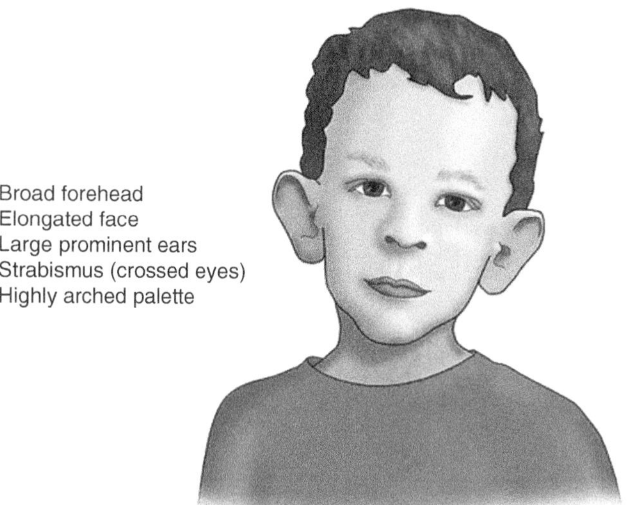

62 Huntington's disease

Background

Huntington's disease (HD) is a progressive, incurable neurodegenerative disorder. It can affect movement, learning, emotion, and cognition, sometimes resulting in dementia.

Epidemiology

Prevalence is approximately 1 per 10 000 individuals.

Genetics

HD is inherited in an AD manner, associated with an expansion in the expressed CAG tract in exon 1 of the *HTT* gene on chromosome 4. With paternal transmission, anticipation is observed, with the CAG repeats often increasing from generation to generation. CAG codes for glutamine – Q in the single-letter notation for amino acids. HD is the most important of several 'High-Q' disorders in which proteins carrying an abnormally large polyglutamine tract undergo abnormal interactions with other proteins in the cell.

Healthy individuals will carry two copies of the *HTT* gene, each containing CAG trinucleotide repeats in the normal range. If there is an expanded number of CAG repeats in one copy of the gene, this can give rise to disease.

Number of CAGs	Effect
≦26	Normal, stable
27–35	Intermediate allele
36–39	Reduced penetrance allele
≧39	Huntington's disease allele

Individuals with a HD allele are very likely to experience some of the symptoms of HD from their 40s. Those with a smaller 'reduced penetrance' allele may develop some HD features significantly later in life (i.e. 60s or later). Carriers of an intermediate allele will not develop symptoms of HD, but the intermediate allele is unstable and can undergo further expansion on being passed to the next generation – so carriers of an intermediate allele can have children who are themselves at risk of HD.

Individuals who carry a very large expansion of the CAG tract (50+ repeats) may present in childhood or adolescence with Juvenile HD. This rare condition has different clinical features, including rigidity and seizures.

Although HD is a single gene disorder and fully penetrant when the expansion size is above 39 CAG repeats, there is not always a clear family history of HD in individuals who turn out to have this condition. Adoption, family breakup, misdiagnosis as another condition (often Parkinson's disease or dementia) are all reasons for the lack of such a history.

Pathophysiology

The protein product of the normal *HTT* gene is essential for normal development and it has been shown that double knockouts of this gene are incompatible with life. The Huntingtin protein has roles in many cellular functions including signalling and metabolic regulation.

Expansion in the CAG tract in the gene results in a longer run of glutamines in the protein product. This causes the protein to adopt a different shape (misfold). The long polyglutamine tracts from different HTT molecules can align with other to form oligomers, and ultimately aggregates. The misfolded protein can interact with other proteins in ways that differ from normal HTT. Such interactions may trigger apoptosis and neurodegeneration. It is unclear whether cytotoxicity is due to the misfolded protein, its oligomers, the larger aggregates, or possibly a combination of some of these.

The main cellular focus of neurodegeneration in HD is the medium spiny projection neurones in the striatum. Substantial loss of these has already occurred by the time that gene carriers experience symptoms. As the disease progresses, there is neurodegeneration more widely in the brain (Figure 62.1).

Symptoms and clinical features

Typically, symptoms begin the fourth or fifth decade of life, although the age of onset correlates inversely with the size of the underlying gene expansion. HD can present in a variety of ways:

- **Mood:** HD patients may have episodes of depression, sometimes serious enough to warrant admission to a psychiatric hospital. Such episodes can predate any diagnosis of HD.
- **Movements:** Involuntary, rapid movements of the limbs, trunk, and face. These become progressively more severe and widespread affecting the whole body. As the disease progresses, unsteadiness can lead to falls. Many patients choose to use a wheelchair at this stage. Later still, the hyperkinetic features of HD are superseded by much reduced movement.
- **Cognition and memory:** The insidious onset of symptoms in HD can include cognitive decline and memory problems. These can manifest as declining performance at work, increasing rigidity of thinking and adherence to routine. Tasks requiring extensive multitasking such as driving become progressively more difficult for patients with HD.

Diagnosis

The above clinical features may enable a clinical diagnosis of HD, but there are some rare conditions which mimic it, such as some of the spinocerebellar ataxias (SCA 1,2,3, 17), and also dentatorubral-pallidoluysian atrophy (DRPLA).

Diagnostic genetic testing, i.e. examining the repeat size of an individual with symptoms suggestive of HD, provides important confirmation.

Clinical Genetics and Genomics at a Glance, First Edition. Edited by Neeta Lakhani, Kunal Kulkarni, Julian Barwell, Pradeep Vasudevan, and Huw Dorkins.

Figure 62.1 Gross neuropathological findings in HD. The most striking feature is loss of volume of the striatum in the basal ganglia, but neurodegeneration is more widespread as the disease progresses.

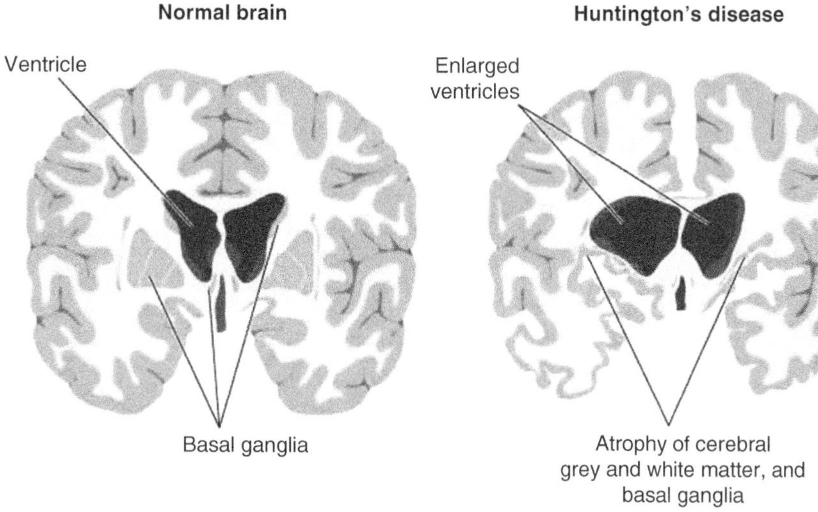

Management

To date treatment options have been limited and directed towards symptom relief:

- Antidepressants such as selective serotonin reuptake inhibitors can be useful, as may antipsychotics.
- Dopamine depleting agents have been used to manage the abnormal movements but can cause depression.
- Social support of patients and their families is crucial in this chronic disease.

First- and second-degree relatives of a person with HD will be at 50 and 25% risk of having inherited the expanded HD allele, respectively. They have the option of *presymptomatic* genetic testing to determine their own genetic status. Only a minority (up to about 1 in 4) of individuals at risk choose to have such a test. Reasons for this are covered elsewhere (see the 'Genetic testing in neurodegenerative diseases' box in chapter 60). With the advent of potentially effective treatments for HD, demand for such testing may increase.

In cases where there is an affected grandparent and a diagnosis is sought in a foetus at risk, although the parent themselves do not wish to know their status, either 'exclusion' or 'non-disclosure' testing techniques may be utilised.

HD runs its course over 15–20 years, with progressively worsening disability. The main cause of death is bronchopneumonia.

The future

There is an intensive effort to develop treatments to address the neurodegenerative process, rather than just the resultant symptoms. Antisense oligonucleotides (ASOs) have been developed to depress levels of mRNA for huntingtin. Given the important functions of normal Huntingtin, it is desirable to achieve selective knockdown of the expanded allele encoding the abnormal protein. The safe delivery of these ASOs into the CNS has been demonstrated in early trials, but this is yet to result in a safe, effective treatment. Other approaches in development include possible CRISPR-based gene editing. Cell-based therapies using induced pluripotent stem cells or neural progenitor cells for transplantation are being considered, possibly in combination with a gene editing stage.

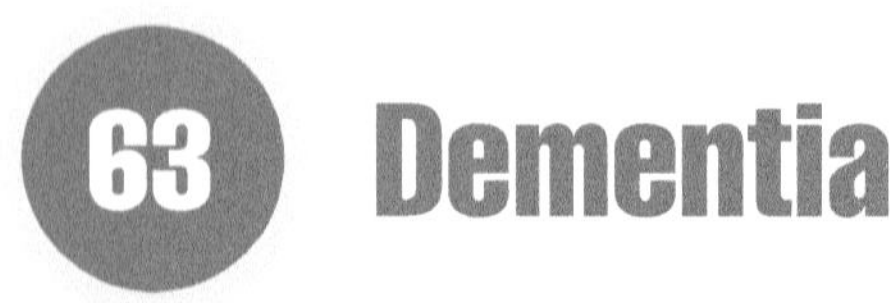

63 Dementia

Background

With an ageing global population, dementia is a major public health challenge. It is characterised by progressive cognitive decline. Abnormal forms of certain proteins accumulate in the brain. This precedes neurodegeneration, which may not be detectable until several years after the process has started.

Epidemiology

Approximately 5% of the population over 65 in many countries may be affected with dementia, while over the age of 85 this proportion reaches 1 in 5. Most instances of dementia are sporadic cases. Below the age of 65, approximately half of all cases of dementia are due to either Alzheimer's disease or vascular dementia. Over that age, the proportion due to these two causes reaches 80%.

Genetics

Alzheimer's disease is most often sporadic, although there are genetically determined susceptibilities. This is distinct from familial Alzheimer's disease.

Consideration of which abnormal protein is important in causing the dementia enables a molecular classification – the three major groups being amyloidopathies (e.g. Alzheimer's disease – sporadic or familial), tauopathies (e.g. frontotemporal dementia, FTD), and prion diseases (e.g. familial Creutzfeldt-Jakob disease, familial fatal insomnia).

Pathophysiology

Genes which contribute to susceptibility to sporadic Alzheimer's disease include apolipoprotein E (ApoE). The ε4 allele confers a threefold increased risk of Alzheimer's disease in Caucasians who carry one single copy, while the risk for ε4 homozygotes is increased eightfold. Multiple other susceptibility loci have been found on GWAS. Individually, these have less impact and are not used in clinical risk assessment.

Less than 5% of instances of Alzheimer's disease is due to a pathogenic variant in a penetrant single gene. These are usually inherited as dominant traits. Important examples include the amyloid precursor protein gene *APP* and the Presenilins (1 and 2); other monogenic forms of Alzheimer's disease have been described but are much rarer.

FTD is rarer (prevalence 1 in 10 000) but a higher proportion (25%) of this disorder has a genetic basis. Three important genes associated with FTD are *MAPT, GRN*, and *c9orf72*. The range of gene variants in *MAPT* associated with FTD includes missense and splice site alterations, but in *c9orf72*, the molecular pathology is different, being an expansion of a hexanucleotide repeat.

Symptoms, clinical features, and diagnosis

- Memory impairment is progressive and can be accompanied by difficulties – in word retrieval, with skilled motor tasks, in recognising people and objects, and in the planning and execution of tasks. Changes in personality early in the disease may be suggestive of FTD.
- It is important to exclude other causes of cognitive decline – many of which are treatable – before making a diagnosis of dementia. These include chronic infections (e.g. HIV, syphilis), endocrine disease (thyroid or parathyroid), chronic alcohol or drug misuse, depression, and deficiencies of vitamins (B12, thiamine). Intracranial pathology such as tumours, bleeds, or hydrocephalus should also be considered, while a history of cardiovascular disease may suggest vascular dementia.
- CADASIL is a rare syndrome of migraine, transient ischaemic attacks or strokes, and dementia – cerebral autosomal dominant arteriopathy with subcortical infarcts and leukoencephalopathy.
- Brain imaging is important to define the extent and pattern of cortical damage. MRI or CT are the standard modalities used but more functional studies such as SPECT can be useful to identify regional perfusion defects, e.g. in FTD. The use of ligands that bind to cerebral amyloid deposits is an alternative approach.
- Strictly speaking, a diagnosis of Alzheimer's disease is based on histopathological findings such as neurofibrillary tangles and senile plaques, but clinical findings supported by investigations to exclude other conditions (above) usually permit the diagnosis to be made with reasonable certainty.

Genetic testing

Early age of onset and a positive family history make it more likely that an individual with dementia carries a relevant pathogenic gene variant. The modified Goldman scoring (G.S.) system ranks such information thus:

1 Family history suggestive of autosomal dominant inheritance – ≥3 people affected in 2 generations, linked by 1 first-degree relative
2 Three or more affected members in a family but not linked as above
3 One affected relative with onset of dementia <65
3.5 One affected relative with onset of dementia >65 and
4 No known family history of dementia

Gene panel testing should be offered in Alzheimer's disease when there is a strong family history (G.S. ≤ 2), or a sporadic case with young age of onset (<60). When the patient has FTD, the presence of additional features such as motor neurone

Clinical Genetics and Genomics at a Glance, First Edition. Edited by Neeta Lakhani, Kunal Kulkarni, Julian Barwell, Pradeep Vasudevan, and Huw Dorkins.

disease/amyotrophic lateral sclerosis, or the behavioural variant of FTD will warrant genetic testing in sporadic cases. For FTD with primary progressive aphasia (PPA) or corticobasal syndrome, genetic testing is appropriate when there is a sufficiently strong family history (G.S. < 3).

Genetic testing could be considered when the age of onset of Alzheimer's disease is somewhat later (60–65), or in older symptomatic individuals with a family history of early onset disease (G.S. = 3).

Sometimes a clinical presentation will enable testing of a single gene, e.g. Huntington's disease, or a prion disease but in most cases, a gene panel is required, not least because the phenotypes associated with variants in individual genes can overlap.

Presymptomatic genetic testing can be offered to families in which a definitely pathogenic variant has previously been identified. As always, such presymptomatic testing should be undertaken carefully, following established protocols for neurodegenerative disease. In the absence of any effective therapy, only a minority of those at risk will wish to clarify their genetic status.

Management

Anticholinesterase drugs can improve memory and function for a limited period of time in patients with Alzheimer's disease, but not FTD. Medical and social support of patients with dementia, and their families, is important.

The future

Drug therapies are under development to target a number of processes that ultimately lead to neurodegeneration. The expression of an abnormal gene product, resulting in a misfolded protein, may be silenced through the use of an allele-specific oligonucleotide. Inhibition of the processing of amyloid precursor protein is another strategy, as is the development of monoclonal antibodies against amyloid. For GRN, trials of *GRN* gene replacement are underway.

64 Parkinson's disease

Background

Parkinson's disease (PD) is a progressive neurodegenerative disease, which gives rise to a movement disorder.

Epidemiology

PD is a disease of older age, with a median age of onset of approximately 60, and an approximate prevalence of 150–180 per 100 000. The prevalence of PD increases with increasing age. Younger-onset PD is also recognised, with 5% of cases beginning before the age of 40. PD is commoner in males than females, the lifetime risks being 2.0 and 1.3%, respectively.

Genetics

Most PD is not associated with the presence of underlying pathogenic gene variants, although there can be familial aggregation of cases. Up to about 10% of patients with PD may carry disease-causing variants in one of a number of genes. Of these, variants in three genes confer autosomal dominantly inherited susceptibility – these are alpha-synuclein (*SNCA*), leucine-rich repeat kinase (*LRRK2*), and glucocerebrosidase (*GBA*). Incomplete penetrance and variable expression are features of the dominantly inherited variants. Variants in three others confer PD susceptibility in a recessive manner – parkin RBR E3 ubiquitin-protein ligase (*PRKN*), PTEN-induced kinase (*PINK*), and parkinsonism-associated deglycase (*DJ1*). *PRKN* gene variants are associated with rare juvenile parkinsonism.

Multiple loci have been identified on GWAS that may be associated with PD risk. These are not currently used in clinical genetic testing.

Pathophysiology

The cause of idiopathic PD is not understood. It is believed that oxidative stress caused by the production of free radicals in the basal ganglia may be a cause of neuronal cell death, most strikingly in the example of MPTP poisoning. It is possible that exposure to environmental chemicals such as manganese and carbon monoxide may also give rise to parkinsonism in this way.

Certain drugs may induce parkinsonism in patients, e.g. antipsychotics with dopamine (DA) receptor-blocking activity.

Death of dopaminergic neurones in the substantia nigra is the key feature of PD; however, the neurodegeneration progressively becomes more widespread within the brain. An important neuropathological feature is the presence of Lewy bodies. These are neuronal inclusions comprising alpha-synuclein and ubiquitin. Lewy bodies first appear in the brain stem but subsequently appear in the brainstem and the cortex.

Symptoms

Cardinal features of PD are (i) bradykinesia, (ii) a resting tremor, (iii) rigidity, and (iv) postural instability. Not all patients will present with all four – the later emergence of postural instability favours a diagnosis of PD. No resting tremor may be seen in up to a fifth of patients. A number of other syndromes can mimic PD, so *absence* of features such as cerebellar signs and gaze palsies can also support PD as the correct diagnosis (Figure 64.1).

Clinical features and diagnosis

PD remains a clinical diagnosis, based on the symptoms listed above. Typically, the disease begins asymmetrically.

PD patients face progressive disability due to motor dysfunction and depression. The development of swallowing difficulty is a major risk factor for death, because of the risk of aspiration. Apart from pneumonia, other consequences of reduced mobility such as urinary tract infection, and – later in the disease – the results of falls, all contribute to increased mortality.

As the disease progresses, a significant proportion (30%) of PD patients will develop dementia. While some of this may reflect the age profile of the PD patient population, and the presence of other causes of dementia, e.g. Alzheimer's disease or cerebrovascular disease, much of the dementia is the consequence of PD itself.

The presence of atypical features necessitates consideration of alternative diagnoses, including dementia with Lewy Bodies, multiple system atrophy, and progressive supranuclear palsy. Genetically determined conditions that can overlap with PD included Huntington's disease and Wilson's disease, and in these cases, specific genetic testing should be considered with informed consent.

Management

Pharmacological therapy targeting the deficiency of dopaminergic signalling in the nigrostriatal pathway remains the mainstay of treatment. L-DOPA is a precursor of DA which, unlike the latter, can cross the blood–brain barrier. It is subsequently converted to DA in the brain. Other drug treatments include DA receptor agonists (e.g. apomorphine), and drugs which inhibit the breakdown of DA by monoamine-oxidase B (selegiline) or catechol-o-methyl-transferase (entacapone).

Drug therapy provides symptomatic relief but does not address the underlying neurodegeneration. To address the latter, grafting of suitable neurones has been attempted. This has attendant problems associated with the source of such material, and also the age of the PD patient population. Embryonic cells have been used in the past – now stem-cell-based treatment is being developed.

Clinical Genetics and Genomics at a Glance, First Edition. Edited by Neeta Lakhani, Kunal Kulkarni, Julian Barwell, Pradeep Vasudevan, and Huw Dorkins.

Deep brain stimulation (DBS) involves the placement of electrodes in the basal ganglia. It is used for younger patients (below the age of 70) to treat dyskinesias and tremor. DBS is an adjunct to, but not a replacement for, dopaminergic drug therapy.

Patients can benefit from physiotherapy, speech therapy, and occupational therapy to reduce disability.

PD can run a very variable course, with typically 10–20 years between initial diagnosis and death.

The future

Genetic testing has not been routinely undertaken in PD, not least because of its limited clinical utility. Individuals with a clear dominant family history and younger onset disease are more likely to have been offered testing, as have patients of specific ethnicities such as African Berber or Ashkenazi Jewish, in which there is a higher frequency of *LRRK2* and *GBA* variants. The targeting of such testing may mean that the contribution of pathogenic gene variants to sporadic PD has been underestimated.

Genetic testing is likely to be offered more widely in PD as evidence accumulates that knowledge of a patient's genetic status may help predict course of the disease. For example, non-motor features of PD may be less apparent in carriers of *LRRK2* or *PRKN* gene variants.

Homozygotes or compound heterozygotes for pathogenic variants in *GBA* can have Gaucher disease, a treatable disorder, which in mild form may present in adult life to a neurologist.

The emergence of clinical trials of treatments for PD targeted at individuals with changes in specific genes is likely to stimulate increased demand for genetic testing. It is too early to say whether such a 'precision medicine' approach will yield any therapeutic benefits in PD.

Figure 64.1 Clinical features of Parkinson's disease.

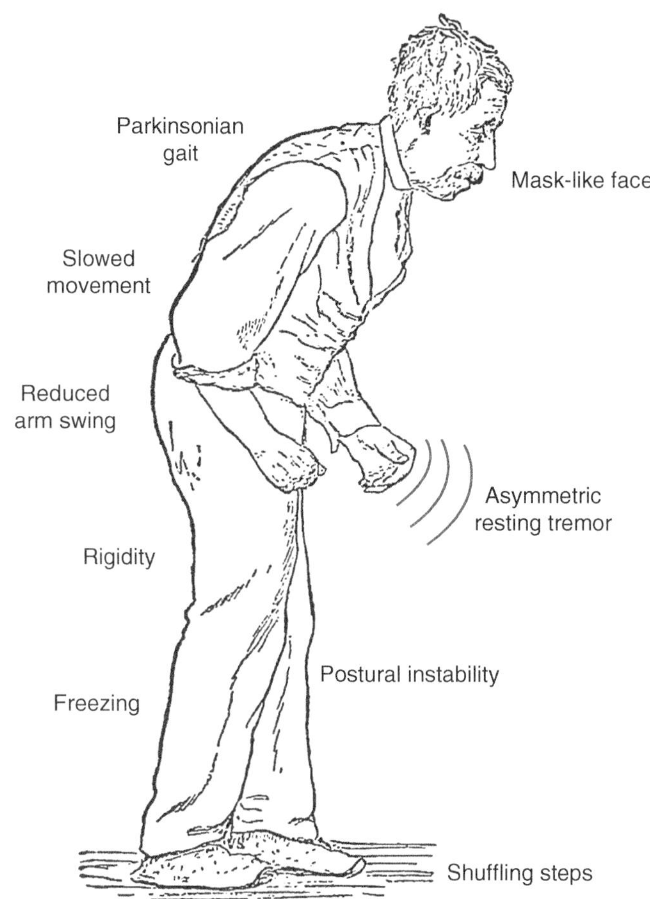

65 Myotonic dystrophy

Background

Myotonic dystrophy (DM) is a progressive multisystem genetic condition characterised by progressive muscle weakness and wasting, myotonia (prolonged muscle contractions causing difficulty relaxing certain muscles), cataracts, and arrhythmias. It is the most common inheritable neuromuscular disorder. There are two types of myotonic dystrophy:

- **Myotonic dystrophy type 1 (DM1):** also known as 'Steinert's disease'.
- **Myotonic dystrophy type 2 (DM2):** also known as proximal myotonic myopathy.

Epidemiology

DM1 is estimated to have a prevalence of 1 in 8000 in Western Europe and 1 in 100 000 in Japan. The incidence is 1 in 500 in areas such as Quebec due to 'founder effects'. The prevalence of DM2 varies in different populations, although is reported to be more common in Germany, Eastern Europe, and Finland.

Genetics and pathophysiology

DM1 and DM2 are repeat expansion disorders and are inherited in an AD manner. DM1 is caused by triple-repeat expansion of 'CTG' in the non-coding region of the *DMPK* (myotonic dystrophy protein kinase) gene located on chromosome 19q13.3. The *DMPK* gene is responsible for the production of myotonin kinase, which is present in skeletal muscle. Individuals usually have 5–37 CTG repeats. Individuals with 38–49 repeats are said to have a 'premutation' allele and are asymptomatic, although their children are at risk of having expanded repeats. Those who have 50 or more CTG repeats have symptomatic disease; this can range to the 1000s. This is associated with full penetrance, extreme variability, and anticipation (the condition becomes worse through generations due to an increase in triplet-repeat size). If females have clinical signs or symptoms, there is a potential for greater expansion and an increased risk of having a child with congenital myotonic dystrophy (a more severe form of DM). Congenital DM is most likely to have been maternally inherited.

DM2 is caused by a CCTG repeat expansion in the *CNBP* (*ZNF9*) gene located on chromosome 3q21. *CNBP* (*ZNF9*) encodes for zinc finger protein 9. The number of repeats in pathogenic expansion for DM2 range from 75 to 11 000 repeats. Unlike DM1, the number of repeats does not correlate with age of onset or disease severity.

Symptoms and clinical features

Signs and symptoms of DM can begin at any age but often begin in the second or third decade of life (Figure 65.1). Symptoms overlap and may include:

- Muscle weakness and wasting
  - Muscle weakness in DM1 initially affects the distal upper limbs leading to difficulty with fine dexterity tasks of the hand and also involves the legs (leading to a foot drop), face, and neck.
  - Muscle weakness in DM2 usually affects the proximal and axial muscles, particularly the neck and hip flexors.
- Myotonia gives rise to the 'grip myotonia' sign caused by involuntary muscle contraction with delayed relaxation. The onset of myotonia in DM2 is usually in the third to fourth decade of life.
- Myalgia and stiffness
- Posterior subcapsular cataracts
- Conduction disturbances and tachyarrhythmias
- Other symptoms may include endocrine abnormalities, gastrointestinal symptoms similar to those of irritable bowel syndrome, and daytime sleepiness.
- Characteristic facial features include a long face.

Top Tip: In the history, ask about any signs of hands 'locking up'. This may be when opening a door, using a can opener, or holding a hand. If you shake an affected individual's hand, they may have a delayed grip release (grip myotonia). Tapping of the thenar eminence may elicit myotonic contraction.

Symptoms of DM2 may be milder than those of DM1.

Congenital DM is thought to be a variation of DM1. Symptoms are present from birth and may include severe generalised weakness, hypotonia, respiratory compromise, bilateral talipes, and intellectual disability. Reduced foetal movements with polyhydramnios are often reported in the antenatal period.

Diagnosis

- Molecular testing includes targeted analysis of the CTG trinucleotide repeat in the *DMPK* gene and CCTG repeat in the *CNBP* gene via PCR or Southern Blot.
- Non-molecular testing that can aid diagnosis includes electromyography (EMG), creatinine kinase levels, and muscle biopsy.

Management

There is no cure for DM and treatment is usually centred around monitoring expected complications of the condition. This includes:

- Cardiorespiratory monitoring for arrhythmias and sleep disordered breathing.
- Physiotherapy and moderate exercise training to maximise muscle and cardiorespiratory function (avoiding over exertion which may lead to more rapid disease progression).
- Early reporting of worsening vision to treat cataract formation.
- Occupational therapy involvement for assistive devices for muscle weakness and home adaptation.

Clinical Genetics and Genomics at a Glance, First Edition. Edited by Neeta Lakhani, Kunal Kulkarni, Julian Barwell, Pradeep Vasudevan, and Huw Dorkins.

- Speech and language therapy for dysphagia and aspiration.
- Certain anaesthetic agents and medications such as statins should be avoided.
- Medications such as gabapentin, pregabalin, non-steroidal anti-inflammatory drugs, and tricyclic antidepressants may be used for treatment of myalgia.

The future

Although no cure exists, advances in basic and translational research are paving the way for the development of novel therapeutic interventions aimed at targeting the faulty pathways, for example via inhibition of the molecule CDK12 (and thereby preventing the transcription of faulty RNA).

Figure 65.1 Clinical features of Myotonic Dystrophy.

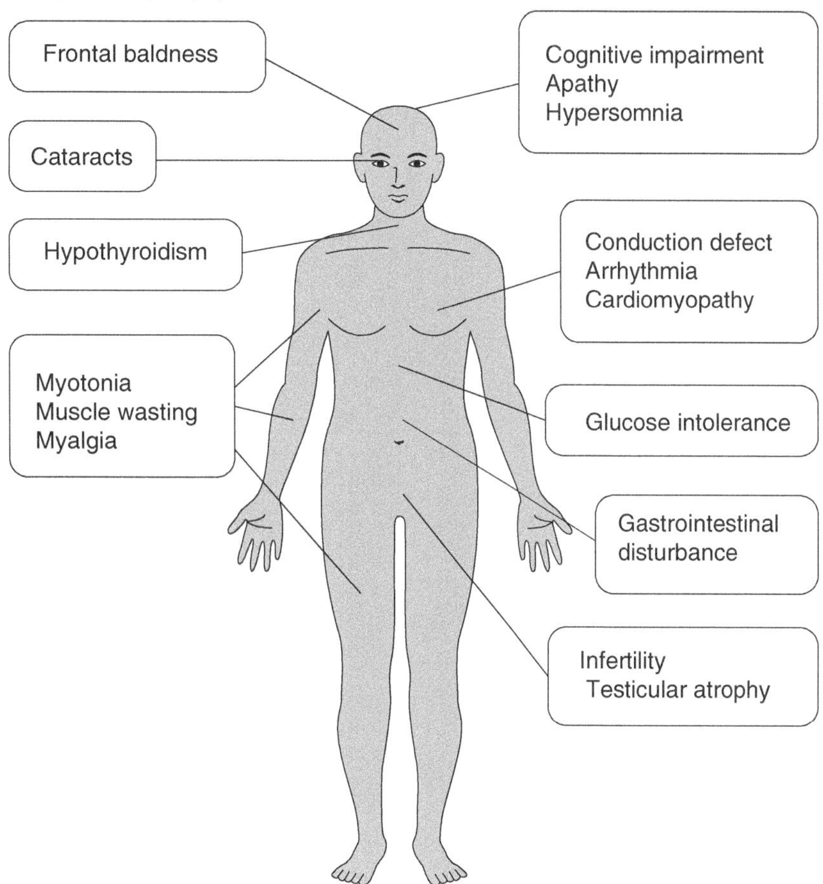

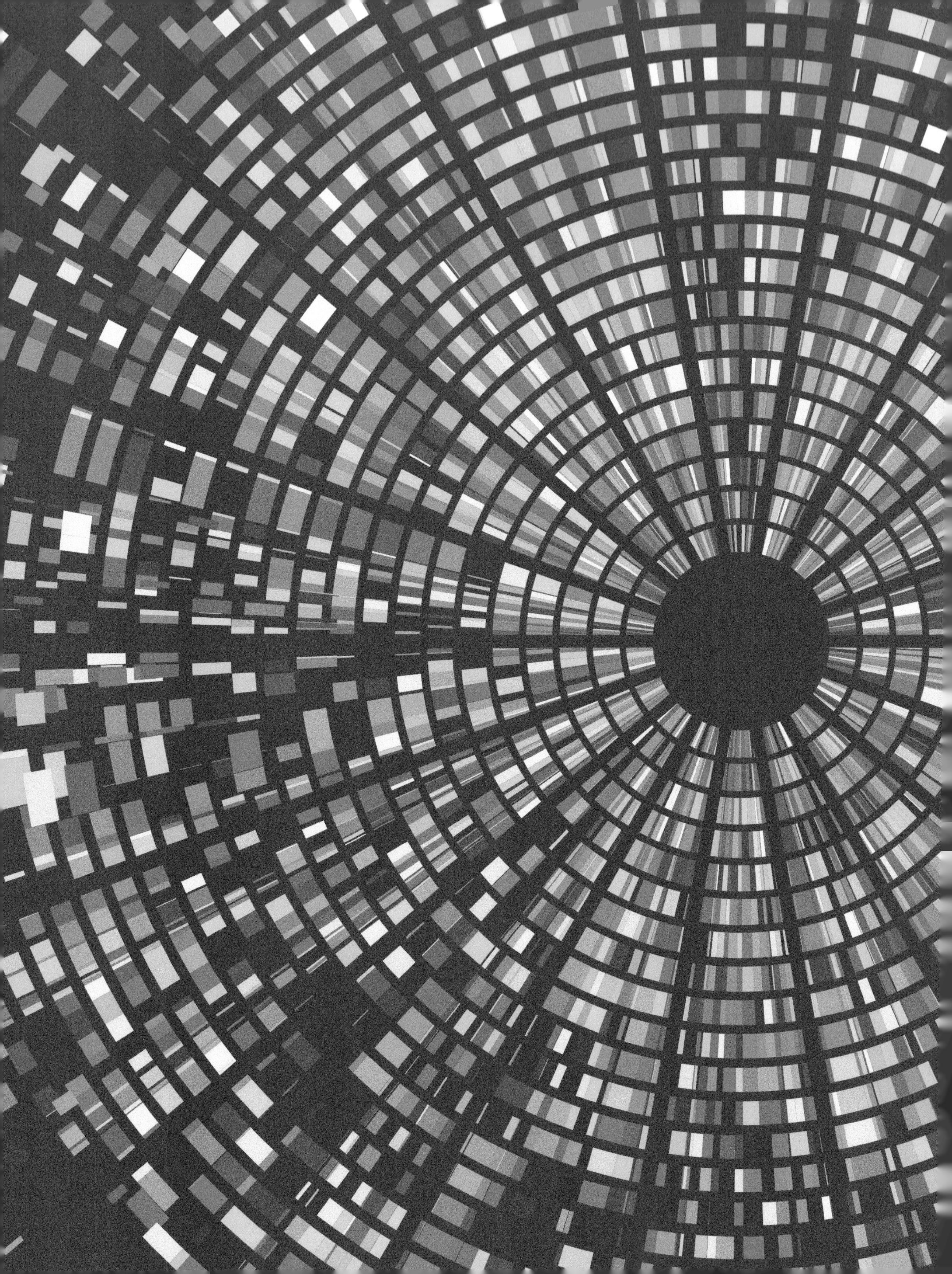

Paediatrics and Obstetrics

Chapters

66 Foetal anomaly screening

This section covers the foetal anomaly screening programme currently adopted in the UK, with particular emphasis on detailed anomaly scan screening in the second trimester. Screening by ultrasound scan has been an integral part of foetal anomaly screening for over 50 years. It is thought that up to 3% of foetuses have structural anomalies. Detection of these anomalies by imaging, together with genetic and biochemical testing, yields more accurate information for families regarding prognosis and future decision-making in the pregnancy.

First trimester screening

The first trimester combined test is performed from 11 weeks and 2 days to 14 weeks and 1 day of gestation. This test considers maternal age, NT (nuchal translucency) measurement, biochemical tests (including free beta hCG, Human chorionic gonadotrophin; and PAPP-A, Pregnancy associated plasma protein A), and gestational age (calculated by crown rump length, CRL via antenatal ultrasound scan). This test is performed to assess the risk of a pregnancy being affected by Trisomy 13 (Patau syndrome), 18 (Edwards syndrome), or 21 (Down syndrome).

Second trimester quadruple test

This test is performed at around 16 weeks of gestation and is the nationally recommended strategy for second trimester screening. It is offered to women who book late for first trimester screening or when NT measurement cannot be obtained in the first trimester. This test considers maternal age and four biochemical markers measured between 14 weeks plus 2 days and 20 weeks of gestation; these include AFP (alpha fetoprotein), hCG (Human chorionic gonadotrophin), uE3 (Unconjugated oestriol), and Inhibin-A.

Antenatal ultrasound scan

Ultrasound scanning is generally considered safe, effective, and non-invasive technique for foetal imaging. Pregnant women being cared for by the UK's NHS are offered two scans during pregnancy. The first is the dating scan, which is offered between 8 and 12 weeks of gestation, and is designed to determine the gestational age and to identify single or multiple pregnancies. This scan measures the crown rump length (CRL), which when correlated with the gestational age is an important test to guide further interventional prenatal diagnostic testing via techniques such as Chorionic Villus Sampling (CVS) or Amniocentesis.

The second scan is the high-resolution foetal anomaly scan, which is usually performed in the second trimester – usually between 18 and 20 weeks and 6 days of gestation. This is performed according to the NHS Fetal Anomaly Screening Programme (FASP) ultrasound scan base menu and foetal cardiac guidelines. It is recommended that this screening pathway is completed by 23 weeks (plus 0 days) of pregnancy. The ultrasound scan base menu includes the following 6 measurements: (i) Head circumference; (ii) Trans-cerebellar diameter; (iii) Coronal view of lips and nasal tip; (iv) Abdominal circumference; (v) Femur length; (vi) Sagittal view of spine (sacrum and skin covering).

Foetal echo includes the situs, four chamber view, and outflow tract views (right, left, and 3 vessel/trachea view). If congenital heart disease is suspected, a specialist foetal echo by a paediatric cardiologist is recommended. In general, the 20-week scan looks for anomalies of the brain, spinal cord, face, heart, bones, kidneys, and abdomen.

There are 11 conditions screened as a minimum for in England between 18 and 20 weeks and 6 days (see Table 66.1).

On occasion, certain scan findings that occur in normal foetuses are found in an increased frequency in foetuses with specific disorders. These are known as 'soft markers' and include echogenic bowel, echogenic foci in the heart, choroid plexus cysts, mild ventriculomegaly, and shorter long bones. These can be associated

Table 66.1 Conditions screened in England between 18 weeks and 20 weeks and 6 days.

Conditions	Detection rate (%)
Anencephaly	98
Open spina bifida	90
Cleft lip	75
Diaphragmatic hernia	60
Gastroschisis	98
Exomphalos	80
Serious cardiac anomalies includes the following: • Transposition of the great arteries (TGA) • Atrioventricular septal defect (AVSD) • Tetralogy of Fallot (TOF) • Hypoplastic left heart syndrome (HLHS)	50
Bilateral renal agenesis	84
Lethal skeletal dysplasia	60
Edwards syndrome (Trisomy 18)	95[a]
Patau syndrome (Trisomy 13)	95[a]

[a] Detection rates will be reviewed once sufficient data is received following implementation of screening as part of the combined screening strategy.
Source: Adapted from: https://www.gov.uk/government/publications/fetal-anomaly-screening-programme-handbook

Clinical Genetics and Genomics at a Glance, First Edition. Edited by Neeta Lakhani, Kunal Kulkarni, Julian Barwell, Pradeep Vasudevan, and Huw Dorkins.

with foetal aneuploidy. However, it is important to note that the majority of foetuses with soft markers turn out to be normal, and it is important that parents are reassured about this statistic.

When scan anomalies are detected, parents are counselled based on the findings, and genetic testing is offered as indicated depending on the anomalies following discussion with the clinical genetics specialist and other members of multidisciplinary team. In certain cases, foetal MRI scanning is offered; this is especially helpful in central nervous system anomalies, particularly neuromigrational anomalies of the brain.

67 Prenatal diagnostic testing and preimplantation genetic diagnosis

Prenatal diagnostic testing

Prenatal interventional testing includes chorionic villus sampling (CVS) and amniocentesis. Both of these tests carry a risk of miscarriage (about 1 in 100). There are some sources quote lower risks, however, this is operator dependant.

CVS tests are performed from approximately 11 weeks of pregnancy. They involve taking a small sample from the chorionic villi; these are derived from the trophoblast – the extraembryonic part of the blastocyst – and consist of cytotrophoblast and syncytiotrophoblast (that is shared with embryonal cells). This test is performed either transabdominally or transvaginally.

Amniocentesis is performed from approximately 16 weeks of pregnancy. This involves taking a small amount of the amniotic fluid (10–20 ml) that surrounds the baby and contains foetal skin cells and cells from the foetal gastrointestinal and genitourinary tracts.

For structural anomalies identified by second trimester scanning, when interventional prenatal testing is undertaken (i.e. CVS or amniocentesis), QF-PCR (Quantitative fluorescent polymerase chain reaction) or FISH analysis (fluorescence in situ hybridization) can be performed alongside chromosomal microarray (CMA) testing, which is the first line investigation. QF-PCR or FISH analysis provides results within 24–48 hours for certain abnormalities (for example, common trisomies and sex chromosome anomalies). CMA testing takes about 10–14 days to generate a result.

CMA has many advantages over traditional G-banding karyotype analysis, as it can detect many submicroscopic rearrangements known as microdeletion or duplications. Some of these deletions and duplications produce variable clinical phenotypes; however, many of these submicroscopic rearrangements are likely to be benign. Many are of uncertain or unknown clinical significance and can lead to challenging prenatal counselling and clinical decision-making scenarios. These require careful consideration of various factors and require multidisciplinary team input to provide informed advice to the parents. It is also important to note that deletions or duplications are found in approximately 6% of pregnancies with a structural anomaly (and 1% without any structural anomaly).

Non-invasive prenatal testing (NIPT) includes free foetal DNA (ffDNA) testing, which can be performed after confirming the stage of pregnancy, taking place from approximately nine weeks of gestation. ffDNA is genetic material that comes from the foetus but can be detected in the mother's blood during pregnancy. NIPT is used for detecting trisomies (such as T21, T18, or T13) or sex-chromosome aneuploidies (such as like Turner syndrome (45,X0) or Klinefelter syndrome (47, XXY)). Non-invasive prenatal diagnosis (NIPD) is for testing single gene conditions.

As part of the new NHS-genomic medicine service and national test directory in England, NIPD includes testing for many conditions, including cystic fibrosis, congenital adrenal hyperplasia, Apert syndrome, Crouzon syndrome, alongside many skeletal dysplasias (such as Achondroplasia). Prenatal rapid exome sequencing (sequencing of the coding part of more than 20 000 genes) is currently being offered in many centres in England (known as 'R21' in the National Test Directory) for foetal anomalies with a likely monogenic disorder. This is performed using a nationally agreed panel of genes known to cause genetic conditions and utilises 'Trio' testing (i.e. using samples from both parents and the foetus) to aid rapid diagnosis alongside the clinical features and family history.

Ethics

Ethical issues are very common in the prenatal diagnostic setting and include concepts such as clinical utility, informed consent, confidentiality, patient autonomy, best interest, and balance of risks versus benefits. Termination of pregnancy for foetal abnormalities is always a difficult issue for both families and professionals alike. What constitutes a 'serious abnormality in the foetus' is hard to define or ascertain. In general, the four basic pillars of biomedical ethics are followed when making a decision. Involvement of clinical ethics committees is also very helpful in complex and ethically challenging scenarios.

In the era of genomic medicine, it is recommended that tests are offered, are clearly indicated on the basis of clinical findings, existing investigation results, and family history – rather than simply because a technologically advanced test is available – as interpretation of the results can be complex in many cases. It is also important that patients and families are appropriately counselled, including provision of all of the relevant information, options, implications, and limitations of prenatal diagnostic testing. Effective and efficient communication with families is key to managing these delicate, time limited, situations, and it is pertinent to involve parents early in the decision-making process to achieve optimum maternal and foetal health outcomes.

Preimplantation genetic diagnosis

In comparison to prenatal diagnosis, preimplantation genetic diagnosis (PGD) is carried out on embryonic cells before pregnancy is established. It harnesses techniques such as in vitro fertilization (IVF) or intracytoplasmic sperm injection (ICSI). Once the development of the embryo has occurred to the 8-cell stage, one cell (blastomere) is removed for molecular cytogenetic or molecular genetic analysis to detect or exclude either a specific unbalanced chromosomal translocation or the detection or exclusion of a known pathogenic alteration related to a monogenetically inherited condition.

PGD is funded nationally by the NHS for patients living in England (differing from IVF, which is often funded regionally). Before PGD is considered, couples must fulfil certain criteria (Table 67.1). Fulfilment of these criteria enables up to three cycles of NHS funded PGD. This funding ceases if they have a healthy child, are not responding to treatment, or no longer fit the eligibility criteria. For couples ineligible for NHS funding, self-funded treatment is available.

Clinical Genetics and Genomics at a Glance, First Edition. Edited by Neeta Lakhani, Kunal Kulkarni, Julian Barwell, Pradeep Vasudevan, and Huw Dorkins.

Table 67.1 Mandatory criteria for couples seeking NHS funded PGD.

- Treatment to start before the female partner is 40.
- Female partner must have a body mass index (BMI) of more than 19 and less than 30.
- Both partners must be non-smokers.
- Couples must not already have an unaffected child.
- Couples must have been in relationship for a year.
- Couples must live at the same address.
- Couples must have had genetic counselling locally.
- Testing occurred in an accredited laboratory.

PGD can be a complicated and protracted process, with many considerations during its course, including through times of uncertainty and emotional highs and lows. The length of time PGD takes depends on a number of factors, including the genetic condition PGD is being used for, funding, and the availability of DNA samples from family members. Couples will likely attend around four or five appointments for each cycle. There are some risks associated with PGD treatment for the woman, including the chance of multiple pregnancies, as well as the small chance of ovarian hyper stimulation syndrome (OHSS).

In the United Kingdom, the Human Fertilisation and Embryology Authority (HFEA) plays a key role in regulating preimplantation diagnosis, and centres that carry out this procedure must obtain a licence. The legislation varies in other counties. To offer a safe and effective service, a multidisciplinary team is established, including specialists in in vitro fertilisation, clinical geneticists, genetic counsellors, cytogeneticists, and molecular biologists. With appropriate regulation and use, PGD can offer families the possibility to allow future family members to be disease free.

68 Edwards' syndrome

Background

Edwards' syndrome (trisomy 18), was originally described by Edwards et al in April 1960 as a trisomy and delineated to chromosome 18 in 1961. It is a common chromosomal disorder due to the presence of an extra chromosome 18, either full, mosaic trisomy, or partial trisomy 18q. It causes a mutisystemic condition that leads to abnormalities in foetal formation. In utero, many of the features described below can be identified and therefore has high detection rates as part of the NHS Foetal Anomaly Screening Programme (FASP), is associated with abnormalities in multiple sites.

Epidemiology

Edwards' syndrome is the second most common autosomal trisomy after Down syndrome (trisomy 21). It occurs in approximately 1 : 5000 births and however due to the high frequency of fetal loss and pregnancy termination after prenatal diagnosis, the rate is likely higher.

Genetics

Trisomy 18 occurs when a person has three copies of chromosome 18 rather than the usual two (Figure 68.1). Most cases are not inherited and occur de novo. It is suggested that the extra chromosome is present because of nondisjunction. In parent-of-origin studies the extra chromosome appears most often of maternal origin, the result of an error during the segregation of chromosomes in meiosis or postzygotic mitosis. In the minority of cases in which the extra chromosome has a paternal origin, the error is the result of a postzygotic error. The cause of nondisjunction is unknown. Several mechanisms may occur:

- **Full trisomy 18:** 3 copies of chromosome 18 in all cells (46XX +18) (Figure 68.1)
  - 90–95% occur via non-disjunction
  - More common in advanced maternal age
  - Most severe; affected individuals may not survive birth and may not live past first birthday
- **Mosaic trisomy 18** (46XX/47XX+18)
  - Rare: 5–10% cases (1 in 20)
  - Third copy of chromosome 18 is only in some cells (mix of normal and cells with trisomy)
  - Milder; some babies with this form may live till adulthood
- **Partial trisomy 18**
  - Very rare: <1% cases (~1 : 100)
  - Only a portion of the third copy of chromosome 18 is present in cells (rather than the whole extra chromosome 18)
  - Usually due to translocation
  - Phenotype depends on how much chromosome 18 is present in cells

Pathophysiology

The additional genetic material from the third copy of chromosome 18 disrupts normal development.

Symptoms and clinical features

Features vary between individuals (Figure 68.2). The majority of affected individuals have:

- Small for gestational age
- Cardiac defects: VSD, ASD, tetralogy of Fallot
- Broad forehead/nose
- Severe intellectual impairment
- Fingers: camptodactyly, overlapping digits, nail hypoplasia

Other features include:

- Prominent occiput
- Microcephaly
- Low set/malformed ears
- Micrognathia
- Small mouth
- Palpebral fissures
- Broad nose
- Cleft lip and palate, high palate
- Rocker bottom feet (prominent calcaneus)
- Clenched fists
- Malformations of internal organs (diaphragmatic hernia, omphalocoele, kidney, and ureter abnormalities)

Diagnosis

Diagnosis of trisomy 18 is usually made antenatally. First trimester non invasive screening based on maternal age, serum markers and scan findings demonstrates high sensitivity for diagnosis of trisomy 18. A risk is given to the parents and the option for invasive testing offered.

Serum markers: the levels of human chorionic gonadotropin, unconjugated estriol, and alpha-fetoprotein are significantly lower in pregnancies with trisomy 18 compared to unaffected pregancies. Scan findings: the most common scan finding detected in the late first/early second trimester is the increased nuchal translucency thickness and the absence or hypoplasia of the nasal bone. Adding the evaluation of reversed flow in the ductus venosus and the tricuspid valve regurgitation, increases detection rates significantly . Other some structural anomalies can be detected by ultrasound screening during the first trimester; omphalocele (21%), abnormal posturing of the hands (6%), megacystis (4%) abnormal four-chamber view of the heart (4%) Early-onset fetal growth restriction (26%).

Antenatally if an increased risk is identfied, an amniocentesis or chorionic villus sampling (CVS) can be undertaken to make a definitive diagnosis. The option of non-invasive prenatal testing using cell-free fetal DNA in maternal plasma can also me used

Clinical Genetics and Genomics at a Glance, First Edition. Edited by Neeta Lakhani, Kunal Kulkarni, Julian Barwell, Pradeep Vasudevan, and Huw Dorkins.

Figure 68.1 Trisomy 18.

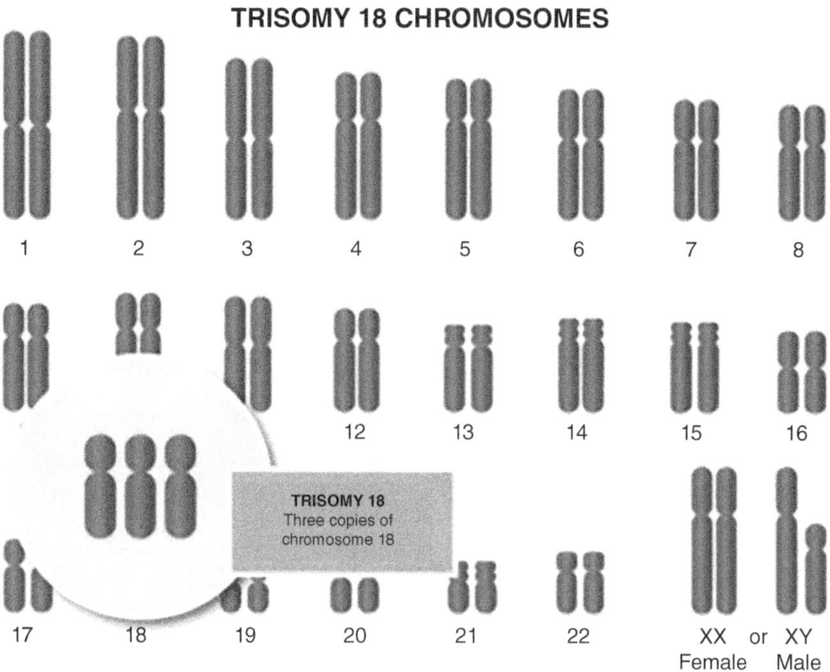

(97.4 sensitivity and 99.95% specificity). After birth, confirmation can be made using a rapid FISH, which will confirm trisomy 18 within 72 hours. A follow up array CGH is will identify mosaicism and partial trisomies.

Management

Many ethical issues surround the care and management of infants and children with Edwards' syndrome. Management decisions should centre on the best interests of the child, while also considering parental opinions.

Counselling is an important part of management. If an antenatal or neonatal diagnosis of Edwards' syndrome is made, families will need support and counselling. Uncertainty about the outcome should be discussed, alongside decisions regarding resuscitation, intensive care, and any potential surgery.

For full trisomy 18, care should focus on comfort care and making memories. Cardiac defects may not be suitable for surgery as prognosis maybe guarded. Partial and Mosaic Edwards have a better prognosis and hence management may include a multidisciplinary team approach to tackling the challenges these children may have.

If Edwards' syndrome is due to an unbalanced translocation, both parents should undergo chromosomal analysis. It may be that the translocation in the infant occurred de novo, but a balanced translocation may be found in one of the parents. This has significance for future pregnancies. Other family members may also be affected. Screening and/or prenatal diagnosis should be offered for future pregnancies accordingly. For full Edwards' syndrome, the risk of recurrence in a future pregnancy is higher than the general population risk and estimated as less than 1%. The risk may be higher if a parent carries a balanced translocation.

Figure 68.2 Physical features of an infant with trisomy 18.

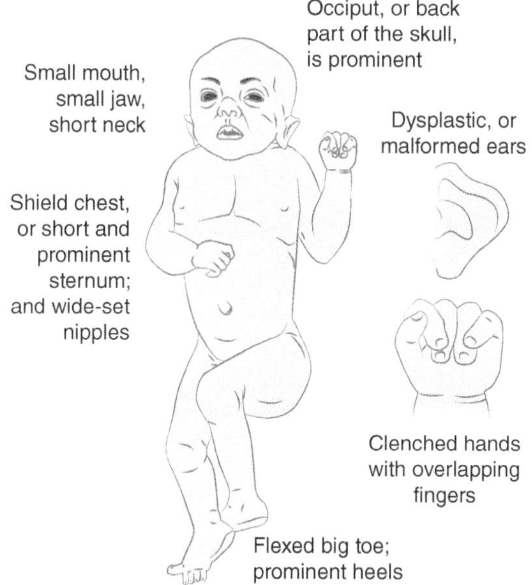

The future

While there is no cure, refinements in aspects of management (for example, paediatric cardiac surgery) has improved life expectancy.

69 Patau syndrome (trisomy 13)

Background

Patau syndrome (trisomy 13) was first described by Dr Patau in 1960. Approximately 50% of pregnancies diagnosed with Trisomy 13 at 12 weeks will end in miscarriage or stillbirth.

Epidemiology

Trisomy 13 occurs in approximately 1 in 10 000–20 000 live births in the United Kingdom. It is the third most common autosomal trisomy after trisomy 21 (Down syndrome) and trisomy 18 (Edwards' syndrome). It is more common in mothers of advanced maternal age (>35) due to non-disjunction.

Genetics

Most cases are not inherited and occur as de novo alterations. In trisomy 13 occurs, an affected individual has three copies of chromosome 13 instead of the usual 2 (see Figure 69.1). Three main types exist:

- **Full trisomy (46XY + 13) (Figure 69.1):** Accounts for 90% of cases. Three copies of chromosome 13 in all cells.
- **Mosaic trisomy 13 (46XY/47XY + 13):** Accounts for 5% of cases. Three copies of chromosome 13 exist in some cells.
- **Partial trisomy 13:** Very rare (<1%). Only a portion of the third copy of chromosome 13 is present in cells (rather than the whole extra chromosome 13). This usually occurs due to a Robertsonian translocation.

Pathophysiology

The extra copy of chromosome 13 affects normal embryonic development and causes prechordal mesoderm fusion defects. Altered fusion causes midline defects often incompatible with life. This may result in miscarriage, stillbirth, or dying shortly after birth.

Symptoms and clinical features

Trisomy 13 causes severe intellectual disability alongside multiple physical abnormalities (that may cause a threat to life) (Figure 69.2). Partial and mosaic phenotypes show a variable expression of the features. Common features include:

- Cardiac defects: Particularly ASD, but also VSD, tetralogy of Fallot, double outlet right ventricle (DORV)
- Microphthalmia/anophthalmia
- Abnormal pelvic bone shape
- Abnormal fontanelles/cranial sutures
- Bilateral single palmar crease

Other features include:

- Cleft lip/cleft palate (Figure 69.3)
- Hypotonia, seizures, apnoeas
- IUGR, failure to thrive, feeding difficulties
- Sloping forehead, microcephaly, micrognathia
- Small/malformed/low-set ears, pre-auricular skin tags
- Clenched hands, post-axial polydactyly, other limb abnormalities

Figure 69.1 Trisomy 13 (Patau syndrome).

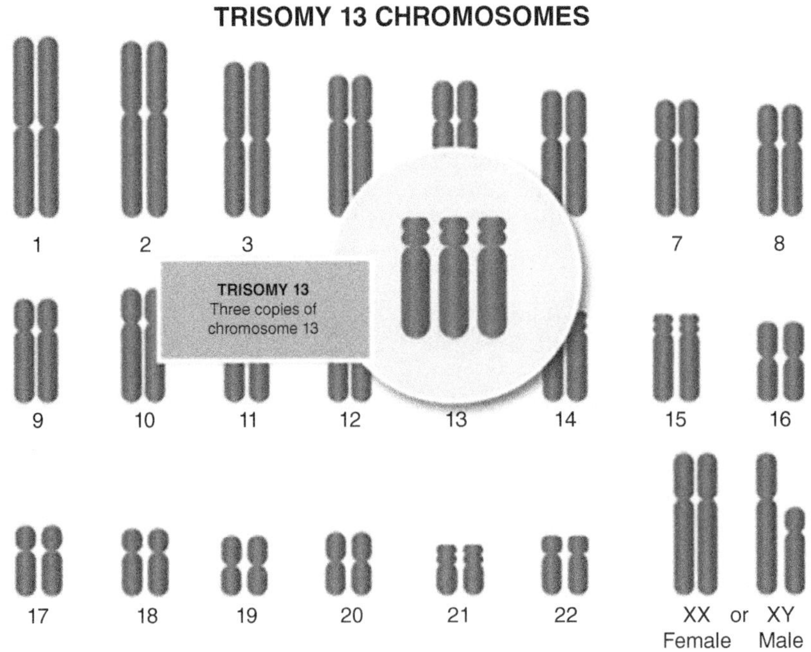

Clinical Genetics and Genomics at a Glance, First Edition. Edited by Neeta Lakhani, Kunal Kulkarni, Julian Barwell, Pradeep Vasudevan, and Huw Dorkins.

Figure 69.2 Clinical features of Patau syndrome.

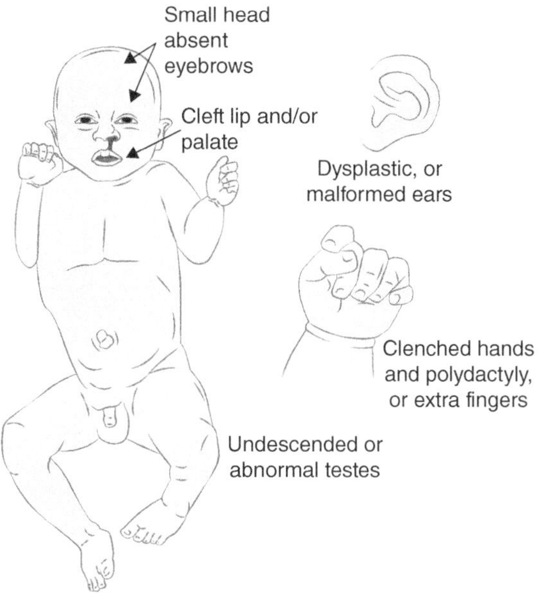

Figure 69.3 Infant with Patau syndrome.

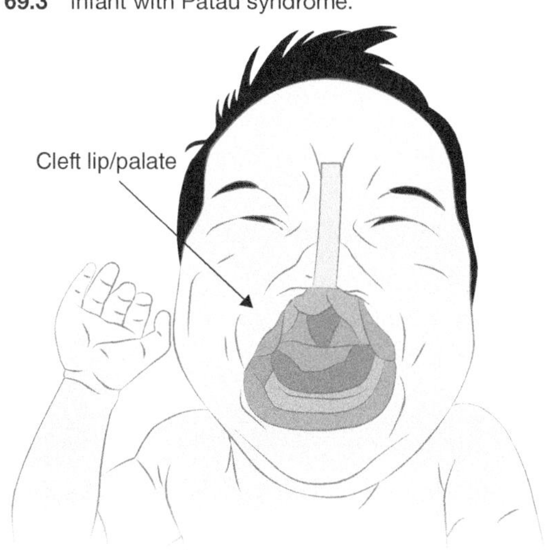

- Alobar holoprosencephaly (failure of the brain to divide into right and left hemispheres, resulting in the loss of midline structures
- Congenital talipes equinovarus, rocker-bottom feet
- Genitourinary defects, including cryptorchidism
- Abdominal defects including omphalocoele, hypospadias, hernias

Diagnosis

Often the initial indication of trisomy 13 is an increased fetal nuchal translucency (FNT), noted at the first scan. Part of the first-trimester screening also includes the measurement of free beta subunit or total human chorionic gonadotropin (B-hCG) and pregnancy-associated plasma protein-A (PAPP-A). Both of which are decreased in trisomy 13. Combined these can predict an increased risk of trisomy 13 and the offer of invasive confirmative testing.

Antenatal diagnosis can be performed with amniocentesis or chorionic villus sampling (CVS). Non-invasive pre-natal testing may be performed by fetal-free DNA analysis. Postnatally, FISH can detect trisomy 13 followed by a confirmatory karyotype. Microarray analysis will confirm a partial or mosaic trisomy 13.

Management

Overall, trisomy 13 has a very poor prognosis. Historically, over 80% did not survive past the first month of life, and 90% did not survive to 1 year, with median survival being 7–10 days in liveborn affected individuals. Prognosis is better with Mosaic and unbalanced translocations. With improved neonatal care, more recent studies have reported survival rates at 11.5% at 1 year and 9.7% at 5 years. Intensive care and surgical treatment for full trisomy 13 remains controversial.

For children that survive, complications ensue that must be addressed, including respiratory difficulties, feeding difficulties, cardiac failure, and poor vision and sight. Treatment is therefore focused on symptom management, alongside providing comfort for those.

Parents must be counselled regarding future pregnancies. Most cases of full trisomy 13 occur by chance (i.e. are de novo), hence recurrence risk for full trisomy is low (less than 1%). Recurrence risk may be higher if a parent has a balanced translocation or partial trisomy.

The future

There is no cure, with treatments focused on addressing the various issues that arise. Improved treatments have resulted in improved survival rates.

70 Williams syndrome

Background

Williams-Beuren Syndrome was first identified by Dr John Williams in 1961 and reported by Dr A.J Beuren in 1962. It is a rare genetic neurodevelopmental disorder.

Epidemiology

Occurs in approximately 1 : 18 000 cases in the United Kingdom. Both sexes are affected equally.

Genetics

WS is caused by a heterozygous 1.5- to 1.8-Mb deletion of the Williams-Beuren syndrome critical region (WBSCR) on chromosome 7q11.23, presenting with a 100% penetrance. The deletion size is similar across most individuals with WS and leads to the loss of one copy of 25–27 genes on chromosome 7q11.23.

The majority of cases are secondary to a de novo deletion of this region, with rarely an affected parent inherited in an AD - manner.

Some genotype-phenotype correlation has been documented and has led to a better understanding of the pathophysiology of the condition.

Pathophysiology

25–28 continguous genes are noted in the WBSCR, and smaller/larger deletions have allowed for some genotype - phenotype correlation to be delineated. The resulting multisystemic phenotype has some cardinal features that include, but are not limited to, cardiac abnormailites (of note supravalvular stenosis), intellectual disability and hypersociability.

CLIP2, ELN, GTF2I, GTF2IRD1, and *LIMK1* are some of the genes that are deleted. Loss of the *ELN* gene is associated with connective tissue abnormalities and cardiac disease. Deletions *CLIP2, GTF2I, GTF2IRD1*, and *LIMK1*, amongst others, may account for the behavioural and cognitive difficulties. *GTF2IRD1* deletion may account for the distinctive facial features.

Symptoms and clinical features

- The facial gestalt of WS is unique: young children typically have a small head, full cheeks, smooth philtrum, micrognathia, prominent ears, small under-developed teeth, large mouth, broad nasal bridge, anteverted nares (Figure 70.1)
- Vision and hearing difficulties
- Cardiac abnormalities: supra-valvular aortic stenosis

Figure 70.1 Clinical features of Williams syndrome (include broad forehead, bitemporal narrowing, peri-orbital fullness, stellate iris, short nose and broad nasal tip, wide mouth and full cheeks).

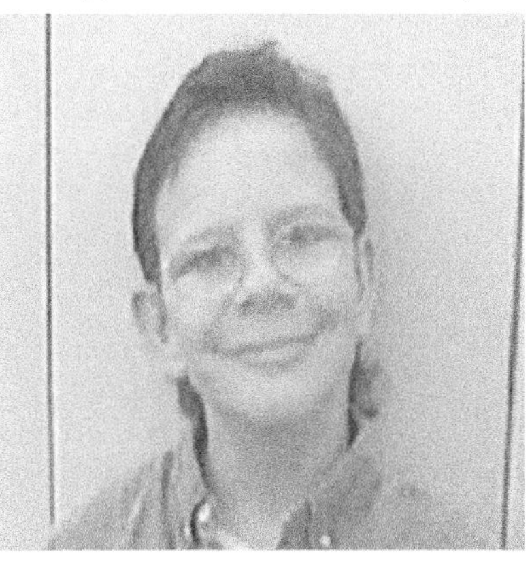
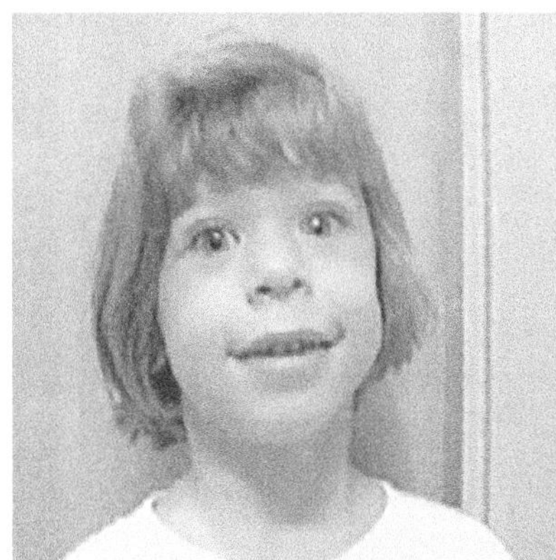
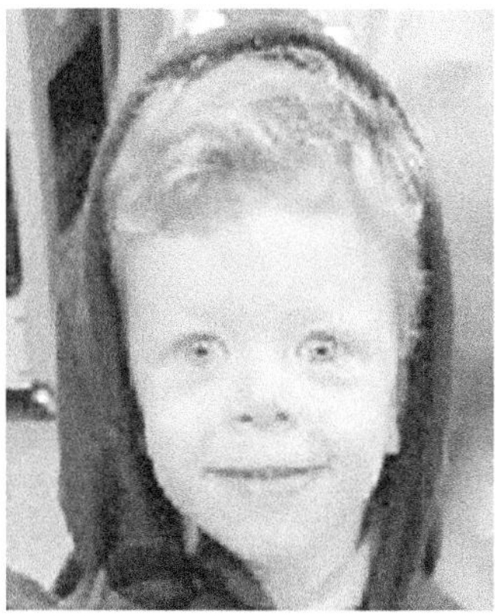
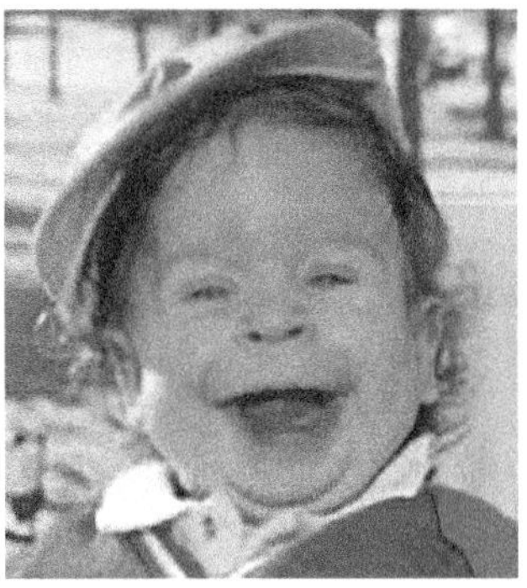
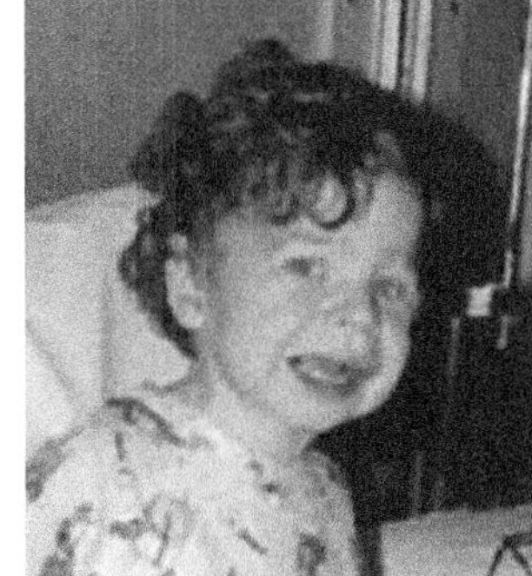
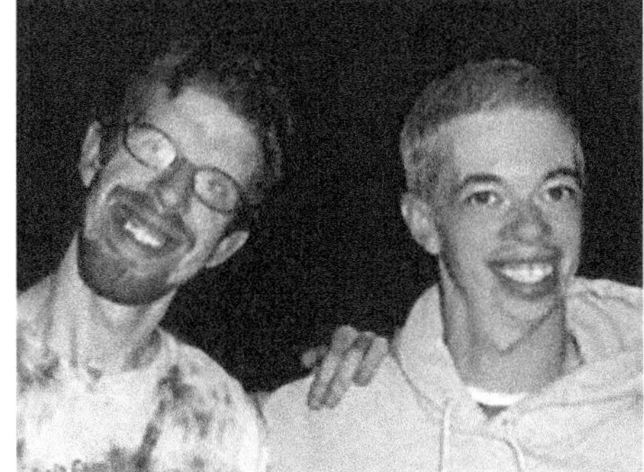

Source: E.A. Nikitina/A.V. Medvedeva/G.A. Zakharov/E.V. Savvateeva-Popova/Acta Naturae.

Clinical Genetics and Genomics at a Glance, First Edition. Edited by Neeta Lakhani, Kunal Kulkarni, Julian Barwell, Pradeep Vasudevan, and Huw Dorkins.

- Endocrine abnormalities: hypercalcaemia, hypothyroidism, early puberty
- Poor growth/feeding difficulties
- Connective tissue abnormalities, including hypotonia and hyperextensible joints
- Development: delayed milestones, friendly, outgoing, talkative personality, short attention span, easily distracted, variable learning difficulties

Diagnosis

Diagnosis is made by genetic testing to identify the microdeletion. Determining the copy number of sequences can be done including chromosomal microarray (CMA) or targeted deletion analysis by fluorescence in situ hybridization (FISH). Other investigations include:

- Blood levels of calcium
- Hearing and vision screen
- Echocardiogram and ECG for cardiac abnormalities

Management

This is via a multidisciplinary approach. Genetic counselling is required when making a diagnosis. Aspects of care include:

- Endocrinology: Manage hypercalcaemia, hypothyroidism, growth difficulties, early puberty
- Early intervention services for developmental and behavioural problems: Occupational therapy/physiotherapy/speech therapy/special education team
- Hearing and vision screening
- Dentists: Address dental abnormalities, including malocclusion
- Feeding support, dietician involvement
- Cardiac surgeons: Address congenital cardiac abnormalities

Prognosis: 80% of affected individuals have cardiovascular abnormalities requiring surgery. Morbidity is usually due to arteriopathy and congenital heart disease. Children with Williams syndrome can survive to adulthood and live semi-independently to independently, including the ability to work.

Future pregnancies: Most cases of Williams syndrome are de novo, although some are inherited in an AD fashion, hence counselling must be offered for future pregnancies. However, the recurrence risk is low for unaffected parents with a child with Williams syndrome, and prenatal testing is therefore rarely indicated.

The future

Ongoing research will help improve the care of affected individuals, including via improved diagnostics and better management of developmental/behavioural problems to improve function and quality of life.

71 DiGeorge syndrome

Background

The features of DiGeorge syndrome were first described in 1828, but it was not formally reported by Dr Angelo DiGeorge until 1965. This condition is caused by the absence of a small part of chromosome 22, resulting in the poor development of several body systems. The term 22q11.2 deletion syndrome covers what were once thought to be separate conditions, including DiGeorge syndrome, velocardiofacial syndrome, and other disorders with the same genetic cause, although features may vary slightly.

Epidemiology

Occurs in 1 in 4000–6000 live births. 22q11.2 deletion is likely to be more common than previously reported given that some individuals remain undiagnosed due to mild features.

Genetics

Each person has two copies of chromosome 22, one inherited from each parent. In 22q11.2 deletion syndrome, one copy of chromosome 22 is missing a segment that includes an estimated 30–40 genes. Many of these genes haven't been clearly identified and aren't well-understood.

The deletion of genes from chromosome 22 usually usually de novo in 90% cases; 10% are inherited, usually in an AD fashion.

Pathophysiology

The features of this syndrome vary and show significant inter and intra famililal variation affecting many systems of the body. Characteristic signs and symptoms may include birth defects such as congenital heart disease, defects in the palate/velopharyngeal insufficiency, learning disabilities, distinct facial features, and recurrent infections due to altered T cell-mediated response that in some patients is due to an absent or hypoplastic thymus.

Symptoms and clinical features

DiGeorge Syndrome is easy to remember with the mnemonic 'CATCH-22'.

- **Conotruncal cardiac anomalies:** Truncus arteriosus, tetralogy of Fallot, interrupted aortic arch
- **A**bnormal facies
- **T**hymic hypoplasia – absent thymus
- **C**left palate
- **H**ypocalcaemia
- **22**q11.2 microdeletion

Clinical features therefore include:

- Heart murmur and cyanosis (due to a cardiac defect)
- Frequent sinopulmonary infections due to T-cell deficiency (from thymic aplasia)
- Characteristic facial features: micrognathia, low-set ears, wide-set eyes, narrow groove in the upper lip, cleft palate (or other problems with the palate) (Figure 71.1)
- Delayed growth, difficulty feeding, failure to gain weight or gastrointestinal problems
- Breathing problems
- Hypotonia
- Signs of hypocalcaemia (muscle twitching, spasms)
- Hormonal problems (from an underactive parathyroid)
- Delayed development (delay in rolling over, sitting up, or other infant milestones)
- Delayed speech development or nasal-sounding speech
- Learning delays or disabilities: ADHD, autism, behavioural problems

Figure 71.1 Facial features of DiGeorge syndrome (upslanting and narrow palpebral fissures, prominent nasal bridge, small mouth).

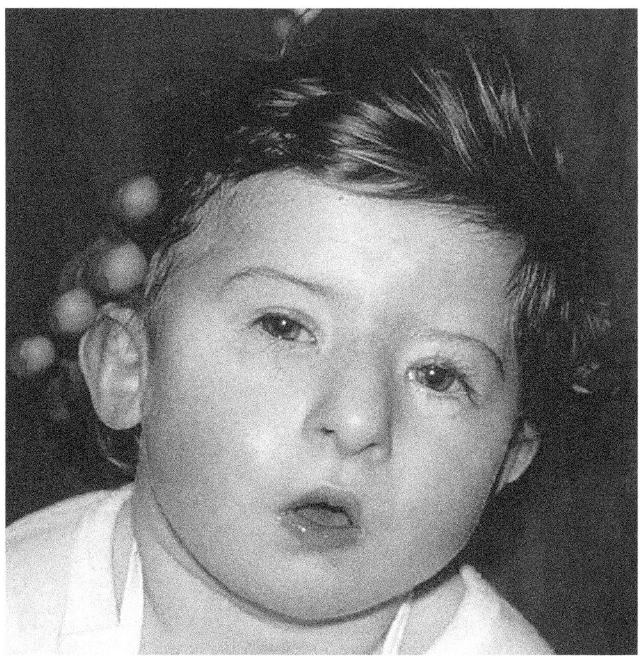

Source: Prof Victor Grech/Wikimedia commons.

Diagnosis

Diagnosis of complete DiGeorge syndrome is made based upon the characteristic clinical features. Newborn screening using a number of tests can help confirm the diagnosis:

- Blood tests for FISH and microarray can detect the 22q microdeletion
- Echocardiogram can identify the cardiac defects
- **Immunological tests:** T- and B-cell lymphocyte subsets, flow cytometry, immunoglobulin levels and vaccine titres (to evaluate response to vaccines)
- Serum calcium, parathyroid, and phosphate levels

Clinical Genetics and Genomics at a Glance, First Edition. Edited by Neeta Lakhani, Kunal Kulkarni, Julian Barwell, Pradeep Vasudevan, and Huw Dorkins.

- Chest x-ray for thymic shadow evaluation (helpful but not diagnostic)
- Ultrasound for possible renal and genitourinary defects

Management

Affected individuals require multidisciplinary care, including involvement of cardiologists, immunologists, endocrinologists, surgeons, and clinical geneticists, with overarching support from a paediatrician and therapists to manage the associated problems including feeding and growth issues, hearing and vision problems, and other related medical conditions. Management must consider the following:

- Immunodeficiency should be carefully evaluated and treated. Prompt antibiotics/antivirals for infections.
- Consider surgery for cleft palate to improve feeding and speech, and cardiac surgery for congenital cardiac defects. Temporary tracheostomy may be required. Gastrostomy may also be required for feeding.
- Early intervention services, speech therapy, occupational therapy, physiotherapy for children with delayed development
- Calcium and vitamin D supplementation as required

Prognosis: Fewer than 1% of patients with 22q11.2 microdeletion have complete DiGeorge syndrome, the most severe subtype, with a very poor prognosis (may not survive to two years). Most of patients with DiGeorge syndrome do not have a defined prognosis as it is highly dependent on the severity of all the associated features that each affected child has. DiGeorge syndrome may be underdiagnosed, and many undiagnosed adults thrive with undetectable congenital anomalies and minor intellectual and/or social impairment.

Future pregnancies: 90% cases are de novo, so there is a low risk of recurrence in future pregnancies. In 10% cases, the 22q11 deletion is passed on to the child by an affected parent (possibly undiagnosed with mild features) in an AD-manner, where there is a 50% recurrence in siblings.

The future

Thymus tissue transplants are not commonplace, with limited long-term data on their use. Stem-cell transplants have not been proven to be effective at replenishing T-cell supplies. Refinements in surgical treatments have improved the outcomes following cardiac or ENT surgery. Early therapy support, for example with speech and language services, has improved the overall development of affected children.

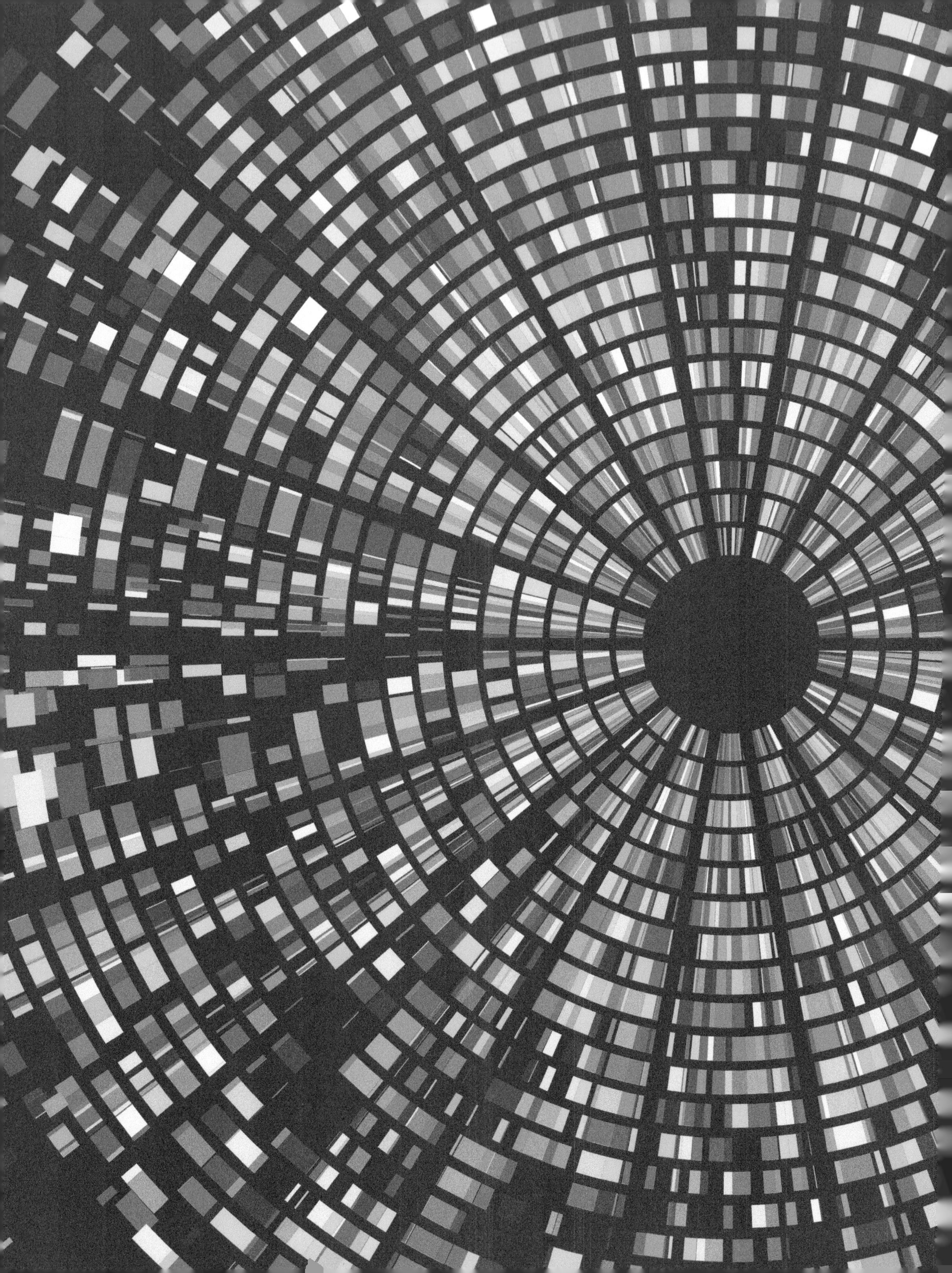

Oncology

Chapters

72 Introduction to cancer

What is cancer?

Cancer is the loss of balance between cell growth, differentiation, and death, leading to uncontrolled proliferation of cells and malignant growth. All cancers are 'genetic', in that they are caused by a pathogenic variant of a gene (also known as an *alteration or mutation*, although the latter term may have negative connotations for patients). These may either be picked up throughout life as an undetected error during cellular division (*somatic* alterations) or, less commonly, they may be *inherited* through the germline from one/both parents. There are various ways in which genetic changes can lead to carcinogenesis, described in detail in the seminal work 'Hallmarks of Cancer' (Hanahan and Weinberg 2011). In the vast majority of cases, cancer is a collection of multiple genetic alterations in a group of cells occurring throughout life with increasing malignant potential, for example causing sustained proliferation, avoidance of immune system, angiogenesis, invasion through the basement membrane, and then metastases (distant spread) (Figure 72.1). Some genes require a single-allele alteration (e.g. oncogenes → proliferation), whereas others require both alleles to be altered (e.g. tumour suppressor genes → loss of control of proliferation) [see 'Two-Hit hypothesis' in the *Retinoblastoma* section]. Patients with a germline alteration start life with a greater risk of cancer because a predisposing alteration is already present in *all* cells; therefore, if/when further alterations occur, they are more likely to become malignant.

Risk factors

One in two people in the United Kingdom will be diagnosed with some form of cancer in their lifetime. The risk for each individual is a complex interaction of *genetic* and *environmental* factors. In general, environmental factors can be thought of as anything that could either damage a cell and increase the risk of genetic alterations that may escape detection (e.g. inflammation, radiation, virus, toxins), or increase the number of replications (e.g. age, hormonal stimulation). Age and gender are the strongest predictors of cancer risk. Worldwide, smoking and viruses (human papilloma, Epstein Barr, and hepatitis B and C) are major risks, but with Westernisation of diets and vaccination programmes, obesity is becoming an increasing factor. Studies have suggested that at least 40% of cancers are potentially preventable with lifestyle modifications. These include cessation of smoking (oral, parotid, pharnyx, lung, oesophageal), reduction of obesity (breast, bowel, endometrial, renal, liver), and alcohol abstinence (liver, oesophageal, breast, bowel, oral and stomach cancers).

The effect of Westernisation was classically described in Japanese migrants that moved to Hawaii and lowered their gastric cancer risk as they ate less raw fish but developed higher rates of bowel cancer. More recently, higher breast cancer rates have been described in South Asians living in Leicester than the indigenous population. This suggests familial and environmental factors underpin a significant proportion of cancer in a polygenic model (Figure 72.2).

While a familial cancer susceptibility increases an individual's risk, it is important to note that lifestyle factors are important in modifying risk. An example is a lifetime risk of lung cancer of 25% (rather than 13%) in *BRCA2* alteration carriers that smoke. This is important when counselling relatives.

Cancer rates and screening

Cancer rates are rising due to increased life expectancy, better reporting (coding), and greater exposure to risk factors. However, improved diagnosis through early detection and screening have also had a major impact (breast, bowel, and cervical). Screening programmes for other cancers have been considered, but the evidence

Figure 72.1 Hallmarks of cancer: Biochemical factors and cell processes that are involved in cancer development.

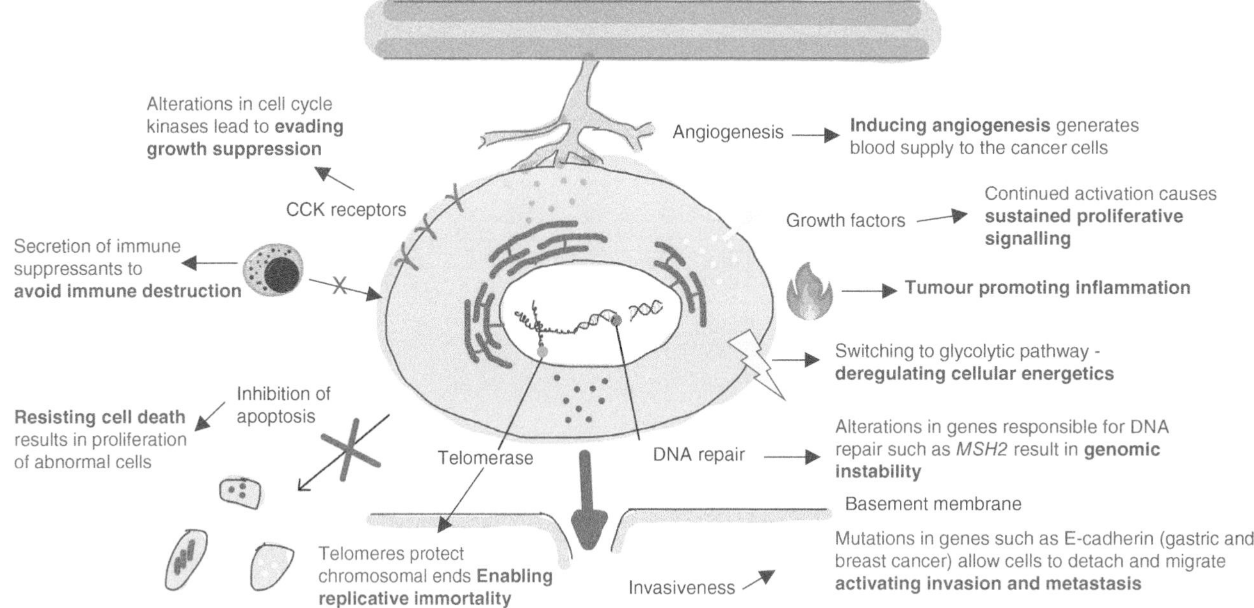

Clinical Genetics and Genomics at a Glance, First Edition. Edited by Neeta Lakhani, Kunal Kulkarni, Julian Barwell, Pradeep Vasudevan, and Huw Dorkins.

Figure 72.2 Cancer is a result of multiple hits in multiple pathways. A single alteration does not cause cancer; however, if undetected it can predispose to further alterations.

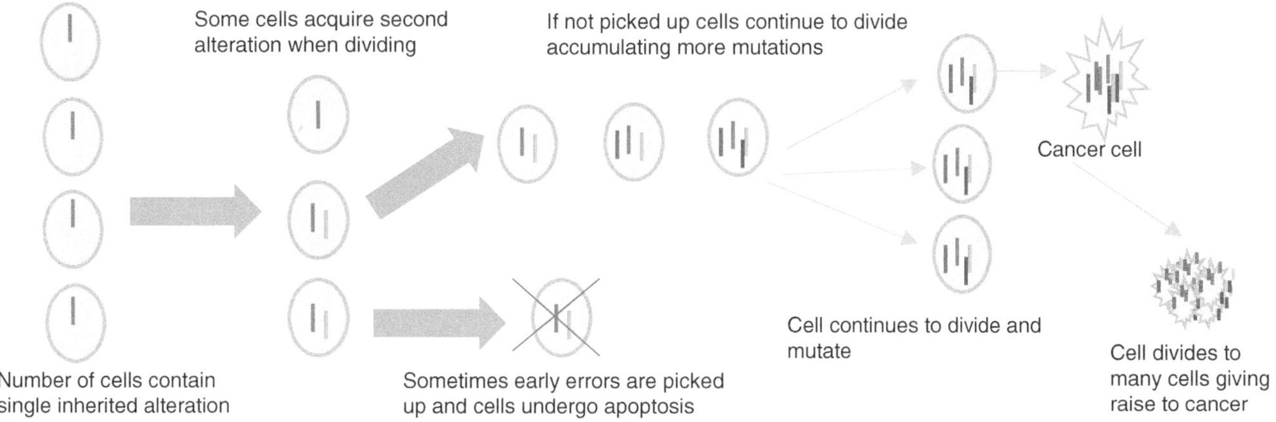
Some cells acquire second alteration when dividing
If not picked up cells continue to divide accumulating more mutations
Cancer cell
Cell continues to divide and mutate
Number of cells contain single inherited alteration
Sometimes early errors are picked up and cells undergo apoptosis
Cell divides to many cells giving raise to cancer

suggests they do not always result in improved survival or improved public health. This may be due to either dual pathology that impacts prognosis, or the wider long-term effect of management interventions on health or the prevalence of indolent disease that would have not caused significant morbidity or mortality if left untreated. This is particularly the case for prostate cancer; treatment can be associated with a high risk of impotence and incontinence, yet malignant cells frequently identified on post-mortem are rarely recorded as a main or contributing cause of death. Familial cancer susceptibility is considered a good candidate for screening programmes due to more aggressive disease, early age of onset, and often multiple or bilateral disease with rapid malignant tumour doubling rates. Unfortunately, falsely reassuring scans/tests can occur, as can over-detection/treatment; patients should be informed of these risks. The challenge for the clinical geneticist is to identify those individuals and families that may be at risk due to an inheritable alteration.

Family history

When taking a family history, it is important to be aware of consanguinity, misreporting of cancer diagnoses, ethnicity, non-penetrance, paternal transmission, and specific syndromic patterns of disease. Consanguinity mostly increases the risk of autosomal recessive (AR) disorders. This is rarely a major factor in Mendelian familial cancer susceptibility as this is usually inherited in an autosomal dominant (AD) fashion. However, there are rare AR disorders that may become more frequent in consanguineous offspring; for example, a recessive polyposis syndrome, and homozygous (the same alteration in both alleles) or compound heterozygous alterations (two different alterations in the same gene, one inherited from each parent) of mismatch repair associated with a very high risk of childhood lymphatic tissue tumours, leukaemia, and brain tumours.

Patient reporting of familial disease is rarely factitious to gain access to screening but may not necessarily be accurate either due to family secrets or hearsay, estranged relatives, relatives living abroad, or uncertain primary tumour origin. Brain and liver tumours are often secondary to another primary tumour (i.e. a metastasis), which may not be known to the unaffected at risk relative. Confirming diagnoses and histology is therefore recommended and may indicate specific cancer syndromes. Some populations are associated with higher rates of particular cancers either through specific alterations that are more common due to a limited gene pool (e.g. Ashkenazi population and *BRCA* alterations) or ethnic differences (e.g. African Caribbean men and prostate cancer).

Most familial cancer syndromes are usually associated with higher cancer rates for carriers of alterations (penetrance), although actual risk calculation may be more complicated. In some conditions (particularly endocrinological cancer syndromes), imprinting may result in unaffected generations (one of the two inherited copies of the genes (alleles) being preferentially expressed by parent of origin due to promoter methylation). Additionally, *BRCA1* and *BRCA2* alterations are associated with a higher risk of breast, ovarian, prostate, pancreatic, and lung cancers, but as men do not have ovarian tissue and much less breast tissue, it is possible that familial breast cancer susceptibility may be missed through the paternal line.

Genetic testing

Familial risk assessment is increasingly calculated either using secondary or tertiary care departmental triage systems or computer models such as the breast and ovarian cancer risk predictor – BOADICEA and CanRisk. These take time and resources to use; a simplified approach is to use a '321 model', with referral to Genetics services for at-risk relatives if there are *three* affected relatives with a single or linked cancer type (e.g. breast or breast and ovarian), across *two* generations with at least *one* diagnosed <50 years, and consider referral if *two* of these are present.

When a patient with a cancer diagnosis is offered a germline genetic blood test to determine the cause (diagnostic testing), this may clarify the risk of developing similar disease in the future both to them and their relatives. It is therefore important that this process is not rushed as it may have significant psychological and medical implications for the future. Diagnostic testing is becoming more common as part of the rise of genomic medicine alongside tumour alteration analysis and somatic testing and is being integrated into routine clinical practice in surgical and oncology clinics through a process called *mainstreaming*. The aim is to design more targeted treatments and improve prognostic indicators through the use of somatic tumour tissue genetic testing and other circulating biomarkers of disease, for example circulating cell-free tumour DNA (cfDNA) and proteomics that may form part of a mathematical algorithm to predict future health (systems biology).

Management

When an inherited alteration is detected, it is possible to test relatives who may have inherited the same alteration (cascade testing). It is generally considered good practice to avoid rushing

Figure 72.3 Simplified diagram showing the actions of some of the proteins that are associated with familial cancers.

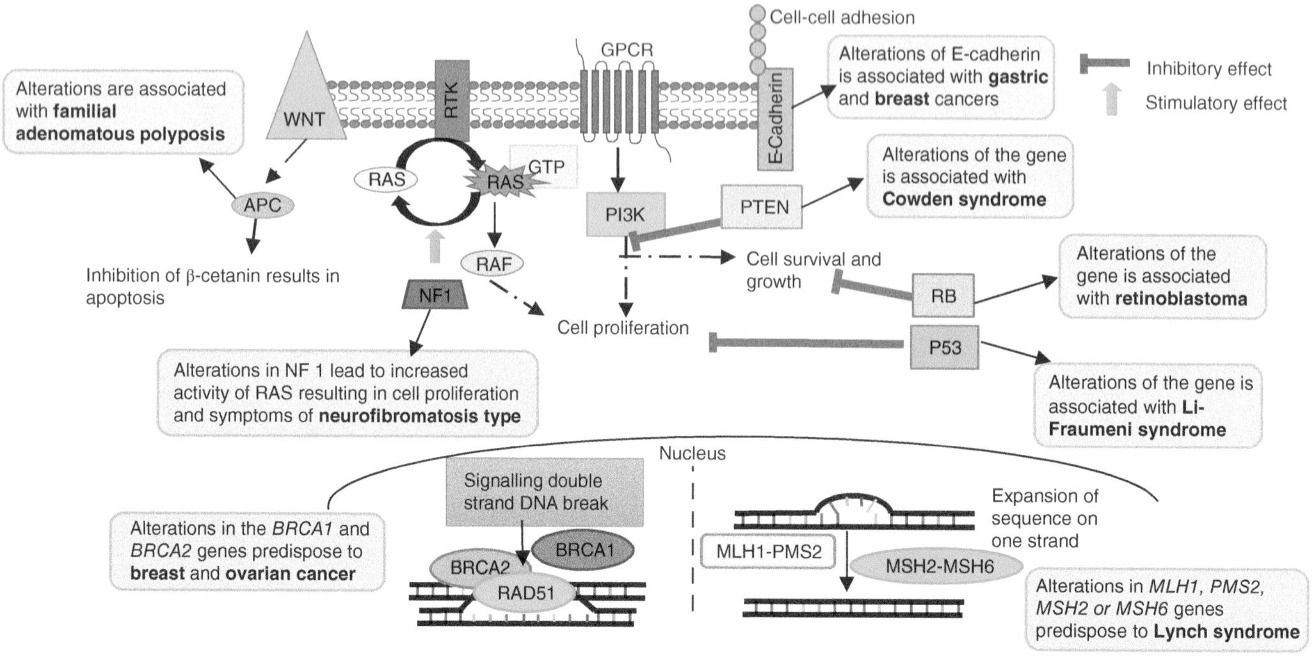

predictive genetic testing in unaffected at-risk relatives if they are otherwise well due to the understandable anxiety that a positive diagnosis can elicit. Testing of children is avoided unless immediate screening or interventions may be required (e.g. MEN2b). Predictive testing is usually arranged around the time that screening or preventative surgery is recommended, or to aid family planning. This is to avoid interfering with family bonding with children, engage adolescents in their own decision making, and because of an understandable desire to go through testing with a hope that the result will be negative and the risk avoided. Support groups can be extremely helpful for families and patients wishing to share their experiences or seek specific advice regarding coping with a familial risk. The impact of predictive genetic testing on life and health insurance is often asked and is regularly re-visited by insurance companies but is rarely an issue for otherwise well individuals within the United Kingdom (where family history is usually used to assess risk) apart from in relation to Huntington disease, but can be a factor overseas.

Apart from lifestyle factors, common tumour prevention strategies include surgical removal of at-risk organs (e.g. mastectomy in *BRCA* pathogenic variants) or chemoprevention (e.g. tamoxifen in breast cancer susceptibility or aspirin in Lynch syndrome). In accordance with cardiovascular risk calculators, active medical preventative intervention management is usually recommended when the risk of an adverse event approaches 1% per year. In the future, this technique may be replaced by gene editing and use of vaccines against genetic instability caused by DNA repair defects.

The following sections describe important familial cancer susceptibility syndromes and important germline mutations associated with cancers (Figure 72.3), how to identify patients that are at risk, and the current and future management options for these patients and families.

Further reading

Hanahan, D. and Weinberg, R.A., 2011. Hallmarks of cancer: the next generation. cell, 144(5), pp. 646–674.

73 Neurofibromatosis

Background

Neurofibromatosis (NF) is a neurocutaneous genetic disorder that predisposes to lesions in the nervous system, skin, and skeleton. The term neurofibromatosis can be used to refer to one of three distinct conditions; three distinct conditions Neurofibromatosis 1 (NF1, also known as Recklinghausen's disease), Neurofibromatosis 2 (NF2), and the more recently recognised Schwannomatosis. Although, these three conditions are referred to under the umbrella term NF, they have clear distinctive features that delineate their differences (Figure 73.1).

Epidemiology

NF1 has a prevalence of approximately 1 in 4000. NF2 is considerably less common (<1 in 40 000).

Genetics

NF is inherited in a single-gene AD fashion. However, up to 50% of cases are due to *de novo* alterations (i.e. no family history). In NF1, the genetic defect (*NF1* on chromosome 17q11.2) is responsible for the protein neurofibromin, which acts as a tumour suppressor. Multiple different types of pathogenic variants (alterations) have been reported. There are not many well-defined genotype–phenotype correlations with specific whole gene deletions being the most well described. In NF2, the implicated gene (*NF2* on chromosome 22q12.2) is responsible for the cytoskeletal protein Merlin (schwannomin) and results in neural tumours.

As with other genetic conditions, NF can demonstrate *somatic mosaicism*; this occurs when the responsible alteration develops post-conception during early embryonic development (Figure 73.2). Consequently, the affected individual has a mix of cells across different tissue types, with and without the genetic alteration for NF. The stage of embryonic development when the alteration occurs determines which cell lines are affected. For instance, it is possible that in the first affected individual, no alteration is detected in the blood but is identified in tumours or other tissues. This is because only tissues that are derived from the original altered cell carry the same gene alteration. If the gonadal tissue is derived from this affected cell-line, the alteration could be inherited by offspring with a more severe phenotype as the alteration will be present

Figure 73.2 Somatic mosaicism commonly seen in first generation for NF1 and NF2. De novo mutation occurs in a single cell, early in the embryonic development. It is present in subset of cells and not necessarily detectable in blood or all tissues.

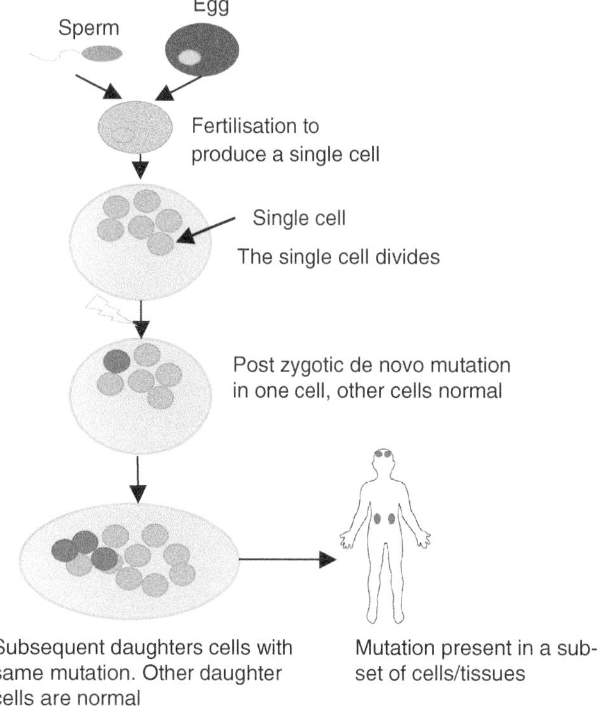

Figure 73.1 Comparison of features of neurofibromatosis type 1 and type 2.

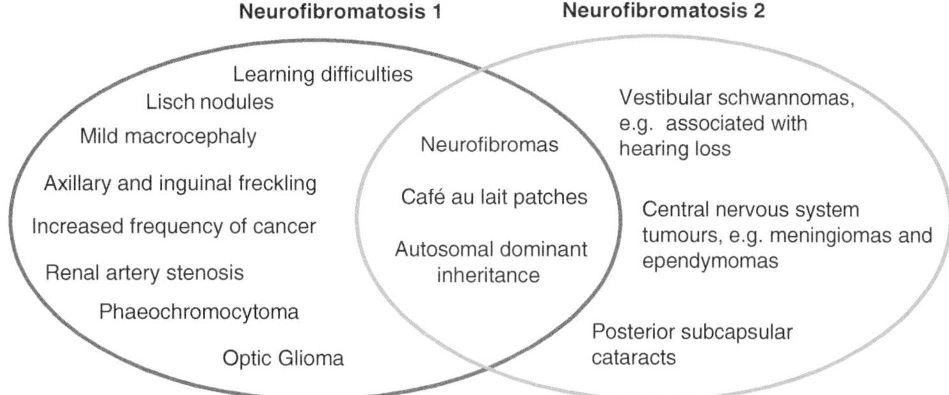

Clinical Genetics and Genomics at a Glance, First Edition. Edited by Neeta Lakhani, Kunal Kulkarni, Julian Barwell, Pradeep Vasudevan, and Huw Dorkins.

in all cells (i.e. from conception). The risk of inheritance is less than the usual 50%, and specialist advice from a clinical geneticist is essential.

Pathophysiology

The leading hypothesis is that the altered genes are responsible for tumour suppression, exampled by *NF1* which codes for neurofibromin, a GTPase-activating protein that negatively regulates RAS/MAPK pathway. Alterations accelerate the hydrolysis of Ras-bound GTP, leading to greater RAS activity, resulting in increased cell proliferation. Tumours are usually benign, but may have local mass effects and carry a risk of malignant transformation.

Symptoms and clinical features

Tumours arising from the neurilemma sheath called neurofibromas are the characteristic feature of NF1. Neurofibromas are common, often develop during adolescence, and can be numerous, cosmetically distressing and painful. Plexiform neurofibromas can occur in major nerves causing rapid growth and pressure effects such as pain or neurological symptoms (e.g. loss of continence, sensation, or power).

NF1 tends to present with multiple café au lait patches in early childhood. Other distinguishing features include macrocephaly, axillary/inguinal freckling, and bone abnormalities (Figure 73.3). Lisch nodules of the iris can be detected by slit lamp to aid diagnosis, although they are benign and have no clinical significance. One-third patients have significant development delay, one third have no learning difficulties, and one third have subtle difficulties such as dyslexia, visuo-spatial awareness problems, or dyscalculia.

The two distinguishing features of NF2 from NF1 are (i) the risk of vestibular schwannomas (known as acoustic neuromas) and (ii) other central nervous system tumours including meningiomas (Figure 73.4) and ependymomas. Vestibular schwannomas present with conductive hearing loss, vertigo, and tinnitus. Cutaneous signs such as café au lait patches or neurofibromas are less common in NF2. Posterior subcapsular cataracts can occur and are particularly relevant given the risk of hearing loss with vestibular schwannomas.

Figure 73.4 MRI of NF2 patient demonstrating large sellar meningioma.

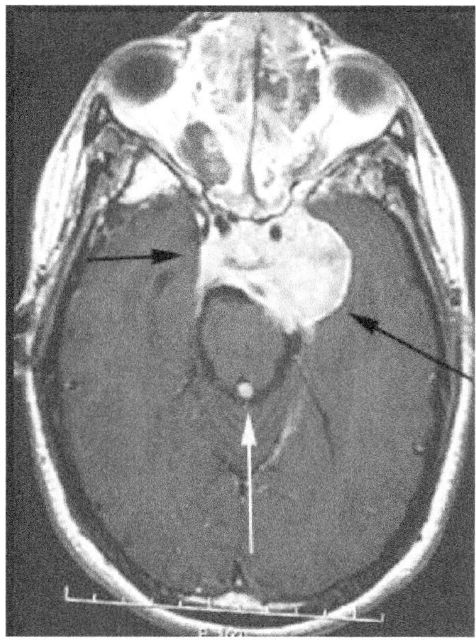

Source: WebMD, LLC.

Figure 73.3 Clinical features of Neurofibromatosis type 1.

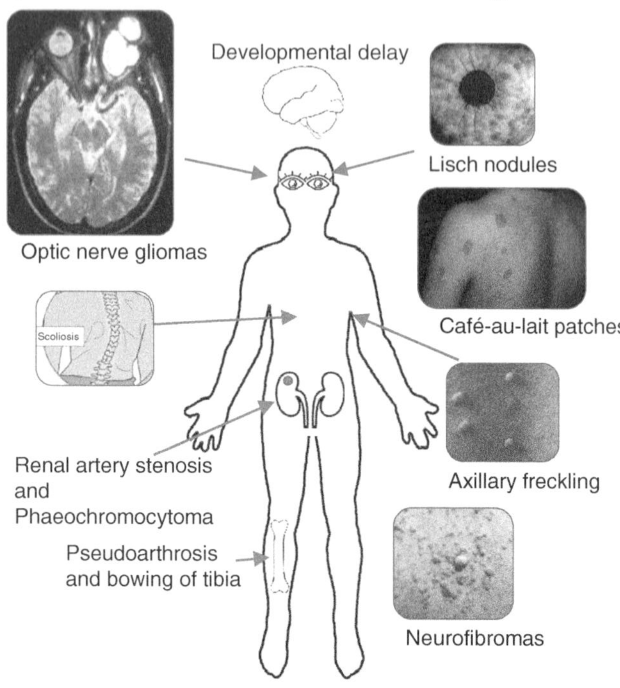

Diagnosis

There are defined diagnostic criteria for NF1 and NF2 (Tables 73.1 and 73.2). Genetic tests are not usually required to confirm a diagnosis but are useful in identifying asymptomatic/at-risk family members and for prenatal counselling/management.

Table 73.1 Diagnostic criteria for Neurofibromatosis type 1.

Neurofibromatosis type 1 diagnostic criteria. Two required for diagnosis
Six of more café-au-lait spots or hyperpigmented macules ≥5 mm and ≥15 mm in pre-pubertal and post-pubertal children, respectively
Axillary or inguinal freckles (>2 freckles)
Optic nerve glioma
Two or more typical neurofibromas or one plexiform neurofibroma
Two or more Lisch nodules or two or more choroidal abnormalities
Sphenoid dysplasia or typical long-bone abnormalities
First-degree relative with NF1

Table 73.2 Diagnostic criteria for neurofibromatosis type 2.

Neurofibromatosis type 2 diagnostic criteria. Any of:
Bilateral vestibular schwannomas
A first-degree relative with NF2 AND • Unilateral vestibular schwannoma OR • Any two of: meningioma, schwannoma, glioma, neurofibroma, posterior subcapsular lenticular opacities
Unilateral vestibular schwannoma AND • Any two of: meningioma, schwannoma, glioma, neurofibroma, posterior subcapsular lenticular opacities
Multiple meningiomas AND • Unilateral vestibular schwannoma OR • Any two of: schwannoma, glioma, neurofibroma, cataract

Management

Many patients with NF1 have few problems, but there is an increased risk of various complications requiring vigilance to screen for tumours and leukaemia. Surgical intervention may be required for pressure symptoms or malignant change. Monitoring includes:

- Annual paediatric review: height, weight, and bone growth
- Assessment of visual acuity and fields, and screening for optic glioma in <7 years.
- Review by educational psychology around school transitions (for learning disabilities)
- Monitoring of blood pressure (for renal artery stenosis and phaeochromocytoma)
- Annual mammogram from 40 to 49 years (due to moderate risk of breast cancer)

Management of NF2 is delivered through specialist multidisciplinary clinics. Specialties involved include audiology, neuroradiology, basal skull, and spinal surgeons, balance teams, specialist nurses, clinical genetics, physiotherapy, and psychology.

Patients with known NF2 or a familial alteration require monitoring via annual audiogram and MRI brain, and spinal MRI every 3–5 years from 10 years of age. Treatment usually involves surgery which can halt disease progression but rarely improves function. Hearing aids are often required. Physiological exercises and cognitive therapies can reduce the distress caused by balance disturbance and tinnitus. An angiogenesis inhibitor, Bevacizumab, is indicated for patients with fast growing tumours.

For both NF1 and NF2, young adults will require education about the variable nature of the disease, and genetic counselling regarding future family planning, prenatal testing, or preimplantation genetic diagnostic testing. For NF1, the internet has many case reports of patients with very severe disease with multiple disfiguring neurofibromas. These are rare but can be upsetting to new patients researching the condition. It is important to stress that a large number of patients with NF1 have relatively few problems.

The future

Numerous novel treatments are currently in trials for treating tumours associated with NF1, including inhibitors of receptor tyrosine kinases that are upstream (capmatinib) or downstream from RAS (MEK inhibitors), and immune-checkpoint inhibitors (e.g. PD-1 and CTLA-4 inhibitors). Following the SPRINT trial, in April 2020, the FDA approved selumetinib (MEK inhibitor) as the first effective treatment for children with NF1 and plexiform neurofibromas that can not be surgically removed. In NF2, further biological therapies are being developed to compliment surgical treatment.

74 Urological cancers

Background

Urological cancers are frequently influenced by environmental factors, but there are rare genetic conditions that may predispose to them. There are four major heritable causes of renal cell carcinoma (RCC): Von Hippel-Lindau syndrome, hereditary leiomyomatosis and renal cell carcinoma (HLRCC), Birt-Hogg-Dubé syndrome, and hereditary papillary renal carcinoma (HPRC). RCC and urothelial cancers are also associated with tuberous sclerosis and Cowden syndrome, Peutz-Jeghers syndrome, Li-Fraumeni syndrome, and Lynch syndrome (Table 74.1).

Genetics

- Pathogenic variants (alterations) in the Krebs cycle gene, fumarate hydratase (*FH* – 1q42.3-43), results in HLRCC; the phenotype is highly variable. Another Krebs cycle gene, SDH (succinate dehydrogenase), is associated with clear-cell renal cancer, phaeochromocytoma, and paragangliomas.
- Birt-Hogg-Dubé is caused by a germline alteration in the folliculin gene (*FLCN – 17p11.2*) and penetrance is high. *FH*, *SDH*, and *FLCN* all act as tumour suppressors and inheritance is AD.
- HPRC is caused by an alteration in the *MET* proto-oncogene (7q31.2), which has high penetrance and AD inheritance.
- Renal tumours are commonly associated with either somatic or inherited deletions/translocations involving the short arm of chromosome 3. Therefore, a karyotype and comparative genomic hybridisation (CGH) of the tumour specimen is recommended.
- **Other urological tumours:**
  - **Wilms tumour** (nephroblastoma) accounts for 6% of paediatric malignancies. Sporadic cases have a very good prognosis. Familial Wilms tumour is uncommon (5%), but can occur as part of heritable syndromes including:
    - Densy-Drash syndrome – rare disorder causing gonadal dysgenesis, mesangial renal sclerosis, and Wilms tumour. Caused by alterations in the tumour suppressor gene Wilms Tumour 1 (*WT1,* on 11p13).
    - WAGR syndrome – Wilms tumour, aniridia (no iris), genitourinary anomalies, and learning difficulty (previously 'retardation', but this is an outdated term). Caused by deletions to chromosome 11p13 (*WT1* and *PAX6* genes).
    - Beckwith-Wiedemann syndrome – overgrowth condition causing hemihypertrophy, macroglossia, visceromegaly, other complications. Caused by variant in Wilms Tumour 2 (*WT2*, chromosome 11p15).
  - **Prostate cancer** is extremely common. Abnormal histology is identified post-mortem in 85% of men >85 years; however, it only contributes to cause of death <10% of these patients. There is considerable clinical challenge regarding early detection and treatment (Figure 74.1), as this is a careful balance between avoiding invasive investigation and unnecessary treatment side effects in cases which will not progress, versus the need for rapid intervention in cases with associated morbidity and mortality. Investigations and treatments can cause anxiety, incontinence, and impotence. Prostate cancer is more common in men of African Caribbean descent, and an affected first-degree relative provides a three-fold increased risk. Known pathogenic genes associated with prostate cancer include *BRCA1*, *BRCA2* and *MMR* genes (Lynch syndrome), and *HOXB13* (chromosome 17, 20-fold increased risk); in these patients annual prostate specific antigen (PSA) screening is recommended from 40 years. PSA monitoring is not of benefit in the absence of a strong family history or specific ancestry. Genome-wide association studies have identified multiple single nucleotide variants associated with prostate cancer; however, the clinical utility of these is unknown. In the future, combined risk scores (lifestyle, family history, single nucleotide variants) will aid risk stratification.
  - **Bladder tumours** rarely have a strong inherited component. Transitional cell carcinomas are occasionally seen in Lynch syndrome, but the majority of tumours have strong environmental components (transitional cell: exposure to dyes/rubber, cyclophosphamide, radiation; squamous: stones/catheters; adenocarcinoma: schistosomiasis).
  - **Testicular tumours** rarely have a Mendelian basis but are more common with positive family history. Cystadenomas are common in Von Hippel-Lindau syndrome; Sertoli-Leydig cell tumours are described in Peutz-Jeghers syndrome.

Pathophysiology

Histologic findings may be pathognomonic of heritable diagnoses. For example, 20% patients with HLRCC develop RCC. Histology typically reveals type 2 papillary RCC, and they tend to be unifocal, aggressive, and metastasise quickly. *Further detail about specific cancers is outlined elsewhere in this chapter.*

Symptoms and clinical features

- Renal cancer has four cardinal features: pain, mass, haematuria, and hypertension. Hypertension alone is not a strong indicator and haematuria is not always an early feature. When haematuria is present in high-risk families, CT urogram is recommended even if not fulfilling the normal 2-week wait criteria due to the high rate of malignancy. There are extra renal manifestations to these conditions (Figure 74.2).
- **RCC with HLRCC:** Multiple and large fibroids occur in women, causing irregular and heavy menstruation, pelvic pain, and complications during pregnancy. Cutaneous leiomyomas are benign papules or nodules.
- Birt-Hogg-Dubé is a hamartomatous disease causing cutaneous hamartomas (fibrofolliculomas) over the face, neck and trunk; pulmonary cysts (predisposing to spontaneous pneumothorax); and RCC in (often multifocal/bilateral, slow-growing, with unusual histology – e.g. hybrid oncocytic tumours.)
- HPRC causes Type 1 papillary RCC, typically bilateral/multifocal, with no known extra-renal manifestations.

Diagnosis

If hereditary renal cancer is suspected, a family history of relevant tumours (with histology) is important; chromosomal or Krebs cycle abnormalities should be considered, and dermatological

Clinical Genetics and Genomics at a Glance, First Edition. Edited by Neeta Lakhani, Kunal Kulkarni, Julian Barwell, Pradeep Vasudevan, and Huw Dorkins.

examination performed. An individual aged <50 years with a renal tumour, or an affected first-degree relative, should be offered genetic counselling and/or testing.

Management

Smoking cessation is key and early detection involves regular abdominal imaging with MRI/CT. Due to its aggressive nature, HLRCC requires annual screening; if a tumour is found, partial nephrectomy is considered, but if there is any doubt over complete removal, a total nephrectomy is preferred. Fibroids may require anti-hormonal medications, analgesia, or surgical removal (myomectomy/hysterectomy). Where possible, cutaneous leiomyomas are managed conservatively.

Screening via MRI/CT can be less frequent in HPRC and Birt-Hogg-Dubé syndrome (2-yearly), and partial nephrectomy is the surgery of choice to preserve renal function. Dermatology input for cryotherapy, surgery, or other interventions may be required for fibrofolliculomas. Pneumothoraces are treated as per standard care.

The future

Improved diagnostic and therapeutic tools (e.g. enhanced imaging such as higher resolution MRI, nanoparticles for drug delivery, wider indications for robotic surgery, tissue engineering) will play a role in improving outcomes for patients with urological cancers.

Table 74.1 Syndromes associated with hereditary renal cell carcinoma.

Syndrome	Gene	Renal cancer type	Other manifestations
Hereditary leiomyomatosis with renal cell carcinoma	*FH*	Papillary – Type 2	Cutaneous leiomyomas Fibroids
Birt-Hogg-Dubé syndrome	*FLCN*	Oncocytic, chromophobe, hybrid	Fibrofolliculomas, lung cysts, pneumothorax
Hereditary papillary renal cancer	*MET*	Papillary – Type 1	
Von-Hippel Lindau syndrome	*VHL*	Clear cell	CNS and retinal haemangioblastomas, phaeochromocytoma, renal cysts, pancreatic lesions
Familial clear-cell renal cancer due to chromosome 3 translocation	*Chr 3*	Clear cell	
Hereditary phaeochromocytoma and paraganglioma	*SDH B/C/D*	Clear cell (distinct phenotype)	Paraganglioma, phaeochromocytoma, gastrointestinal stromal tumour

Figure 74.1 Risk factors for developing prostate cancer GWAS – Genome-wide association study; SNPs - Single nucleotide polymorphisms.

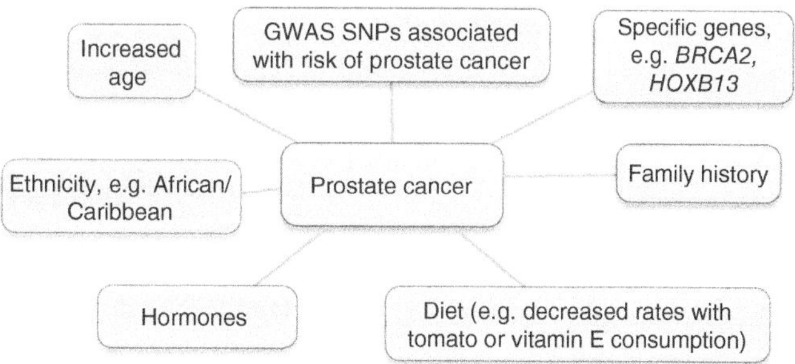

Figure 74.2 Extra-renal manifestations of heritable conditions associated with renal cell carcinoma.

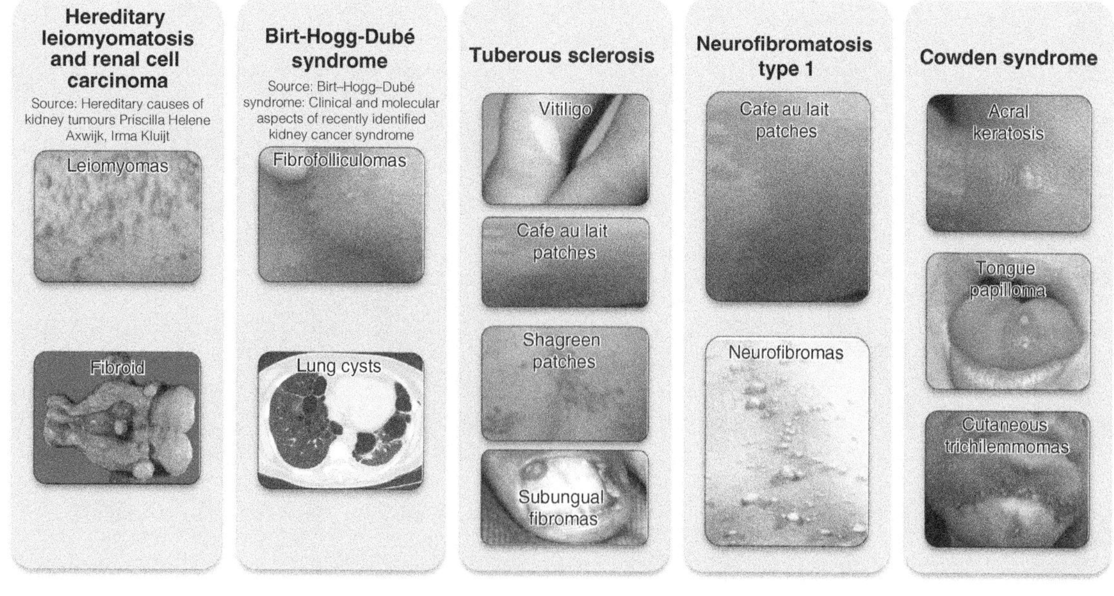

75 Peutz-Jeghers syndrome

Background

Peutz-Jeghers syndrome (PJS) is a cancer predisposition condition characterised by the development of benign neoplasms within the gastrointestinal tract called hamartomatous polyps, significantly increased risk of developing certain types of cancer, and mucocutaneous pigmentation.

Epidemiology

The prevalence of this condition is uncertain; estimates range from 1 in 25 000 to 300 000 individuals. In individuals with PJS, the lifetime risk of developing cancer is as high as 93%.

Genetics

A pathogenic variant (alteration) in the *STK11* gene (*LKB1*) is the most common cause of PJS (located at 19p13.3). It is inherited in an AD fashion; one copy of the altered gene in each cell is sufficient to increase the risk of developing benign polyps and malignant neoplasms, with a 50% risk of passing on the mutation to each offspring (Figure 75.1). Alterations are found in at least 80% of affected families. For the minority of people with PJS that do not have an alteration in the *STK11* gene, the cause of the disorder is unknown. There are no clear genotype–phenotype correlations, although it has been suggested that missense alterations have a greater time-to-first polypectomy or other symptoms than cases of truncating alterations or no detectable alteration. In ~50% of all cases, an affected person inherits an alteration in the *STK11* gene from one affected parent. The remaining cases likely result from new (de novo) alterations in the *STK11* gene.

Figure 75.1 Example pedigree diagram showing family with Peutz-Jeghers syndrome.

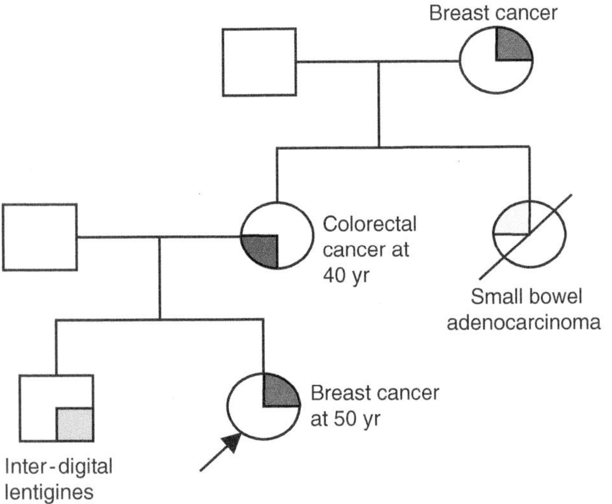

Pathophysiology

The *STK11* gene is a tumour suppressor gene. An alteration in its structure or function disrupts its ability to restrain cell division. *STK11* codes for the enzyme serine/threonine kinase 11, which is important for regulation of cellular polarity, maintaining energy homeostasis, and apoptosis. The resulting uncontrolled cell growth leads to the formation of noncancerous polyps and cancerous tumours in people with PJS. Pathogenic variations in *STK11* are highly penetrant and always show clinical manifestations.

Symptoms and clinical features

- Clinical signs of PJS can be seen in childhood. Features include small, hyperpigmented macular lesions on the lips (Figure 75.2), around and inside the mouth, near the eyes and nostrils, around the anus, and occasionally on the hands and feet (melanocytic macules). They appear during childhood and often fade as the person gets older, but buccal pigmentation often persists into later life.
- Multiple hamartomatous polyps begin to grow in the stomach and intestines during childhood or adolescence (Figure 75.3). Polyps commonly begin to cause symptoms between 10 and 30 years of age and up to 50% of affected people require surgery before the age of 18 years due to a polyp-related complication. Polyps affect the entire gastrointestinal tract but are most prevalent in the small bowel (particularly the jejunum). They have also been reported to grow in the lungs, gallbladder, ureters, and bladder.
- Symptoms from polyps include vomiting, diarrhoea, abdominal pain, intestinal obstruction, bleeding, and associated anaemia. Intussusception – a condition where one section of bowel slides into an adjacent section (see Figure 75.4) – can cause severe pain and intestinal obstruction and requires emergency surgical intervention.
- People with PJS have a very high risk of developing cancer during their lifetime. Cancers of the gastrointestinal tract, pancreas, cervix, ovary, and breast are among the most commonly reported (Table 75.1).

Figure 75.2 Peri-oral lentigines.

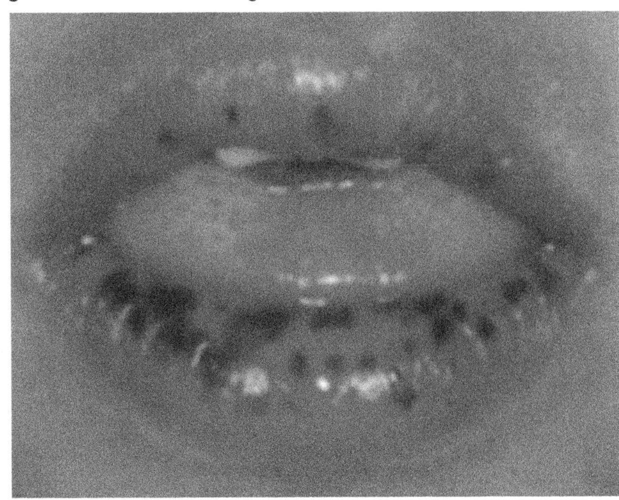

Clinical Genetics and Genomics at a Glance, First Edition. Edited by Neeta Lakhani, Kunal Kulkarni, Julian Barwell, Pradeep Vasudevan, and Huw Dorkins.

Figure 75.3 Large pedunculated polyps in patient with Peutz-Jeghers syndrome.

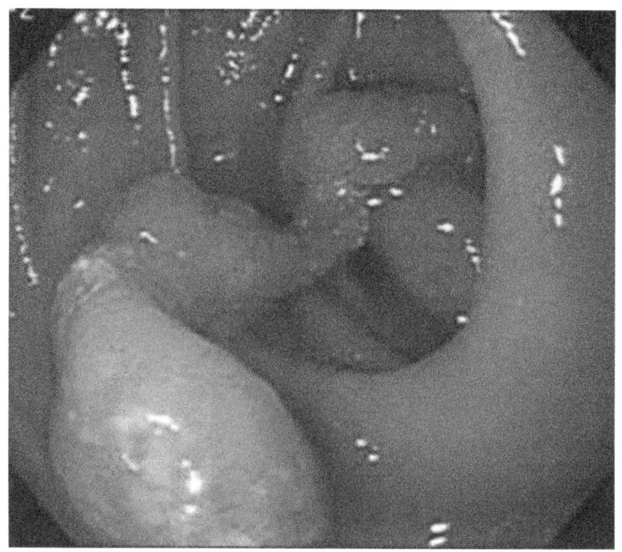

Peutz-Jeghers syndrome associated with renal and gastric cancer that demonstrated an STK11 missense mutation.

Figure 75.4 Intussusception shown via barium enema.

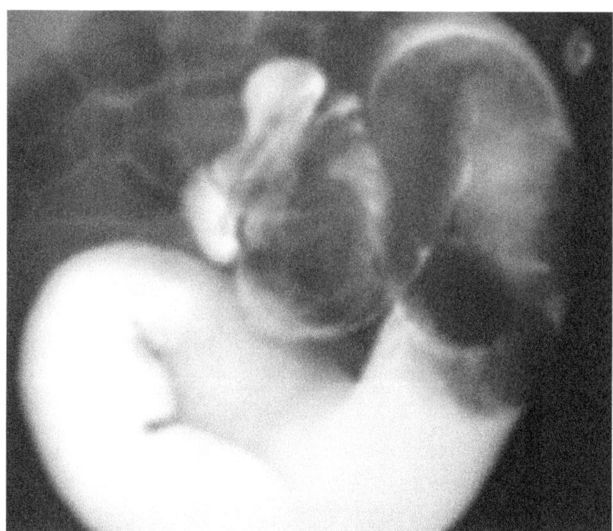

Source: WebMD, LLC.

Table 75.1 Relative and absolute risk of Peutz-Jeghers syndrome associated tumours to age 65.

	Relative risk	Absolute risk (%)
All sites	15	93
Oesophageal	57	0.5
Stomach	213	29
Small bowel	520	13
Large bowel	84	39
Pancreatic	132	36
Breast	25	54
Endometrial	16	9
Cervix	1.5	10
Ovarian sex cord tumours (may be oestrogen secreting)	27	21
Testicular (sertoli)	4.5	9
Lung	17	15

Diagnosis

A clinical diagnosis of PJS can be made if any of the following features are present:

- ≥2 PJS polyps
- Any number of PJS polyps and at ≥1 close relative diagnosed with PJS
- Characteristic hyperpigmented macular lesions and ≥1 close relative diagnosed with PJS
- Any number of PJS polyps and characteristic hyperpigmented lesions

Genetic testing for the identification of pathogenic alterations in the *STK11* gene is recommended if there are characteristic hyperpigmented macular lesions, two PJS polyps found on endoscopy, or a positive family history of PJS.

Management

- There is no definitive cure for PJS. The mainstay of management is surveillance for the development of cancer, removal of large polyps (>1 cm), and symptom control. Investigations are required to establish extent of disease and include upper and lower gastrointestinal endoscopy and small bowel study (MRI or capsule endoscopy), usually started from the age of 8 years.
- Endoscopic polypectomy is performed for removal of polyps >1 cm due to risk of malignant transformation and to reduce side effects of large polyps (intussusception, obstruction, bleeding, and anaemia). Regular screening and polypectomy have been shown to reduce the frequency of emergency surgery and bowel loss.
- Patients with PJS require an extensive screening programme (Table 75.2). If a cancer is found, the treatment is in the standard manner for that particular malignancy. Chemoprotection (e.g. tamoxifen) and risk-reducing mastectomy and hysterectomy with bilateral salpingo-oophorectomy should be discussed with female patients to consider reducing their risk of malignancy.
- For individuals where a pathogenic variant has been identified in an affected family member, prenatal testing and pre-implantation genetic diagnosis is possible.

Table 75.2 Recommended screening for malignancy in patients with Peutz-Jeghers syndrome.

Screening test	Frequency
Full blood count	Annually
Examination of abdomen, pelvis, testes, breasts	Annually
Upper GI endoscopy	3 yearly
Lower GI endoscopy	3 yearly
Small bowel capsule endoscopy or MRI	3 yearly
Breast MRI	Annually from 30 yr
Transvaginal ultrasound and serum CA-125	Annually

The future

There are a few medications that have shown potential in animal models. Celecoxib (COX2 inhibitor) has shown to reduce polyp burden in mice, and mTOR inhibitors (such as rapamycin and everolimus) that inhibit cellular growth and proliferation have also successfully reduced polyp numbers in mice. These may provide future therapeutic interventions for patients with PJS.

76 Von Hippel-Lindau syndrome

Background

Von Hippel-Lindau syndrome (VHL) is a cancer predisposition syndrome that results in malignant and benign neoplasms in various systems of the body. It named after the German ophthalmologist Eugen von Hippel who first described the condition in 1904.

Epidemiology

Prevalence is estimated at around 1 in 53 000 with annual birth incidence of 1 in 36 000. Most (97%) patients have symptoms <65 years of age, with the average age of symptomatic onset being around 26 years.

Genetics

VHL is caused by a pathogenic variant (alteration) within the *VHL* gene at 3p25.3. A small percentage (~3%) have no identifiable alteration. It is inherited in an AD manner with only 20% due to *de novo* mutations. VHL syndrome is an example of the two-hit hypothesis that describes how most tumour suppressor genes require both alleles to be inactivated to cause phenotypic change (see *Retinoblastoma*). While VHL is inherited as AD with one altered gene, as two copies of the *VHL* gene must be altered to cause VHL syndrome, almost all affected individuals eventually acquire an alteration in the second copy of the gene in some cells leading to the features of VHL.

Pathophysiology

More than 370 inherited alterations in the *VHL* gene have been identified in people with VHL syndrome. Mutations in the *VHL* gene inhibit VHL protein production or lead to an abnormal version of the protein. The VHL protein is a classic tumour suppressor; therefore, an altered or missing VHL protein cannot effectively regulate cell survival and division. VHL protein is the key regulator of cellular hypoxia through regulation of HIF (hypoxia-inducible factor). Accumulation of HIF results in enhanced levels of growth factors including vascular endothelial factor, platelet-derived growth factor, and transforming growth factor alpha. Dysregulation of these growth factors result in blood vessel growth (angiogenesis) and uncontrolled cell division leading to the development of cysts and tumours, which can be benign (such as haemangioblastomas) or malignant (such as renal cell carcinoma).

Symptoms and clinical features

VHL syndrome mainly effects three systems: urological, neurological, and endocrine (Figure 76.1). Symptoms and clinical manifestation are determined by the location of the lesions. The presentation is highly variable and can be very distinct even within families; however, four syndrome phenotypes have been described:

- **VHL type 1.** Retinal angioma, central nervous system (CNS) haemangioblastoma, renal cell carcinoma, pancreatic cysts, and neuroendocrine tumours. Characterised by low phaeochromocytoma risk. Truncating or missense pathogenic variants that are predicted to grossly disrupt the folding of the VHL protein are associated with VHL type 1.
- **VHL type 2.** Phaeochromocytoma, retinal angiomas, and CNS haemangioblastoma. It is characterised by a high risk for phaeochromocytoma. Individuals with VHL type 2 commonly have a missense pathogenic variant. VHL type 2 is further subdivided:
  - **Type 2A.** Phaeochromocytoma, retinal angiomas, and CNS haemangioblastoma; low risk for renal cell carcinoma.
  - **Type 2B.** Phaeochromocytoma, retinal angioma, CNS haemangioblastomas, pancreatic cysts, and neuroendocrine tumour with a high risk for renal carcinoma.
  - **Type 2C.** Risk of phaeochromocytoma only.

Diagnosis

VHL syndrome should be suspected in individuals with a family history of VHL, or in patients with any of the common VHL-associated lesions (see Table 76.1). In particular, multiple cysts, retinal/spinal/cerebellar haemangioblastomas, phaeochromocytoma, and renal cell carcinoma in patients under 50 years should be investigated. Diagnosis is via genetic testing. Approaches include single-gene testing, use of a multi-gene panel, and more comprehensive genomic testing with whole-exome or whole-genome sequencing.

Management

There is no universal treatment for VHL, with management involving a MDT approach.

Treatment of manifestations: Surgical intervention is required for most CNS lesions (complete removal of brain and spinal lesions when large or symptomatic). Retinal angiomas may be removed with laser or cryotherapy prospectively; however, optic disc involvement often impedes treatment from being vision-sparing. Renal cell carcinoma requires monitoring and kidney-sparing surgery if/when tumour size or growth is too great. Phaeochromocytomas are removed with partial adrenalectomy when possible. Pancreatic cysts and neuroendocrine tumours should be monitored and may need removal. Endolymphatic sac tumours often require removal to preserve hearing and vestibular function; whilst cystadenomas of the epididymis or broad ligament need treatment when symptomatic or threatening fertility.

Surveillance for prevention of secondary complications: For individuals with VHL syndrome, those with a *VHL* pathogenic variant, and at-risk relatives of unknown genetic status:

- **Starting at age one year:** Annual evaluation for neurologic symptoms, vision problems, and hearing disturbance; annual blood pressure monitoring; annual ophthalmology evaluation.
- **Starting at age five years:** Annual blood or urinary fractionated metanephrines; thin-slice MRI with contrast of the internal auditory canal in those with repeated ear infections.

Clinical Genetics and Genomics at a Glance, First Edition. Edited by Neeta Lakhani, Kunal Kulkarni, Julian Barwell, Pradeep Vasudevan, and Huw Dorkins.

Figure 76.1 Rule of 3 in Von Hippel-Lindau syndrome.

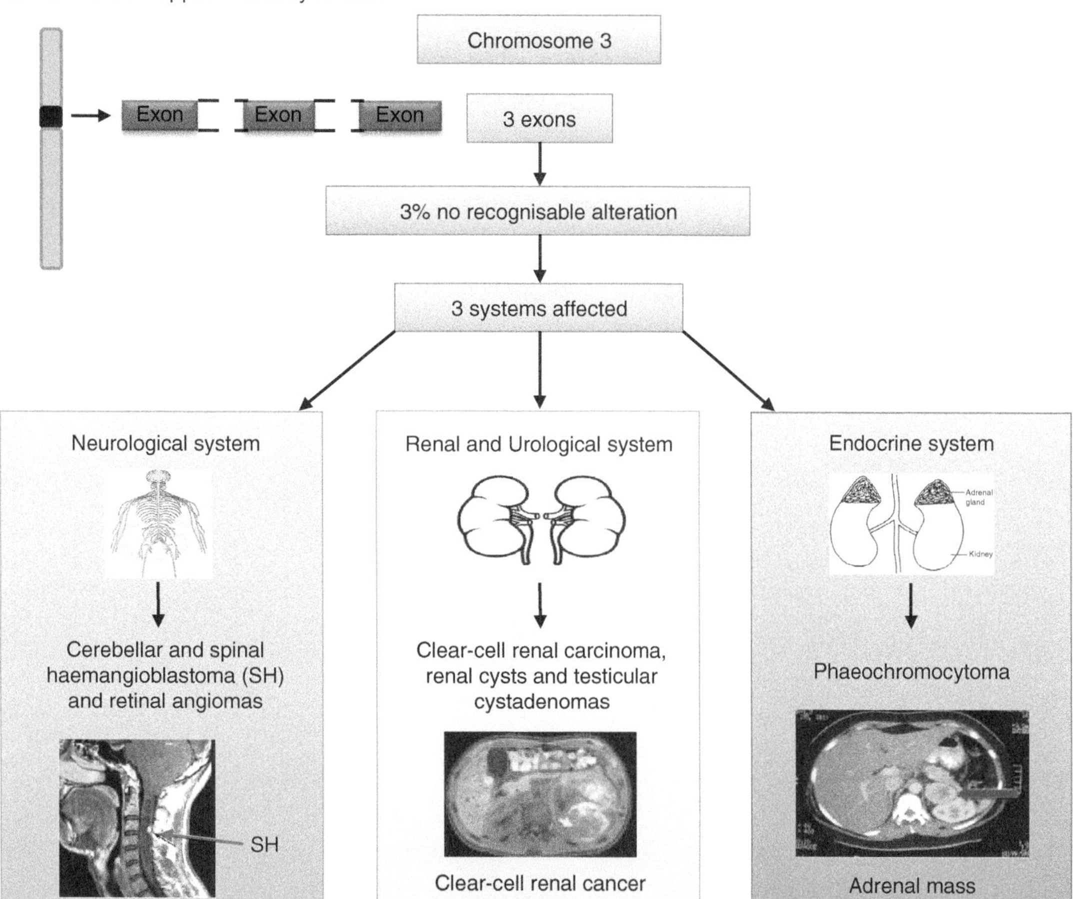

Table 76.1 Common Von Hippel-Lindau associated lesions and symptoms.

Site of Lesion	Symptoms
Retinal haemangioblastomas (frequency: around 60%)	Often the initial manifestation of VHL syndrome. Can cause retinal detachment, glaucoma, macular oedema, and vision loss
Cerebellar haemangioblastomas (up to 70%)	Headache, vomiting, gait disturbances, or ataxia
Spinal haemangioblastomas / related syrinx (up to 50%)	Pain. Sensory and motor loss with cord compression
Renal cell carcinoma (up to 70%)(particularly clear cell) **Multiple renal cysts are very common**	Hypertension, haematuria, mass, abdominal pain. Leading cause of mortality
Phaeochromocytomas (up to 20%)	Can be asymptomatic. Sustained/episodic hypertension, headache, sweating, palpitations
Pancreatic lesions (up to 17%)	Often remain asymptomatic and rarely cause endocrine or exocrine insufficiency. Can cause painless jaundice
Endolymphatic sac tumours (up to 25%)	Hearing loss of varying severity
Cystadenomas of the epididymis (up to 60%)	Rarely cause problems. Bilateral may result in infertility

- Starting at age 11 years: Annual abdominal ultrasound until 16 years.
- Starting at age 16 years: MRI scan of the abdomen annually and MRI of the brain and total spine every one to three years, depending on disease burden.

Pregnancy management: Intensified surveillance for cerebellar haemangioblastoma and phaeochromocytoma during preconception and pregnancy; MRI without contrast of the cerebellum at four months gestation.

The future

There are currently trials investigating tyrosine kinase inhibitors and HIF-2α inhibitors in patients with VHL-associated renal cell carcinoma. Large clinical databases are being formulated that could give more insight into predicting phenotype from the genotype and allow more targeted surveillance and treatments in the future.

77 Inherited bowel cancers

Background

In the United Kingdom, bowel cancer is the third commonest cancer in men and women, with the third highest mortality. There are two common inherited bowel cancer syndromes that account for approximately 3% of all bowel malignancies: Familial adenomatous polyposis (FAP) and Lynch syndrome (also known as hereditary non-polyposis colorectal carcinoma syndrome, HNPCC). Both conditions cause bowel polyps with high malignant potential; regular screening is required. In FAP, the number of polyps is significantly higher and begin developing younger.

Epidemiology

In the general population, 1/14 men and 1/19 women are diagnosed with bowel cancer. Approximately, 10% have a strong inherited component, 5% overall via Mendelian inheritance (Figure 77.1). FAP affects 1 in 10 000, with a nearly 100% lifetime risk of colorectal cancer (CRC). Lynch syndrome is found in 2% of patients with CRC. Those affected have a lifetime risk of 80%, and an associated risk of endometrial cancer (60%), gastric, small bowel, ovarian, urothelial, prostate, pancreatic, and other cancers (Figure 77.2 and Table 77.1).

Genetics

In FAP, and the variant Gardner's syndrome, there is a pathogenic variant (alteration) in *APC* (adenomatous polyposis coli gene, chromosome 5). *De novo* alterations account for 25% of cases, 20% of which display somatic mosaicism (*see Neurofibromatosis*).

Lynch syndrome is caused by the inheritance of an alteration in a mismatch repair gene (MMR): *MLH1* or *MSH2* (90%), *MSH6* (10%), or *PMS2* (rarely). There are some known genotype–phenotype correlations; for example individuals with *MSH6* alterations have lower CRC but higher endometrial cancer risk. Lynch Syndrome is associated with a high risk of ovarian and endometrial adenocarcinoma, that can sometimes have a endometrioid histology. It is also associated with another form of genomic instability called microsatellite instability due to inaccuracy in copying repeat sequences throughout the genome that can cause abnormalities in other cancer driver genes. Finding this in Lynch syndrome tumours can help define potential benefit of 5-FU or immunotherapy.

These are highly penetrant AD conditions. A rare AR type of polyposis syndrome is caused by alterations in the *MUTYH* gene. Other inherited conditions associated with CRC include Peutz-Jeghers, Bloom, and hyperplastic polyposis syndromes.

Table 77.1 Risk of common cancers in Lynch syndrome compared to the general population.

	Risk of cancer in Lynch syndrome	Risk of cancer in the general population
Colorectal cancer in males:		
By 50 yr	45%	
Lifetime risk	80%	7%
Colorectal cancer in females:		
By 50 yr	20%	
Lifetime risk	40%	5%
Endometrial cancer:		
By 50 yr	10%	
Lifetime risk	50%	2%
Gastric cancer	5%	1–2%
Ovarian cancer	10%	1.4%
Pancreatic cancer	2%	1%
Urothelial tract cancer	10%	1–3%
Prostate cancer	10%	5%
Central nervous system	3%	0.7%
Small bowel cancer	1%	<0.003%

Figure 77.1 Proportion of bowel cancer with familial inheritance pattern.

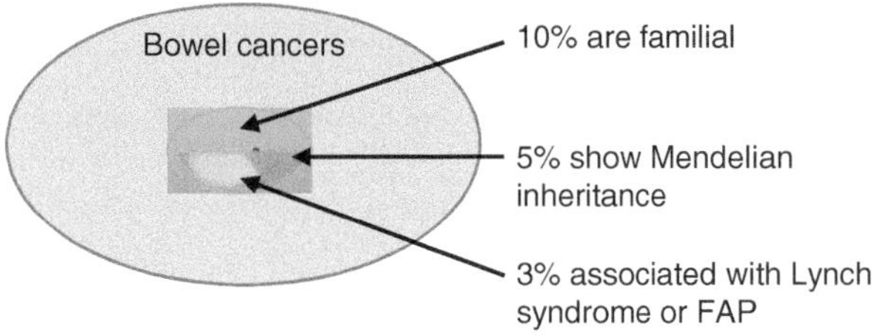

Figure 77.2 Lynch syndrome pedigree with three affected individuals across two generations, and gynaecological tumours.

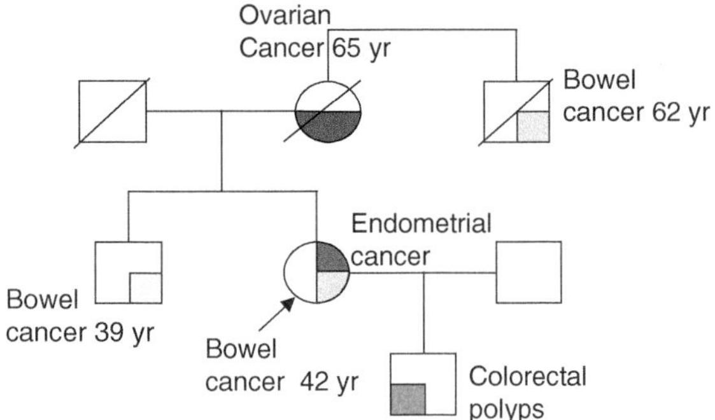

Pathophysiology

Dysfunction of MMR genes implicated in Lynch syndrome lead to the accumulation of alterations across the genome, especially in the microsatellite repetitive sequences (short DNA sequences

Clinical Genetics and Genomics at a Glance, First Edition. Edited by Neeta Lakhani, Kunal Kulkarni, Julian Barwell, Pradeep Vasudevan, and Huw Dorkins.

susceptible to mutations during replication), creating a molecular phenotype termed microsatellite instability (MSI). MSI is evidence of genomic instability and increased risk of carcinogenesis. *APC*, a tumour suppressor, usually controls beta-catenin as part of the WnT signalling pathway preventing cellular proliferation. APC dysfunction results in hundreds to thousands of polyps developing in the bowel and eventually, one or more almost inevitably become malignant.

Symptoms

Adenomas are generally asymptomatic and only cause symptoms if large or bleeding. FAP and sporadic tumours are mostly left-sided, presenting with altered bowel habit and/or rectal bleeding. Lynch syndrome is frequently associated with right-sided bowel tumours as the wider lumen means bowel habits may be unaltered and bleeding hidden within stool; consequently, lesions are easily undetected when curative. Symptoms include weight loss, abdominal discomfort, or anaemia-related (Figure 77.3).

Extraintestinal manifestations: FAP causes congenital hypertrophy of the retinal pigment epithelium (CHRPE) in 50%, which is uncommon in the general population (5%). Patients with Lynch syndrome may develop other tumours; for example irregular menstruation or post-menopausal bleeding in endometrial cancer.

Diagnosis

FAP is diagnosed if endoscopy shows >100 colonic adenomas; attenuated-FAP (less severe subtype with an approximately 70% lifetime risk for CRC) is diagnosed if 10–100 adenomas are found (Figure 77.4). Gardner's syndrome is another variant of FAP associated with osteomas, small bowel desmoid tumours/polyps, gastric tumours, epidermoid cysts, and thyroid cancer (Figure 77.5). *APC* gene mutations are tested to confirm diagnosis and screen at-risk relatives.

Testing for Lynch syndrome was classically arranged if an individual had 1 affected first-degree relative and FAP was excluded, or according to the Amsterdam Criteria (3,2,1 rule) (Figure 77.6):

- ≥3 relatives with Lynch-associated cancer
- across 2 generations
- 1 diagnosed <50 years

Currently, NICE recommends all CRC tumour tissue is assessed for MSI or MMR proteins, and germline testing is offered to those found to be high-risk for Lynch syndrome.

Genetic testing for FAP and Lynch syndrome is recommended for any patient diagnosed with CRC <30 years, or where there is a significant history of additional polyps or family history of similar tumours in accordance with the national test directory.

Figure 77.4 Multiple polyps seen on endoscopy with FAP.

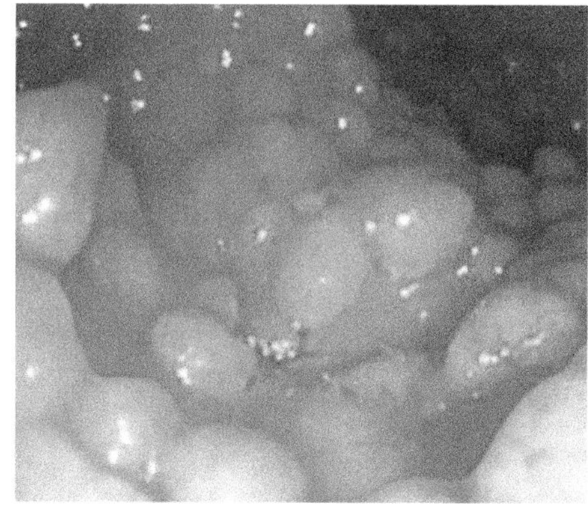

Source: Caoimhin74 / Wikimedia Commons / CC BY-SA 3.0.

Figure 77.5 Features of Gardner syndrome.

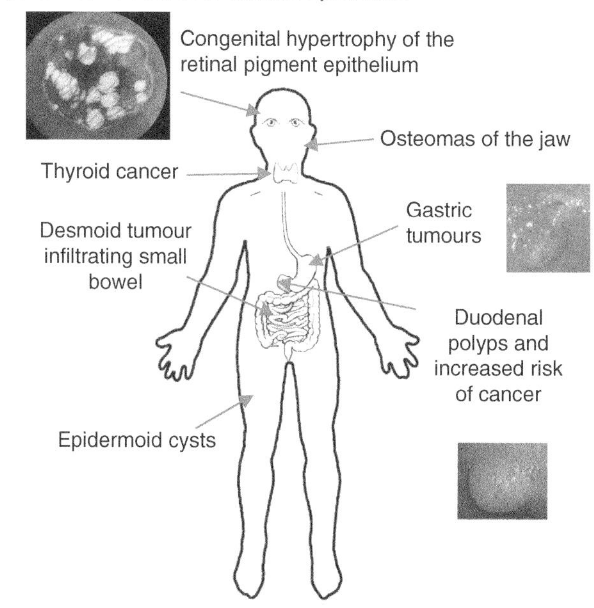

Figure 77.6 Cancers associated with Lynch syndrome.

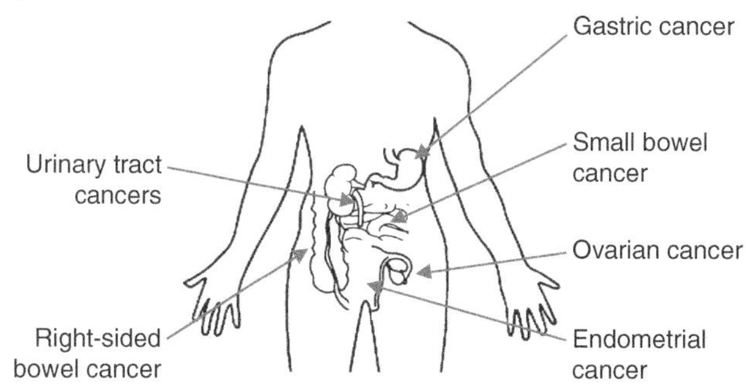

Figure 77.3 Differences in presentation of left- and right-sided bowel tumours.

Right-sided bowel cancer
Associated with Lynch syndrome

- Signs and symptoms of iron-deficiency anaemia
- Weight loss
- Lethargy
- Right-sided abdominal mass
- Occult bleeding
- Abdominal distension and bloating

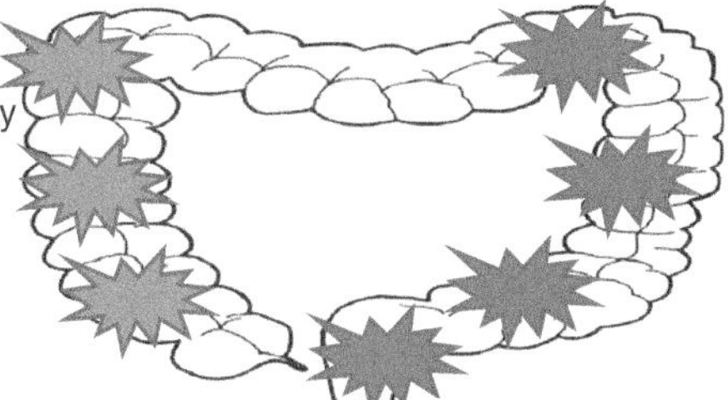

Left-sided bowel cancer
Associated with FAP and sporadic cancers

- Blood in stool
- Change in bowel habits
- Tenesmus
- Left-sided abdominal mass
- Bowel obstruction
- Signs and symptoms of iron-deficiency anaemia
- Weight loss
- Lethargy

Management

Management of FAP and Lynch syndrome involves cascading of risk to relatives, awareness of risk of other tumours, and subsequent screening. Bowel screening leads to an earlier diagnosis of tumours but screening for gynaecological tumours has less evidence; prenatal and pre-implantation genetic diagnosis.

- In Lynch syndrome, regular colonoscopy (1–2 yearly) starting at 25–35 years is recommended. If CRC is detected a subtotal colectomy is often performed. For women, risk-reducing prophylactic hysterectomy and bilateral salpingo-oophorectomy should be discussed after completing their family. Daily aspirin (150–300mg, weight dependent) has been shown to reduce 5-year risk of cancer by 60%, but can worsen asthma, cause gastritis, and increase risk of gastrointestinal bleeding.
- Individuals at risk of or with a confirmed diagnosis of FAP require annual colonoscopy from 10 to 12 years until the polyp load becomes too high for endoscopic removal and surgery is recommended (e.g. colectomy). Upper gastrointestinal endoscopy should take place every 1.5 years from 25 years due to the risk of gastric/duodenal adenomas. Support groups are invaluable.
- In patients with high familial risk but no genetic alteration 5-yearly screening colonoscopy from 40 years is advised; one-off colonoscopy at 55 years is recommended in moderate-risk patients. Current advice in first-degree relatives at risk of familial bowel cancer is to consider daily aspirin.

The future

Studies are ongoing to evaluate the safest effective dose of aspirin for patients with Lynch syndrome and to clarify the benefits and harms. There is also promising research in development of a vaccination against tumour neoantigens, that develop due to MSI, to stimulate an anti-tumour immune response.

78 Inherited upper gastrointestinal cancers

Oesophageal cancer

Oesophageal cancer is the 14th most common adult cancer in the United Kingdom. Prognosis is poor, with 1-year survival of <50%, and 5-year survival of 15%. Oesophageal cancers are mostly due to somatic/acquired genetic variants (alterations) associated with environmental factors. There are two main types: squamous cell carcinoma (SCC), associated with smoking and alcohol, and adenocarcinoma, mainly associated with Barrett's oesophagus (chronic reflux causing mucosal metaplasia). Increased risk is conferred by obesity, poor diet, smoking, achalasia, and Plummer-Vinson syndrome (iron deficiency anaemia and oesophageal webs).

Oesophageal cancers associated with inherited conditions:

- **Tylosis with oesophageal cancer (Howel–Evans syndrome):** Rare AD condition caused by alterations to the *RHBDF2* gene (chromosome 17q25.1). Affected individuals have hyperkeratosis of the palms and soles of the feet, and oral leukoplakia. There is also a greatly increased risk of oesophageal SCC, with regular screening required via upper gastrointestinal endoscopy (Figure 78.1).
- **Bloom syndrome:** Rare AR disorder caused by alterations in the *BLM* gene resulting in striking genomic instability. Associated with low birth weight, failure to thrive, characteristic facial features, telangiectatic rashes, and predisposition to numerous cancers at a young age.
- **Familial Barrett's Oesophagus:** Proposed due to familial clustering of cases. Some candidate genes have been identified but no conclusive single-gene variants yet described.

Gastric cancer

Gastric cancer accounts for around 2% of cancers in the United Kingdom (17th most common cancer), although rates vary worldwide (4x greater incidence in Japan). Most cases are sporadic and risk factors include *Helicobacter pylori* infection, a diet high in smoked/salted/pickled foods, smoking, obesity, and rubber exposure. Direct relatives have a 2- to 3-fold increased risk and 10% of gastric cancers have a familial component. Although some gene changes have been identified, shared environmental factors are often the unifying feature of familial cases. Hereditary AD conditions known to increase gastric cancer risk include hereditary diffuse gastric cancer (HDGC), Lynch syndrome, familial adenomatous polyposis, Li-Fraumeni syndrome, and Peutz-Jeghers syndrome. Individuals with Group A blood type have a 20% increased risk of gastric cancer, but the reason is currently unknown; it may not be due to the blood antigens themselves, but rather the genes that are closely linked with them.

HDGC is caused by an inactivating alteration of E-Cadherin (*CDH1*, chromosome 16), a protein involved in cell-cell adhesion; it functions as a tumour suppressor and, due to its role in adhesion, as an invasion suppressor. HDGC is associated with gastric cancer in 70% (median age 38 years), lobular breast cancers (in 50%) and occasionally cleft lip/palate. Due to the risk of missing early stage diffuse gastric cancers, and the high-risk of developing cancer, patients with *CDH1* alteration are recommended to have prophylactic total gastrectomy (Figure 78.2). Annual endoscopic screening looking for pre-cancerous lesions called signet-cells can help guide the timing of planned surgery. Women require breast cancer screening with annual MRIs from 30 years and may consider risk-reducing mastectomy (Table 78.1).

Figure 78.2 Example pedigree with an inherited E-cadherin alteration (*CDH1*).

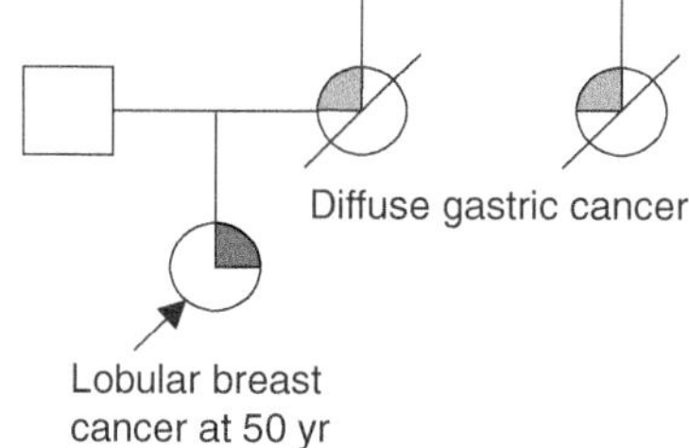

Figure 78.1 Palmoplantar keratoderma (left) and oral leukoplakia (right) seen in Tylosis with oesophageal cancer.

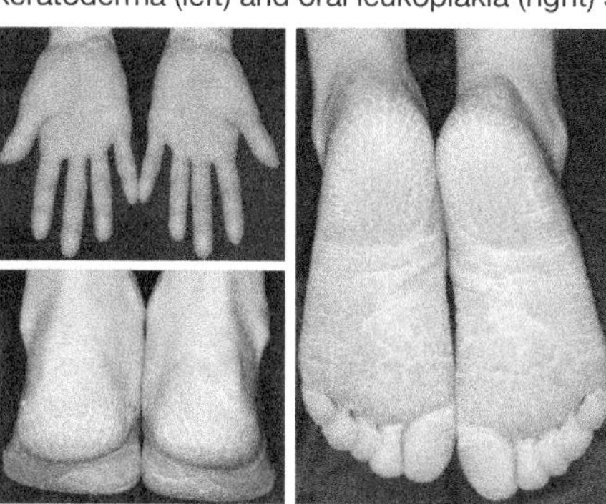

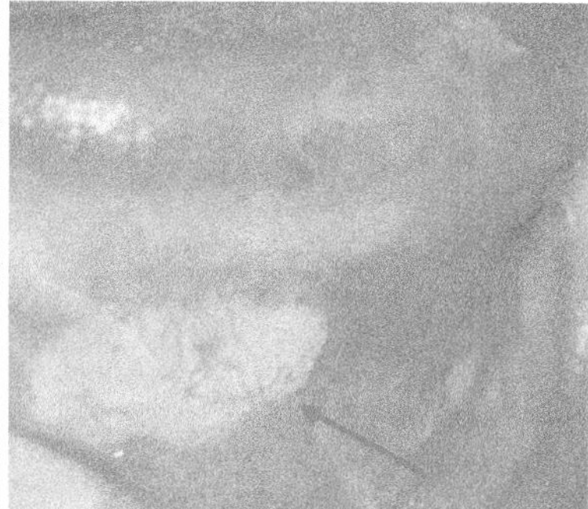

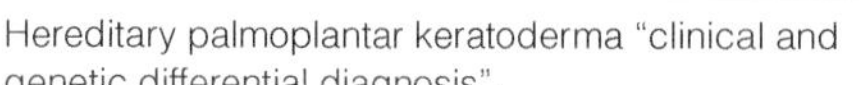
Hereditary palmoplantar keratoderma "clinical and genetic differential diagnosis".

Source: Oral Cancer and Precancerous Lesions.

Clinical Genetics and Genomics at a Glance, First Edition. Edited by Neeta Lakhani, Kunal Kulkarni, Julian Barwell, Pradeep Vasudevan, and Huw Dorkins.

Table 78.1 Genetic screening criteria for hereditary diffuse gastric cancer.

Screening criteria for hereditary diffuse gastric cancer (CDH1)
Families with 2x cases of diffuse gastric cancer among first-/second-degree relatives; one of which was <50 yr
Families with 2x cases of lobular breast cancers among first-/second-degree relatives, with/without diffuse gastric cancer in first-/second-degree relative
Any individual diagnosed with diffuse gastric cancer <35 yr

Liver cancers

The liver is the most frequent site of cancer metastasis. Liver lesions are 40x more likely to be metastatic (commonly bowel, breast, lung cancers) than a primary liver cancer. Hepatocellular carcinoma (HCC) accounts for 2% of cancers. There are cases of familial susceptibility; however, germline monogenic variants have not been established and familial cases are likely multifactorial. The single biggest predisposing factor for HCC is liver cirrhosis (95% of cases progress from cirrhosis). Cirrhosis is an independent risk factor for developing HCC; therefore, as liver disease progresses, so does HCC risk (Figure 78.3).

The biggest causes of cirrhosis are non-alcoholic fatty-liver disease (NAFLD), alcoholic liver disease (ALD), and chronic viral hepatitis infection (Hepatitis C in developed countries and Hepatitis B in developing countries); viral hepatitis particularly predisposes to HCC. These conditions are mostly attributed to environmental factors (diet, exercise, alcohol, blood-borne virus exposure) (Figure 78.4). However, a large degree of inter-individual variability is observed in NAFLD and ALD phenotypic expression – i.e. NAFLD in lean individuals vs. preserved liver function in morbidly obese individuals. Therefore, NAFLD is likely a multifactorial disease caused by a combination of polygenic susceptibility (through genetic modifiers of disease progression and severity) and environmental triggers (Figure 78.5). An example gene found via genome-wide association studies (GWAS) is Patatin-like phospholipase domain-containing protein 3 (*PNPLA3*), which alters adipocyte energy storage/usage and predisposes to NAFLD.

Figure 78.3 CT showing hepatocellular carcinoma.

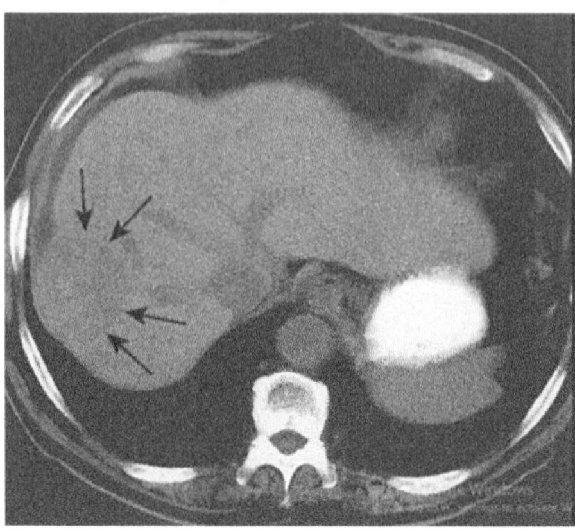

Figure 78.4 Risk factors for hepatocellular carcinoma (HCC).

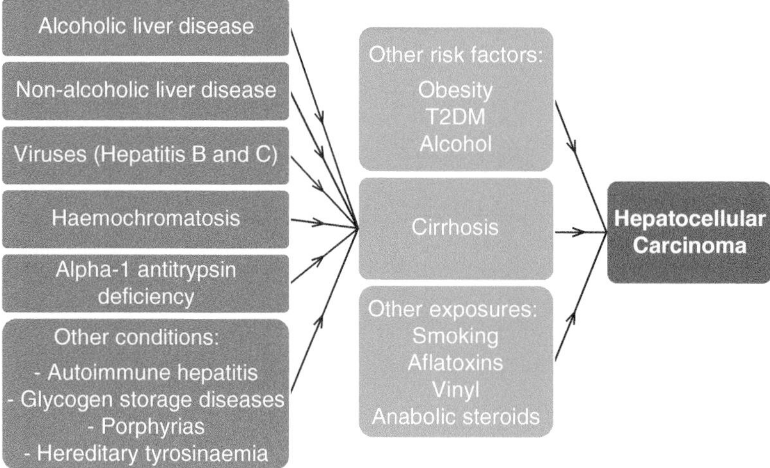

Figure 78.5 Progression of non-alcoholic fatty liver disease.

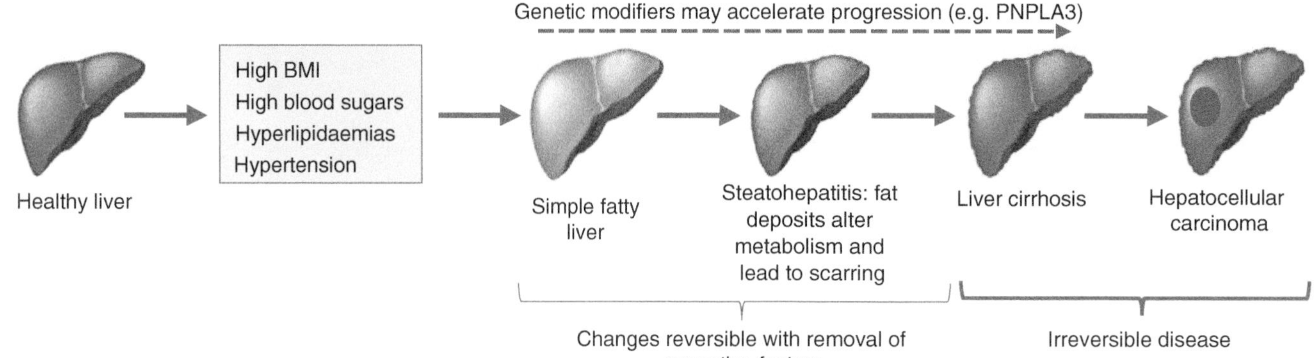

Heritable diseases also lead to liver damage and cirrhosis, including haemochromatosis, alpha-1-antitrypsin deficiency, porphyrias, glycogen storage diseases, and hereditary tyrosinaemia. These conditions indirectly increase the risk of HCC through causing liver damage.

As HCC is multifactorial, it is vital to reduce modifiable risks in patients with familial susceptibility. Patients with any condition that reduces liver function should be counselled to minimise other risks (e.g. alcohol, diet, exercise, diabetic control, smoking). Liver disease caught early is reversible and HCC risk can be reduced. In patients with cirrhosis, 6-monthly alpha fetoprotein (AFP) and ultrasound screening for progression to HCC is required. Surgical resection, radiofrequency ablation, transplant, or systemic pharmacology (chemotherapy) are options.

Pancreatic cancer

The vast majority of pancreatic cancers are sporadic. Inherited genetic variants associated with an increased risk of pancreatic cancer include Peutz-Jeghers syndrome, *BRCA1/BRCA2/PALB2* genes, Lynch syndrome, Li-Fraumeni syndrome, *CDK2NA* linked with melanoma and pancreatic cancer, and familial pancreatic cancers of unknown cause. Patients with early-onset cancers or strong family history require genetic counselling and screening. This is usually invasive (ERCP-endoscopic retrograde cholangiopancreatography) and offered in the United Kingdom through a research project called EUROPAC. It is hoped many inherited cancers will be amenable to screening via tracking of free circulating tumour DNA in plasma. Please see chapter 39 ('Pancreatic cancer') for more details.

79 Inherited breast cancer

Background

Breast cancer is one of the commonest cancers in women. Although germline pathogenic variants (alterations) account for only a small proportion, they can have a major impact on those affected. *BRCA* alterations (breast cancer gene) are the most common high-risk variants, with others including Partner and Localiser of *BRCA2* (*PALB2*), Li-Fraumeni syndrome (high-risk cancer predisposition syndrome), and other moderate-risk genes.

Epidemiology

Lifetime risk in women is 11%. Breast cancer is the second commonest cause of cancer death. 20% of breast cancers have a familial component, but only 5% have a highly penetrant AD gene alteration (Figure 79.1). Women with a *BRCA* alterations have an 80% lifetime risk of breast cancer. Furthermore, 40% of individuals with *BRCA1* and 20% with *BRCA2* alterations develop ovarian cancer; 7% of male breast cancers are associated with *BRCA2* alterations. In addition, 7% of males with *BRCA2* alterations develop breast cancer, and 20% develop prostate cancer (Figure 79.2). The Ashkenazi Jewish community have a particularly high prevalence of *BRCA* alterations due to a *founder effect* (reduced genetic variation caused when a small group establish a new colony).

PALB2 accounts of approximately 0.5% of breast cancers and the lifetime risk of breast cancer in these patients is up to 50%.

Figure 79.1 Proportion of breast cancer associated with familial traits.

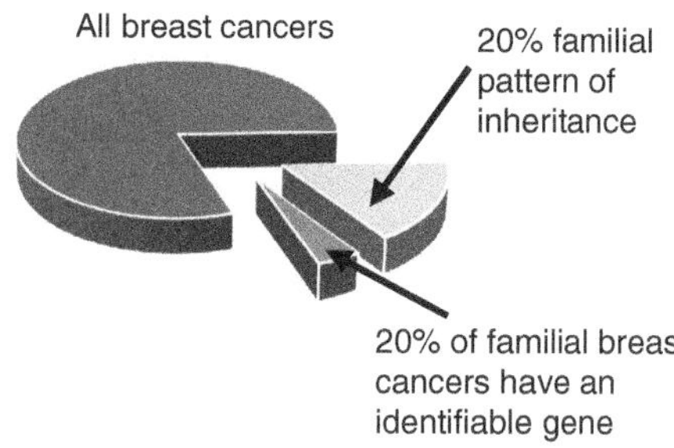

Figure 79.2 Breast cancer and ovarian cancer risk associated with *BRCA* mutation (females).

50% risk by the age of 50
70% risk by the age of 70
80% risk by the age of 80
+ 40% risk of ovarian cancer by the age 80 in *BRCA1*
+ 20% risk of ovarian cancer by the age 80 in *BRCA2*

Li-Fraumeni syndrome affects 1 in 20 000; almost 100% of affected females and 75% of males develop cancer.

Genetics

BRCA1 and *BRCA2* are located on chromosomes 17q21 and 13q13, respectively, and account for over half of known genetic causes of breast cancer. *PALB2* is located on chromosome 16p12. Li-Fraumeni syndrome is caused by a germline alteration in Tumour Protein 53 (*TP53* on 17p13), with 20% of cases caused by *de novo* alterations. *BRCA1*, BRCA2, *PALB2,* and *TP53* are AD tumour suppressor genes.

Peutz-Jeghers (*STK11*), Cowden syndrome (*PTEN*), and neurofibromatosis (*NF*) predispose to breast cancer. Moderate-risk breast cancer susceptibility genes such as *RAD51C, CHEK2*, and *ATM* (ataxia telangiectasia) are also tested in appropriate cases. The E-cadherin gene (*CDH1*) is associated with 50% lifetime risk of lobular breast cancer (and diffuse gastric cancers) (Figures 79.3 and 79.4).

Additionally, high grade serous ovarian cancer can be a feature of germline or somatic alterations in the *BRCA1* or *BRCA2*, as well as germline *PALB2* genes. These tumours often display a characteristic type of genomic instability associated with chromosomal rearrangements, shortening of the end of the chromosomes (telomeres) and loss of the second copy of tumour suppressor genes (called loss of heterozygosity). This genomic instability, called homologous recombination deficiency, is a form of functional genomics and helps define predicted response to drugs that induce double strand breaks in the DNA by impacting on base excision repair.

Figure 79.3 Pedigree showing **high-risk** breast cancer (Three diagnoses with average age <60 years). BC = breast cancer.

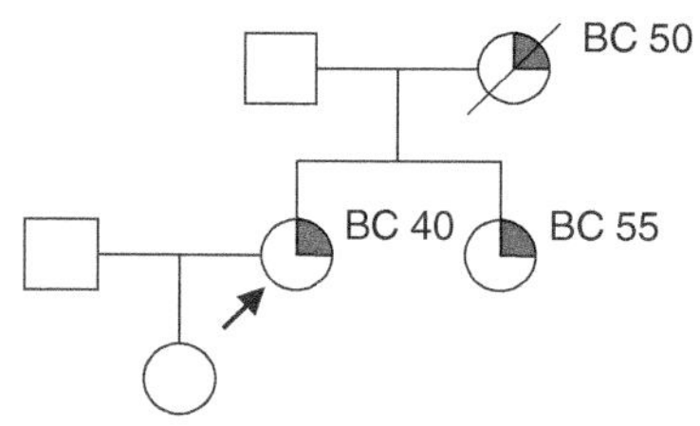

Figure 79.4 Pedigree showing **moderate-risk** family history of breast cancer with two affected relatives with an average age >50 years. BC = breast cancer

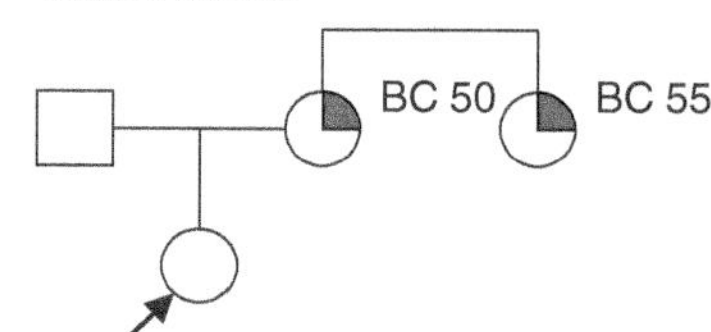

Clinical Genetics and Genomics at a Glance, First Edition. Edited by Neeta Lakhani, Kunal Kulkarni, Julian Barwell, Pradeep Vasudevan, and Huw Dorkins.

Figure 79.5 *BRCA1* and *2* maintain the genomic stability by facilitating double strand break repair through detection and recruitment of other proteins.

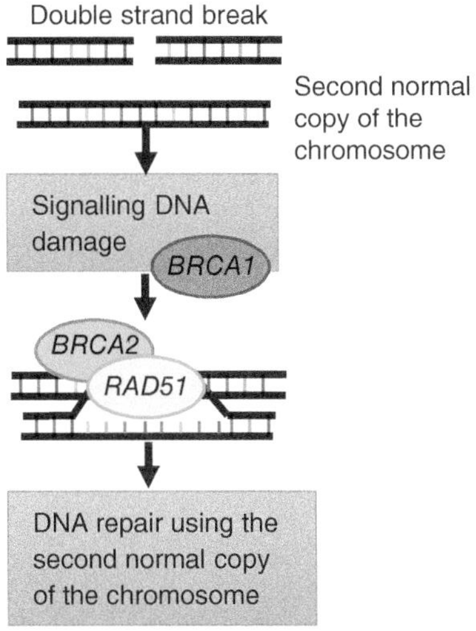

Figure 79.6 Outcomes of double strand break.

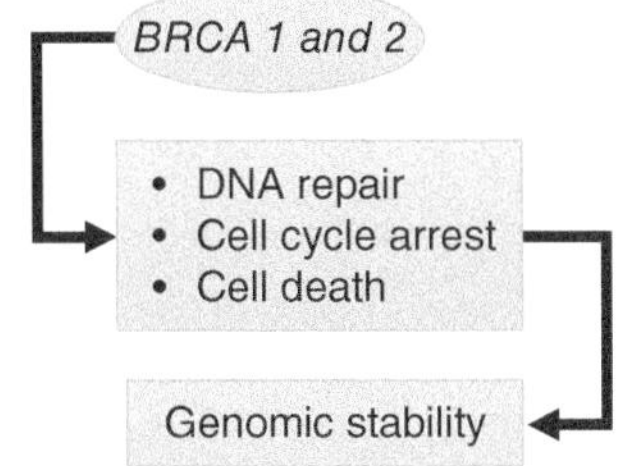

Pathophysiology

BRCA1 and *BRCA2* are important in post-replication DNA repair after a double-strand break, initiating cell cycle arrest or cell death to maintain genomic stability (Figures 79.5 and 79.6). *PALB2* has an important role in *BRCA2* caretaker functions and interacts with *BRCA1*, functioning as a tumour suppressor. *TP53* has been described as the 'Guardian of the Genome' due to crucial roles in activating DNA repair, arresting cell growth by holding the cell in G1 phase, initiating apoptosis, and cell senescence. Loss of *BRCA1*, *BRCA2*, *PALB2*, or *TP53* function increases genomic instability and risk of malignant progression.

Clinical features

BRCA alterations are associated with breast, ovarian, prostate, pancreatic, and lung cancers. Features of breast cancer include breast lump, nipple discharge or inversion, skin changes or pain. Ovarian cancer is often asymptomatic and presents late, with non-specific symptoms of weight loss, abdominal discomfort or bloating.

In Li-Fraumeni syndrome, there is a strong family history of various cancers at young ages (<45 years), in particular sarcomas and breast cancers (see Figure 79.7). Sarcomas can present with pain, a mass, or pressure effects (e.g. compression of peripheral nerves) (Figure 79.7).

Diagnosis

In all patients with breast cancer, a family history should be taken to make a risk assessment for hereditary causes (via the Manchester Scoring System CanRisk or BOADICEA). If there is >10% risk of finding an alteration, then *BRCA1* and *BRCA2* screening should be performed (Figure 79.8). Other genetic tests are considered depending upon family history (e.g. sarcomas, *TP53*). In practice, certain diagnoses trigger a genetic screen due to an accepted >10% risk of alteration, with examples including triple-receptor negative breast cancer in individuals <60 years, and high-grade serous ovarian cancers.

Figure 79.7 Cancers most commonly associated with Li-Fraumeni syndrome.

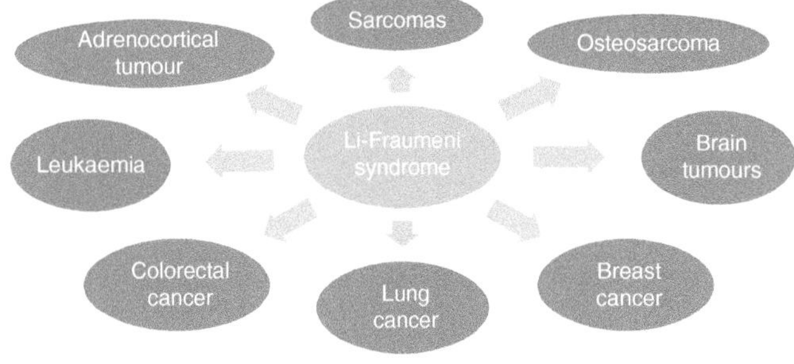

Management

For patients with breast cancer or familial disease, management options include environmental adjustments, screening, pharmacology, or surgery to reduce future risk.

- **Environmental factors:** Hormone replacement therapy increases the risk of breast and ovarian cancer; whereas the combined oral contraceptive pill protects against ovarian cancer but increases breast cancer risk – this should be included in contraceptive counselling. Non-smoking, reduced alcohol consumption, healthy weight, and physical activity should be encouraged.
- **Screening:** All women should be taught 'breast awareness' to encourage regular self-screening. Women at increased risk of breast cancer should have increased surveillance prior and in addition to national screening (Figure 79.8); patients with *BRCA* and *TP53* pathogenic variants require annual MRIs from between 25–30 years and 20 years, respectively.
- **Pharmacology and surgery:** Chemoprevention (tamoxifen) decreases cancer risk (up to 50%) in high-risk patients without breast cancer (e.g. *BRCA* positive), side effects include thromboembolic disease, and endometrial cancer. Risk-reducing prophylactic bilateral mastectomy is the most effective strategy for reducing breast cancer risk (>90% reduction) and should be offered to high-risk patients with the option for breast reconstruction and psychological support. Risk-reducing bilateral salpingo-oophorectomy also significantly reduces ovarian cancer risk, albeit at the cost of surgically induced menopause.
- In patients with breast cancer, a genetic diagnosis influences immediate management decisions: full mastectomy may be preferred to lumpectomy, and PARP-inhibitors (poly (ADP-ribose) polymerase) may be used; these are recently licensed for use in patients with advanced *BRCA*-associated breast cancer and platinum-responsive epithelial ovarian cancers.
- For patients planning a family, pre-implantation genetic diagnosis (PGD) and pre-natal testing are available for *BRCA* and *TP53* genes to reduce inheritance risk.

The future

Studies further assessing the use of PARP-inhibitors in *BRCA*-positive cancers are underway. More sophisticated models are being developed that utilise genomic data (from gene panels to single nucleotide polymorphisms), environmental factors, medications, family history, amongst other sources, to generate personalised risk and management strategies.

Figure 79.8 Approach to genetic diagnosis and management in breast cancer.

STEP 1 Take a three generational family history of cancer of maternal AND paternal line. Ask specifically about red flags:

- Strong family history of breast cancer
- Family history of *BRCA1* or *BRCA2* mutation
- Male breast cancer
- Ashkenazi Jewish descent
- Ovarian cancer
- Early onset or bilateral breast cancer
- Hormone negative breast cancer

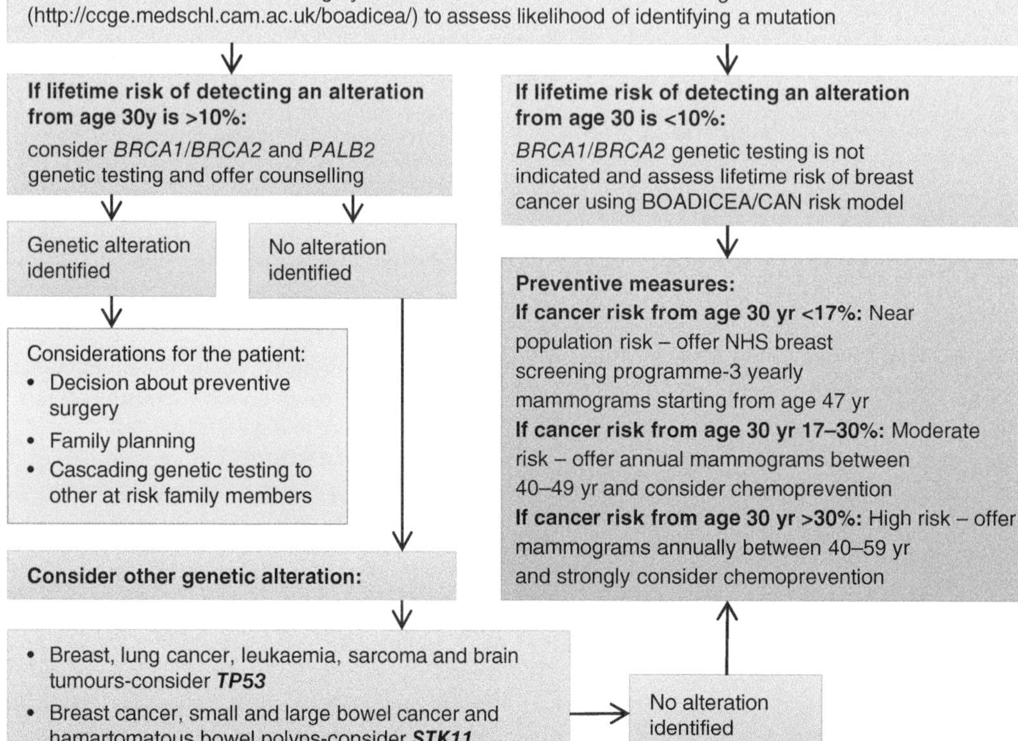

STEP 2 Use Manchester Scoring system or BOADICEA/CAN risk modelling software (http://ccge.medschl.cam.ac.uk/boadicea/) to assess likelihood of identifying a mutation
If lifetime risk of detecting an alteration from age 30y is >10%:
consider BRCA1/BRCA2 and PALB2 genetic testing and offer counselling
Genetic alteration identified
No alteration identified
Considerations for the patient:
• Decision about preventive surgery
• Family planning
• Cascading genetic testing to other at risk family members
Consider other genetic alteration:
• Breast, lung cancer, leukaemia, sarcoma and brain tumours-consider TP53
• Breast cancer, small and large bowel cancer and hamartomatous bowel polyps-consider STK11
• If breast, thyroid, and uterine consider PTEN
No alteration identified
If lifetime risk of detecting an alteration from age 30 is <10%:
BRCA1/BRCA2 genetic testing is not indicated and assess lifetime risk of breast cancer using BOADICEA/CAN risk model
Preventive measures:
If cancer risk from age 30 yr <17%: Near population risk – offer NHS breast screening programme-3 yearly mammograms starting from age 47 yr
If cancer risk from age 30 yr 17–30%: Moderate risk – offer annual mammograms between 40–49 yr and consider chemoprevention
If cancer risk from age 30 yr >30%: High risk – offer mammograms annually between 40–59 yr and strongly consider chemoprevention

80 Retinoblastoma

Background

Retinoblastoma is a rare malignancy of the retina affecting infants. Patients usually have an excellent prognosis, but there is a risk of visual loss. Retinoblastoma was famously investigated by Dr Alfred Knudson who described the 'two-hit hypothesis' that explains the incidence of many hereditary cancers. Furthermore, the implicated *RB1* gene was the first identified tumour suppressor gene.

Epidemiology

Retinoblastoma is rare, but accounts for 3% of childhood malignancies. Incidence is 1 in every 15 000–20 000 live births. Approximately 67% of children are symptomatic <2 years and more than 90% of affected patients are symptomatic <5 years.

Genetics

- The affected gene is *RB1* (13q14); 60% of cases of retinoblastoma are caused by somatic alterations after fertilisation and are not inherited from parents; these are almost always unilateral. The remaining 40% of cases are hereditary and 85% affect both eyes, with 40% developing a further malignancy later in life.
- Hereditary retinoblastoma is AD. In 25% of hereditary cases, the *RB1* pathogenic variant (alteration) is passed down from a parent, the offspring then have a 50% chance of inheriting the gene, and 45% chance of presenting with the retinoblastoma phenotype (due to 90% penetrance). In the other 75% of hereditary cases, the first alteration occurs randomly in a germline cell; in these cases, siblings are unlikely to be affected, but the affected individual may pass the gene onto their offspring.
- **Two-hit hypothesis:** Dr Knudson noticed children with retinoblastoma earlier in life tended to have a positive family history and developed bilateral and multiple disease, in contrast to children who developed retinoblastoma later in life. From this clinical observation, he hypothesised that cells must carry two copies of a gene that prevent tumours (tumour suppressor genes) and for a tumour to occur, an alteration must occur in both copies. These alterations may be inherited or *de novo*. If an individual inherits an alteration in one copy of the gene ('first hit'), then it would only take one cell to randomly develop a somatic mutation ('second hit'), for carcinogenesis to occur. This could be a frequent event and therefore multiple tumours could result. Those who develop a cancer without inherited alterations require two random alterations in the same cell (two hits); this is likely to be uncommon, occur later in life, and the risk of developing multiple tumours by chance is extremely rare (Figure 80.1).

Pathophysiology

RB1 is a tumour suppressor gene. *RB1* encodes the Rb protein which prevents excessive cell growth by binding to and inhibiting E2F, preventing cell cycle progression from G1 (first gap phase) to S phase (synthesis). When DNA is checked for errors and the cell is ready to enter S phase complexes of cyclin and cyclin-dependent kinases (CDK) phosphorylate Rb allowing E2F to dissociate and activate other cyclins to push the cell into S phase. Rb dysfunction leads to dysregulated cell cycle activity, resulting in chromosomal instability, prevention of cellular senescence, and greater risk of carcinogenesis (Figure 80.2).

Symptoms and clinical features

- Retinoblastomas are usually painless and children rarely complain of vision loss (regardless of progressive vision lost). The cardinal presenting sign is leukocoria (white pupil). Strabismus (squint) is also common and can occur prior to leukocoria (Figure 80.3). The eye can become inflamed and swollen, or the pupil can change size (anisocoria) or colour (heterochromia). Less common features include nystagmus, vitreous haemorrhage or resultant hyphaema (blood between cornea and iris), cataract, and glaucoma (Figure 80.4).
- Retinoblastomas can spread locally (extraocular involvement) or metastasise. Signs and symptoms depend on the location, but can cause failure to thrive, vomiting, headaches, and neurological impairment.
- *RB1* is a tumour suppressor, so affected patients are at an increased risk of developing other tumours (19% by 35 years, and a 40% life-long risk). Most common second cancers are sarcomas (particularly osteosarcoma, relative risk up to 500-fold), lung cancer, melanoma, and pineoblastoma/supra-sellar tumours (termed 'trilateral retinoblastoma') (Figure 80.5).

Diagnosis

Retinoblastoma is a clinical diagnosis via ophthalmoscopy. A complete fundoscopic examination of the eye in children may require examination under general anaesthesia. Ultrasound and MRI can reveal extraocular involvement. Genetic testing for the *RB1* alteration is offered to all patients and their families regardless of family history.

As tumour sequencing has become more widely available, it is important to offer this even in unilateral disease. This can help identify alterations within the tumour, which are actually present at undetectable levels in the blood due to mosaicism. Given this, when designing screening plans for at-risk new-born relatives, the family history, germline, and somatic genetic results should be discussed with a specialist centre.

Clinical Genetics and Genomics at a Glance, First Edition. Edited by Neeta Lakhani, Kunal Kulkarni, Julian Barwell, Pradeep Vasudevan, and Huw Dorkins.

Figure 80.1 **Two hit hypothesis;** two mutations are required for loss of gene function. If an individual inherits a single mutation, they are at an increased risk of retinoblastoma as acquiring a second mutation will lead to loss of the tumour suppressor gene.

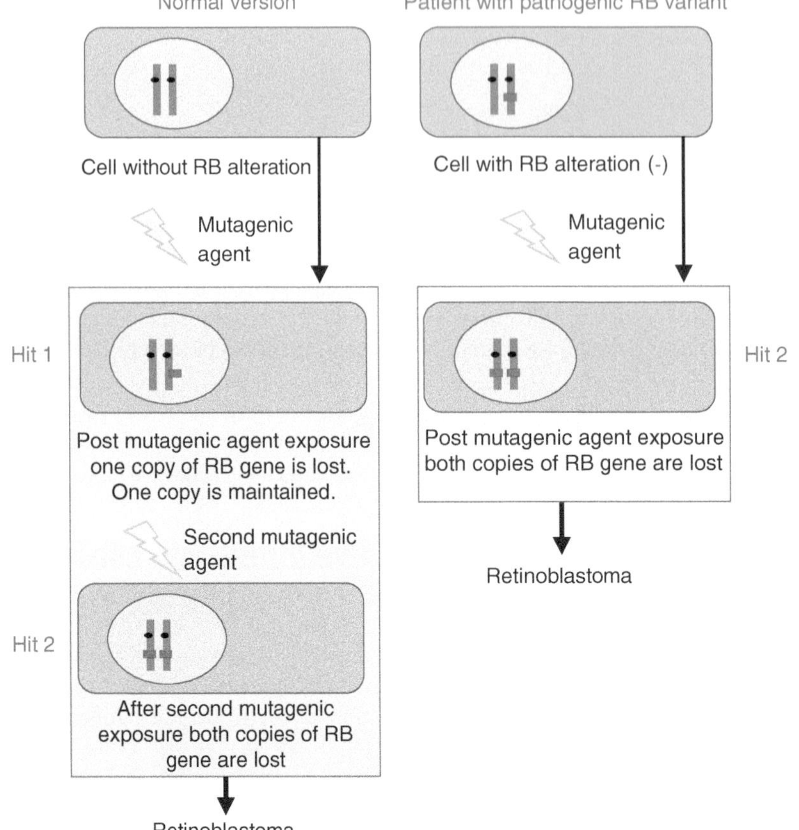
Normal version
Patient with pathogenic RB variant
Cell without RB alteration
Cell with RB alteration (-)
Mutagenic agent
Mutagenic agent
Hit 1
Hit 2
Post mutagenic agent exposure one copy of RB gene is lost. One copy is maintained.
Post mutagenic agent exposure both copies of RB gene are lost
Second mutagenic agent
Retinoblastoma
Hit 2
After second mutagenic exposure both copies of RB gene are lost
Retinoblastoma

Figure 80.2 Role of the retinoblastoma (Rb) protein in cell cycle; The Rb protein acts as a tumour suppressor gene preventing the cell progressing beyond growth 1 phase unless no errors are identified.

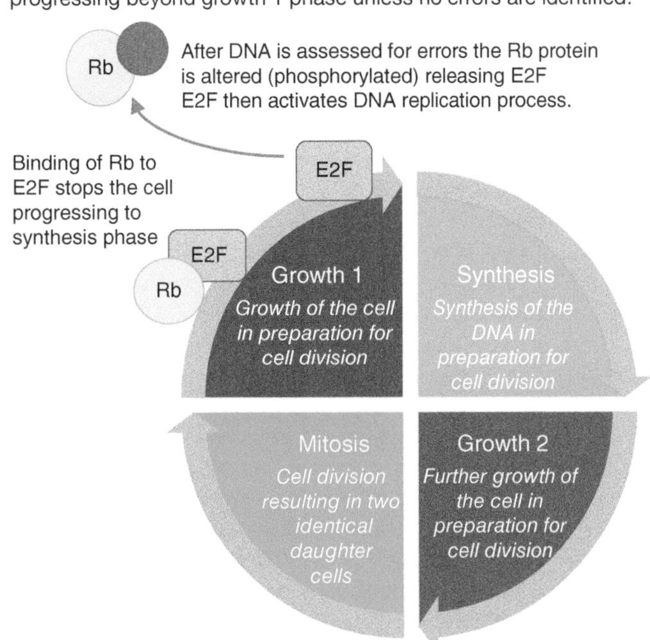
Rb
After DNA is assessed for errors the Rb protein is altered (phosphorylated) releasing E2F
E2F then activates DNA replication process.
Binding of Rb to E2F stops the cell progressing to synthesis phase
E2F
E2F
Rb
Growth 1
Growth of the cell in preparation for cell division
Synthesis
Synthesis of the DNA in preparation for cell division
Mitosis
Cell division resulting in two identical daughter cells
Growth 2
Further growth of the cell in preparation for cell division

Figure 80.3 Fundoscopic images of retinoblastoma.

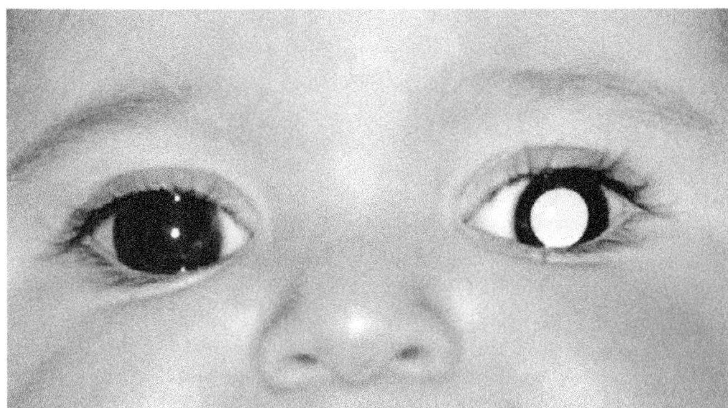

Source: Jane Olver et al. 2014, p. 76 / with permission of John Wiley and Sons.

Management

- Non-surgical treatments are used successful, either independently or in combination. Options include laser treatments, systemic chemotherapy, cryotherapy, brachytherapy, or local chemotherapy using intra-arterial/intra-vitreous delivery. Enucleation (removal of the eye) is required in large unilateral

Figure 80.4 Signs of retinoblastoma.

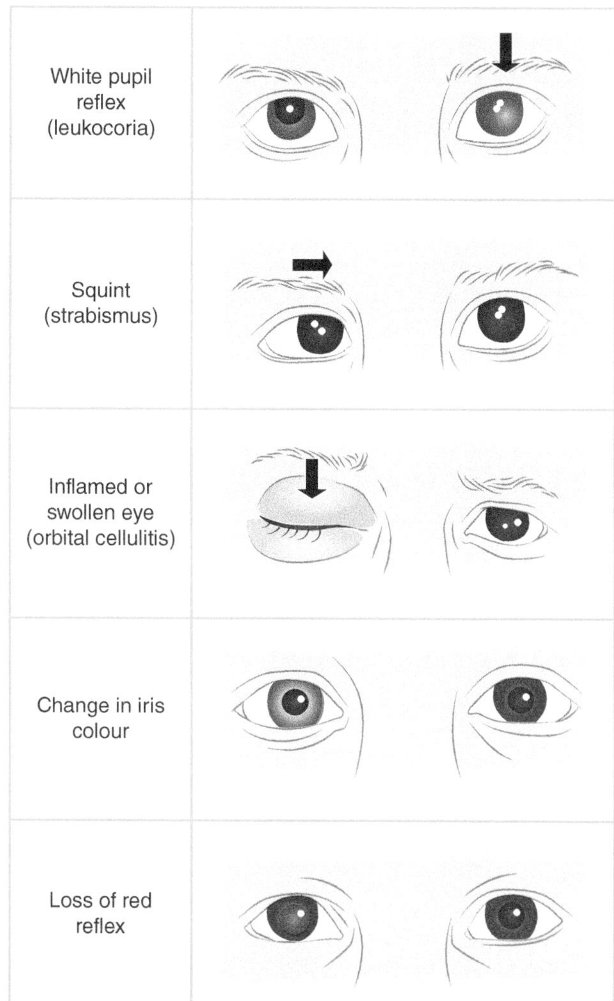

Figure 80.5 Common cancers associated with *RB1* gene alteration.

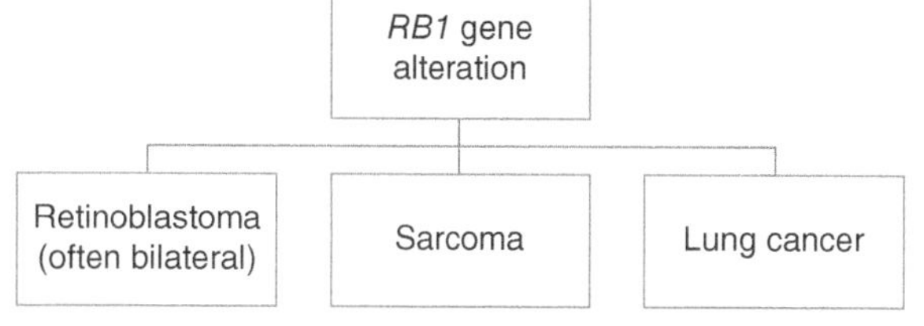

Figure 80.6 Process of pre-implantation genetic diagnosis (PGD).

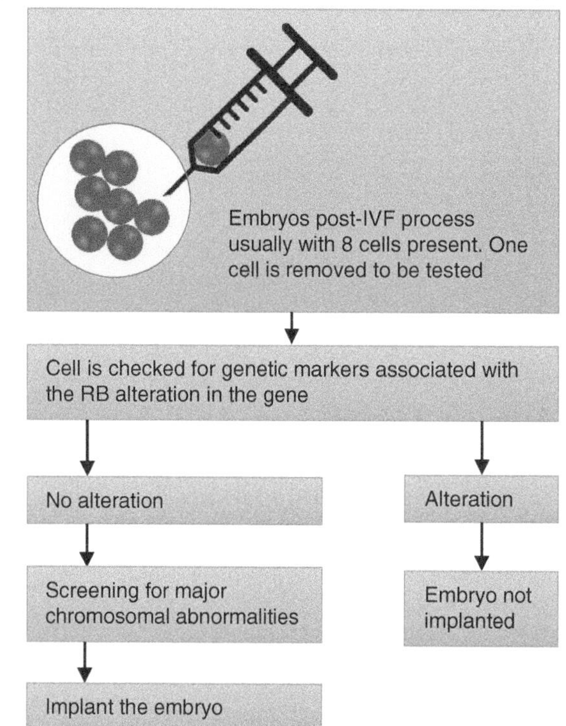

retinoblastomas. Prognosis is excellent; visual prognosis is determined by tumour size and location, with eye preservation often possible with early diagnosis. Metastasis can be rapid and fatal; this is unfortunately more common in lower income countries.

- Infants at risk of inheriting or known to have the *RB1* gene alteration have weekly retinal screening by an experienced ophthalmologist, with screening frequency gradually reduced over the first five years of life.
- A molecular diagnosis of a *RB1* gene alteration provides two main advantages. Firstly, screening at-risk individuals enables earlier diagnosis and treatment that could save vision. Secondly, family-planning advice is offered to reduce the risk of offspring developing retinoblastoma, usually through pre-implantation genetic diagnosis (PGD). PGD involves *in vitro* fertilisation (IVF) techniques and single-cell screening to select an embryo without the *RB1* alteration (Figure 80.6).

The future

Improved chemotherapy regimens continue to be investigated, alongside the use of stem cell transplant. Newer radiation therapy techniques, including intensity modulated radiation therapy and proton beam therapy may help reduce secondary side effects of treatment on adjacent tissues. Other tissue-sparing techniques are also being investigated, including crytotherapy and laser (photocoagulation/thermotherapy). Finally, oncolytic virus therapy is a more novel option under investigation, using a modified virus to target cells without the functioning *RB1* gene.

Multiple endocrine neoplasia

Background

The term multiple endocrine neoplasia (MEN) describes a group of rare neuroendocrine cancer conditions. Affected individuals have a predisposition to multiple cancers in specific neuroendocrine tissues due to a genetic alteration. MEN1 and MEN2 are aetiologically distinct conditions, and MEN2 is further subdivided into MEN2A and MEN2B.

Epidemiology

MEN1 affects between 1 in 20 000 and 40 000 people. MEN2 has a prevalence of 1 in 35 000, of which 95% are the MEN2A subtype and <5% are MEN2B.

Genetics

MEN1 is caused by alterations in the *MEN1* gene (11q13), which encodes for the tumour suppressor nuclear protein menin. MEN1 has AD inheritance and nearly 100% penetrance. There are no known genotype-phenotype correlations.

MEN2 is caused by a pathogenic variant (alteration) in the *RET* gene located on chromosome 10 (10q11.2) containing 21 exons. Genotype-phenotypes correlations have been described: alterations in different exons of the *RET* oncogene are associated with different syndromes, MEN2A is associated with alterations in exons 10 and 11, whereas MEN2B is associated with exons 15 and 16. Transmission is also AD.

Pathophysiology

In MEN1, the two-hit hypothesis can be applied. Although the exact function of menin is unknown, an additional somatic alteration is required to result in carcinogenesis. The resulting neoplasms are usually benign but have endocrine (e.g. hypercalcaemia) and mass effects.

In contrast, MEN2 is caused by the *RET* proto-oncogene that encodes for a membrane tyrosine kinase receptor. This alteration results in *gain* in function (as opposed to *loss* of function with MEN1) leading to uncontrolled growth of cells and tumour formation in affected organs.

Symptoms and clinical features (Table 81.1)

- **MEN1:** The main three features in are primary hyperparathyroidism (90%), pancreatic tumours (70%), and pituitary adenomas (30%) (3Ps) (Figure 81.1). Hypercalcaemia is the most common presenting sign due to hyperplasia of the parathyroid glands. Gastrinomas and insulinomas are the most common pancreatic endocrine tumours. Pituitary adenomas can cause mass effects (headache, bitemporal hemianopia), with other symptoms dependant on the area of the pituitary affected. Prolactinomas are most common, although acromegaly and Cushing's disease can occur (Figure 81.2). Other MEN1-associated tumours include neuroendocrine tumours, lipomas, angiofibromas, collagenomas, meningiomas, leiomyomas, and ependymomas.

Table 81.1 Main features of the subtypes of multiple endocrine neoplasia and the symptoms the features may cause.

	Main features	Cause of symptoms	Symptoms
MEN1 (3x P!)	Parathyroid hyperplasia	Primary hyperparathyroidism → Hypercalcaemia	Polydipsia, polyuria, weakness, constipation, bone pain, renal stones, pancreatitis, depression
	Pituitary adenomas	Prolactinoma	Galactorrhoea, impotence, amenorrhoea, infertility
		Acromegaly (growth hormone)	Coarse facies, sweating, hand and foot growth
		Cushing's disease (ACTH)	Weight gain, myopathy, moon face, many others
		Mass effect	Headache, bitemporal hemianopia
	Pancreatic tumours	Gastrinoma	Peptic ulcers, dyspepsia
		Insulinoma	Hypoglycaemia, sweaty, dizzy
		Non-functioning	Obstruction → jaundice
MEN2A (2x P!)	Medullary thyroid carcinoma	C cell (parafollicular cells) → raised calcitonin	thyroid hard mass, lymphadenopathy, diarrhoea, weight loss
	Phaeochromocytoma	Chromaffin cells → raised catecholamines	Hypertension, palpitations, anxiety, headaches, sweating
	Parathyroid hyperplasia/adenoma	Primary hyperparathyroidism → Hypercalcaemia	Milder than in MEN1
MEN2B (1x P!)	Medullary thyroid carcinoma	C cell (parafollicular cells) → raised calcitonin	More aggressive, presents earlier and more likely to have metastasised than in MEN2A
	Marfanoid habitus and neuromas		Tall stature, arachnodactyly, pectus excavatum, hyperextensible joints
	Phaeochromocytoma	Chromaffin cells → raised catecholamines	Hypertension, palpitations, anxiety, headaches, Sweating

Clinical Genetics and Genomics at a Glance, First Edition. Edited by Neeta Lakhani, Kunal Kulkarni, Julian Barwell, Pradeep Vasudevan, and Huw Dorkins.

Figure 81.1 Endocrine glands commonly affected by MEN.

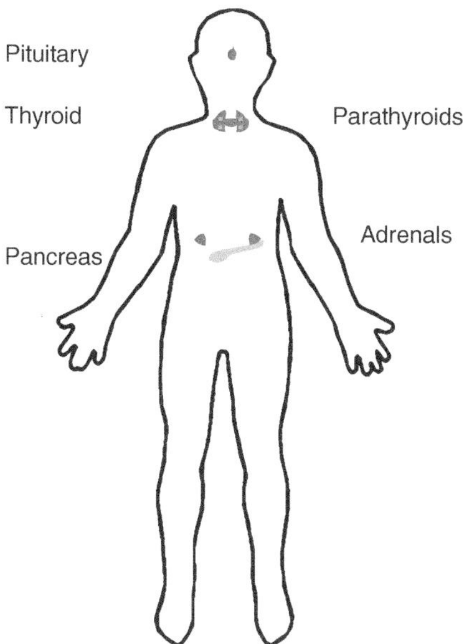

Figure 81.2 Example pedigree diagram showing various presentations of **multiple endocrine neoplasia type 1**: Cushing's syndrome, peptic ulcer perforation (secondary to gastrinoma), galactorrhoea, renal stones secondary to hyperparathyroidism, insulinoma.

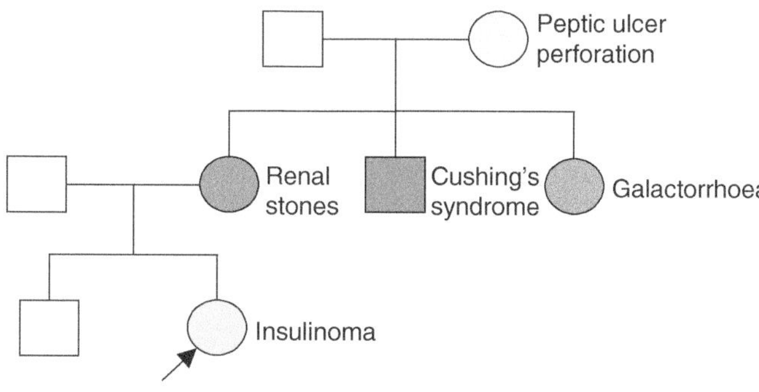

Figure 81.3 Genetic conditions associated with phaeochromocytoma.

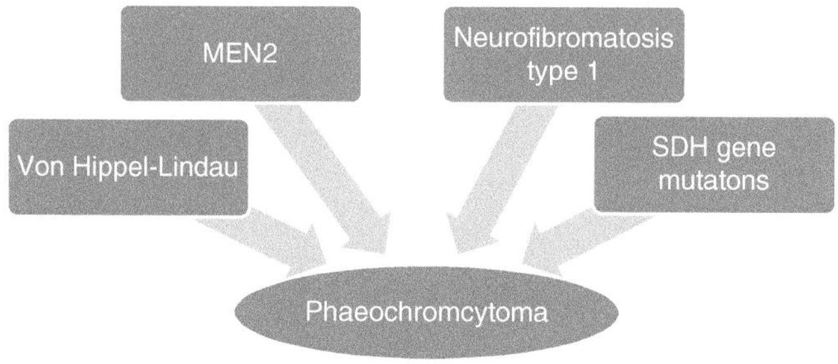

- **MEN2A:** The main three features are medullary thyroid carcinoma (MTC, lifetime risk >90%), phaeochromocytoma (40%), and hyperparathyroidism (20%, usually mild). MTC is a cancer of the C-cells that produce calcitonin. The first sign is often a firm mass in the thyroid or nearby lymph nodes. Diarrhoea is the most frequent systemic symptom. MTC is aggressive and can metastasise quickly. Phaeochromocytoma is a catecholamine secreting tumour of chromaffin cells. It is rare, but 40% of cases are due to Mendelian inheritance (e.g. MEN2, NF1, von Hippel-Lindau syndrome) (Figure 81.3). Familial MTC is considered a subtype of MEN2A; at least 4 members of a family are affected (without other endocrine tumours), the MTC is less aggressive and presents later. Further subtypes include MEN2A with Hirschsprung's disease, and MEN2A with cutaneous lichen amyloidosis.
- **MEN2B:** The main three features are a more aggressive form of MTC that often presents at a younger age, marfanoid habitus, and neuromas, and phaeochromocytoma (50%).

Diagnosis

MEN1 and MEN2 are clinical diagnoses in patients with at least 2 of the main endocrine tumours. Genetic testing should then be utilised to identify a *MEN1* germline alteration or missense alteration of the *RET* gene. Pre-symptomatic genetic testing for *RET* alterations is recommended for all direct relatives of MEN2 patients as this forgoes the need to annual screening for disease.

Tumour screening involves calcium and parathyroid hormone (PTH) for hyperparathyroidism; calcitonin for MTC; catecholamines for phaeochromocytoma; prolactin; IGF-1 for acromegaly; fasting glucose for insulinoma; VIP; imaging including thyroid ultrasound, MRI brain if any suspicion of pituitary adenoma, MRI abdomen for phaeochromocytoma.

Management

Management of MEN requires a MDT approach, including surgeons, oncologists, and endocrinologists.

- MEN1 carriers and at-risk family members require at least annual screening, and affected patients have 6-monthly blood tests and imaging. Surgical removal or medical blockade are the primary treatment for most tumours, depending on tumour size and growth and symptoms. Calcimimetics are used in hyperparathyroidism, bisphosphonates can reduce hypercalcaemia and bone resorption, dopamine agonists can treat prolactinomas, somatostatin is used for acromegaly, and proton pump inhibitors reduce stomach acid production from gastrinomas. Surgical decisions may involve complete or partial removal of the affected gland (e.g. subtotal parathyroidectomy maintains native PTH production but increases the risk of tumour recurrence; whereas total removal requires daily calcium and vitamin D supplements). Adrenocorticotropic hormone (ACTH)- and growth hormone (GH)-producing pituitary adenomas are usually treated with transsphenoidal surgery.
- For patients with MEN2, prophylactic thyroidectomy is recommended as almost all carriers develop MTC. The age of thyroidectomy is influenced by the type of *RET* alteration and calcitonin level (the American Thyroid Association provide defined risk levels). MEN2B will require surgery at an early age, and patients with lower risk alterations may be monitored via annual biochemical surveillance prior to surgery. After thyroidectomy, all patients require life-long thyroid hormone replacement. Phaeochromocytomas are often removed with laparoscopic surgery. Prior to surgery alpha- and beta-blockers inhibit the over production of catecholamines.

The future

Recent data suggests breast cancer to be another MEN1 manifestation and further understanding of *MEN1* and menin may improve screening and targeted therapies. A number of trials are registered to assess alternative therapies for neuroendocrine tumours including tyrosine kinase inhibitors, which are also being investigated for effectiveness in advanced MTC.

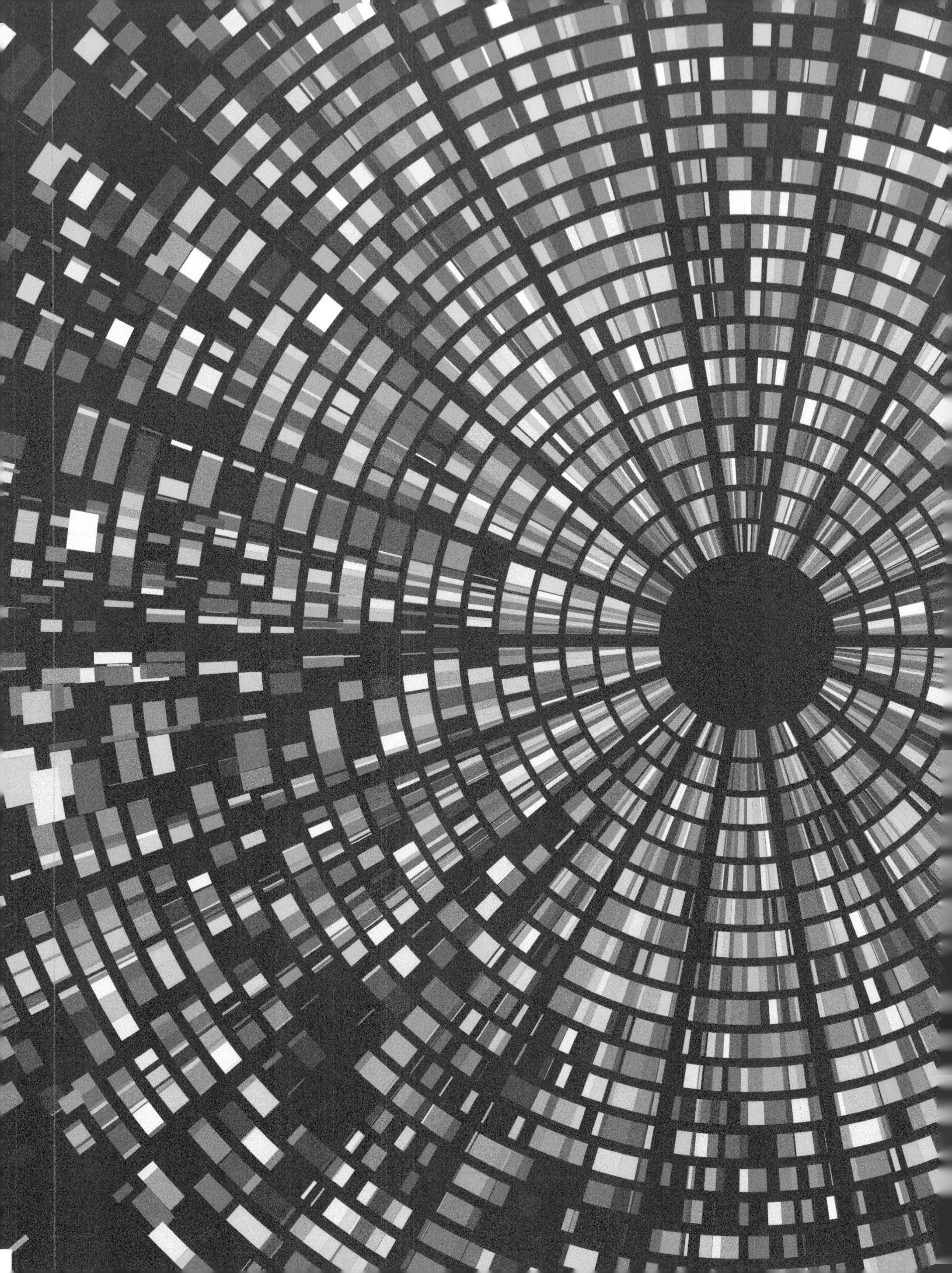

Ophthalmology

Chapters

82 Congenital and childhood cataracts

Background

The word cataract is derived from the Greek word 'cataractos', meaning 'rapidly running water', due to the similarity between the white appearance of rapid running water and mature cataracts.

Aetiology

Cataracts account for about 40% of global blindness. However, the majority are due to age related or senile cataracts. Congenital and childhood cataract (CC) refers to an opacity of the lens of the eye that is present at birth or early in life. It has an estimated prevalence of 3–5 in 10 000, and accounts for 15% of global childhood blindness. The causes can be broadly classified as isolated, chromosomal abnormalities, syndromic, metabolic, endocrinological, traumatic, and infective. The majority of unilateral cataract cases are idiopathic, whereas more than half of bilateral CC have a genetic basis.

In this chapter, we will mainly focus on the genetic causes of cataract, specifically the non-syndromic forms. It is important to highlight that lens opacities can be a part of multi-system genetic disorders (some examples are shown in Table 82.1).

Genetics

CC is a heterogeneous disease with reported alterations in over 100 genes. The modes of inheritance include AD, AR, and X-linked. Approximately a third of CC cases are familial without any systemic and other eye abnormalities.

CC or presenile cataracts can be associated with other eye conditions. Often, they can arise due to anterior segment dysgenesis. *PAX6* mutations is an important cause of CC/pre-senile cataract which also can manifest with pan-ocular phenotypes (aniridia, foveal hypoplasia, and nystagmus). *PAX6* mutations are inherited in an AD manner. Childhood cataracts can also be associated with retinitis pigmentosa and Stickler syndrome.

In OMIM, there are 44 genetic loci associated with CC. In eleven loci, the gene has not yet been identified. Among the known genes, 45% have mutations in lens cyrstallins, 12% in various growth or transcription factors, 16% in connexins, 5% in intermediate filament proteins, membrane proteins, or protein degradation apparatus and in 8% alterations are noted in variety of other divergent genes. There are several mechanisms for the development of CC depending on which genes/pathways are involved. Lack of transcriptional activation results in the failure of development of lens structures and protein components. Cystallin mutations (e.g. *CRYGC*, *CRYGS*) cause abnormal folding of the protein, distorting the compact packing of the molecule or disarray of lens microarchitecture resulting in excessive light scatter compared to wild type. The altered protein is thought to induce the unfolded protein response (serves to reduce stress on the endoplasmic reticulum (ER) when large amounts of denatured, misfolded, or unfolded proteins accumulate within the ER lumen), and thus apoptosis.

Pathophysiology

The lens consists of an outer capsule, epithelium, lens fibres, cortex, and nucleus. The nucleus is composed of embryonic, fetal, infantile, and adult parts, representing the age at which the fibres within them were formed. The transparency and refractile properties of the lens are due to crystallin proteins. Three varieties co-exist (α, β, and γ) and are present at high concentration. They are responsible for 60% of the lens fibre mass. The alterations discussed result in abnormalities in the normal development of the lens structures.

Symptoms and clinical features

Visually significant CC are detected in the newborn checks via a poor red-reflex. CC that develop later in infancy are detected either due to leukocoria (white pupil), change in visual behaviour, nystagmus, or development of strabismus (unilateral cases) (Figure 82.1).

There is significant phenotypic heterogeneity, with significant intra-familial variability described, suggesting the important contributions to genetic and environmental modifiers. Similarly, variable expressivity (i.e. individuals with the same genetic mutation present with varying degrees of disease severity) has been described to be associated with CC.

A thorough history should be taken, including details of any intra-uterine infections, and family history (including any consanguinity), which might point towards a possible genetic aetiology. A full systems review is essential due to the potential multisystem involvement.

Diagnosis

Early diagnosis and intervention is key to preventing blindness. A previous study (in UK) have shown that 66% of children with CC were diagnosed by eight weeks. This emphasizes the significance of the UK Department of Health's inclusion of the red reflex test as part of the neonatal and post-partum six-week health checks. A handheld slit lamp examination allows further classification of CC based on area, degree, and type of opacity seen.

Currently, the most effective genetic testing strategy involves the use of a multigene cataract panel that includes all known CC genes. Single gene testing has been replaced by multigene panels in most scenarios.

Management

Small or paracentral cataracts not affecting vision may be managed by observation. Cataract surgery with intraocular lens (IOL) implant insertion is otherwise recommended for most children once diagnosis is established.

The timing of surgery varies between centres, but the main aim of treatment is to minimise delays in restoring vision and prevent the development of amblyopia and nystagmus. Most experts recommend surgery within the first two months of life.

Clinical Genetics and Genomics at a Glance, First Edition. Edited by Neeta Lakhani, Kunal Kulkarni, Julian Barwell, Pradeep Vasudevan, and Huw Dorkins.

Table 82.1 Syndromic forms of CC and associated systemic disorders.

Chromosomal abnormalities:
- Trisomies (Down (21), Edwards (18), Patau (13) syndrome)
- Monosomies (Turner syndrome)
- Deletions (5p, Cri du chat syndrome)
- Microdeletions (16p13 Rubinstein-Taybi syndrome).

Other systemic disorders:
- Connective tissue disorders (Marfan syndrome, Conradi syndrome, Alport syndrome)
- Dermatological disorders (Cockayne syndrome, incontinentia pigmenti, ectodermal dysplasia)
- Neuromuscular disorders (Alstrom syndrome, myotonic dystrophy)
- Metabolic abnormalities (galactosemia, abetalipoproteinemia, Lowe syndrome, homocysteinuria, Niemann-Pick disease)
- Craniosynostosis/craniofacial defects (Apert syndrome, Crouzon syndrome, Smith-Lemli-Opitz syndrome).

In children with unilateral cataract (or significantly asymmetric bilateral cataracts), intensive post-operative patching of the better seeing eye may be needed to treat amblyopia.

Primary IOL implantation has significant benefits (less amblyogenic risk) compared to secondary IOL implantation or leaving the child aphakic. Most children are made hyperopic, but currently there are no agreed standards. These children will need lifelong bifocals.

Post-operative complications include inflammation and ocular hypertension (leading to glaucoma). Those that do not undergo posterior capsulotomy may require further surgery (due to posterior capsular opacification). The presence of other associated ocular abnormalities (e.g. anterior segment dysgenesis) may complicate surgery and increase post-operative problems.

The future

In 2015, breakthrough *in vitro* and preclinical animal model studies showed that lanosterol treatment was effective in reducing cataract severity and showed increased lens transparency. Lanosterol significantly decreased preformed protein aggregates *in vitro* and in cell transfection experiments. These promising results point towards the possibility of using lanosterol drops as a treatment for cataracts, although human clinical trials are yet to be announced.

Figure 82.1 Paediatric cataract.

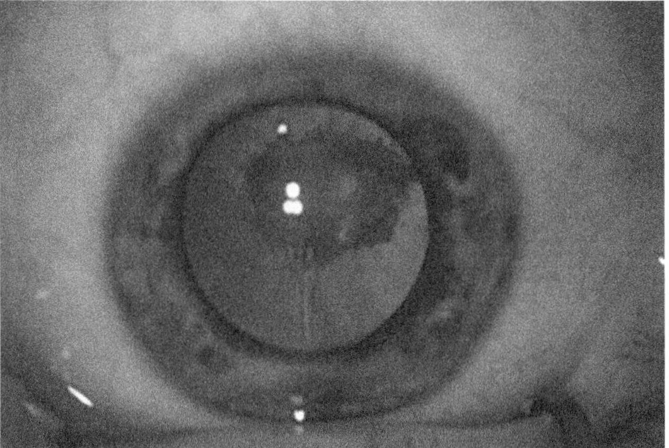

Source: Taken from https://onlinelibrary.wiley.com/doi/full/10.1111/j.1600-0420.2007.01007.x.

83 Colour blindness and achromatopsia

Background

Colour blindness is an umbrella term that encompasses a range of conditions that affect colour vision perception. Red-green defects are commonest, whereas blue-yellow are less common. Acuity is usually unaffected, except in the uncommon condition, monochromacy. Blue cone monochromacy may be considered as a type of achromatopsia – a condition characterised by partial/total absence of colour vision alongside other abnormalities.

Aetiology

Colour blindness affects around 1 : 12 men and 1 : 200 women. Achromatopsia is more uncommon affecting around 1 : 30 000.

Genetics

Short-wave-sensitive opsin-1 gene (*OPN1SW*) is located on chromosome 7 and encodes the blue cone pigment. Allelic variants of *OPN1SW* results in tritanopia (OMIM 190900), which is inherited in an AD manner.

Medium-wave-sensitive opsin-1 gene (*OPN1MW*) and long-wave-sensitive opsin-1 gene (*OPN1LW*) are located on the X-chromosome and encodes the green cone and red cone pigment, respectively. There is only a single red pigment gene; however, the number of green pigment genes vary in number and are arranged in a head-to-tail tandem array with the red pigment gene at the 5′ end. The locus control region (LCR) is a master switch located ~3 kb upstream from the 5′ end of the array and is essential for the expression of both the red and green pigments. Variations in the *OPN1MW* and *OPN1LW* array can result in hereditary red-green colour vision defects (OMIM 303800 and 303900). This mostly manifests in males (in northern Europe: 8% of males and 0.5% females) and is not associated with other ophthalmic or clinical abnormalities.

Pathogenic variants resulting in loss of *OPN1MW* and *OPN1LW* opsin array, hybrid gene formation, inactivating mutations or deletions affecting LCR cause blue cone monochromatism (OMIM 303700). This is inherited in an X-linked manner and mostly affects males.

Alterations of genes involved in the phototransduction cascade (*CNGA3* (OMIM 600053), *CNGB3* (OMIM 605080), *GNAT2* (OMIM 139340), *PDE6C* (OMIM 600827), *PDE6H* (OMIM 601190), and *ATF6* (OMIM 605537)) cause achromatopsia and is inherited in an AR manner. Among these, gene mutations of *CNGB3* and *CNGA3* account for most cases of achromatopsia.

Pathophysiology

The retina contains two main types of receptors that receive light and transmit visual signals: rods and cones. Rods primarily play a role in low light vision, cones in bright light, and for colour. In humans normal colour vision is trichromatic, based on the three populations of retinal cones each with a specific peak sensitivity: 420 nm (blue cones), 530 nm (green cones), and 560 nm (red cones). Although cone photoreceptors only represent 5% of all photoreceptors over the entire retina, they are responsible for high spatial acuity and are concentrated at the foveola. All visual pigments are made up of 11-*cis* retinal (vitamin A aldehyde) and a G-protein receptor called opsin. There are four visual pigments: rhodopsin (in rods) and the three cone pigments. Absorption of a photon of light results in *cis-trans* isomerisation (conversion of 11-*cis* retinal to the all-trans form) and triggers a phototransduction cascade. Different genetic alterations result in specific colour vision loss due to abnormal opsin pigment production, which leads to defective or premature destruction of cones. In achromatopsia, the reaction of cones to light is impaired (only rods are functional), therefore interfering with phototransduction.

Some cases of colour vision are not heritable, instead caused by abnormalities elsewhere in the optic pathway, for example optic nerve or structural visual cortex abnormalities. Acquired colour vision defects may be caused by drugs, including chloroquine or solvents.

Symptoms

Hereditary red-green colour vision and tritan defects often remain undetected as many are not aware of this until they are tested. Blue cone monochromatism and achromatopsia often present with infantile nystagmus (onset within the first six months of life), increased sensitivity to light, eccentric fixation, decreased vision, and poor or no colour discrimination. In achromatopsia, individuals are unable to perceive colours, seeing only black, white, and shades of grey (in incomplete types there may be some colour vision). Individuals also often have hyperopia (far-sightedness) or myopia (short-sightedness).

Clinical features

In hereditary red-green and tritan defects, no abnormalities are noted on clinical and fundus examination. However, colour vision testing will reveal whether the defect is of the protan (red), deutan (green), or tritan (blue) system.

In achromatopsia and blue cone monochromatism, the visual acuity is severely reduced (often 6/60). Pendular nystagmus is often seen, which is conjugate with a low amplitude and high frequency (compared to other infantile nystagmus forms). Examination of pupils may reveal a paradoxical pupillary reaction (initial pupil constriction rather than dilation) when room lights are turned off. Most affected individuals have a normal fundus appearance. Subtle bilateral macular changes such as pigment mottling, narrowing of retinal vessels, or absent foveal reflex have been described. Photophobia is a

Clinical Genetics and Genomics at a Glance, First Edition. Edited by Neeta Lakhani, Kunal Kulkarni, Julian Barwell, Pradeep Vasudevan, and Huw Dorkins.

useful sign in achromatopsia, which becomes more obvious with age.

Diagnosis

Ishihara pseudo-isochromatic plates or Farnsworth-D15 test can be used as a screening test for colour vision (Figure 83.1). Red-green colour vision defects can be detected. However if detailed information on protan, deutan and tritan systems are required the Farnsworth-Munsell 100-Hue test can be used (Figure 83.2).

Both optical coherence tomography (OCT) and electroretinogram (ERG) are useful investigations in achromatopsia and blue cone monochromatism. OCT shows disruption of the inner segment ellipsoid and foveal maldevelopment. ERG will reveal absent cone function and normal rod function. ERG and/or OCT findings together with clinical characteristics is often sufficient for a clinical diagnosis.

Labs utilise either a multigene panel approach, which includes all the achromatopsia genes (*CNGB3, CNGA3, GNAT2, PDE6C, PDE6H, ATF6*) or sanger sequencing of the most common genes associated with achromatopsia (*CNGB3* and *CNGA3*).

Management

There are no treatments or cures for colour blindness or achromatopsia. Underlying causes (i.e. in non-genetic cases) should be addressed. The mainstay of treatment is to optimise vision through the provision of low vision aids (e.g. lenses and glasses with filters to correct deficiencies). As visual acuity develops in early childhood, patients should be offered regular appointments (six-monthly to yearly) for assessment of refractive error and strabismus. Dark/filter glasses or tinted contact lenses may also help reduce photophobia. A clinical trial using a CNTF implant in *CNGB3* mutations showed no evidence of improvement in cone function.

The future

Human gene therapy trials (using Adeno-associated Virus Vector for *CNGB3* and *CNGA3*) are currently ongoing, with promising preliminary data. OCT signs have shown progressive changes over time, suggesting that this could be a progressive disorder where early intervention (within the first decade) with gene therapy may yield the best outcomes.

Figure 83.1 Ishihara chart for colour blindness testing.

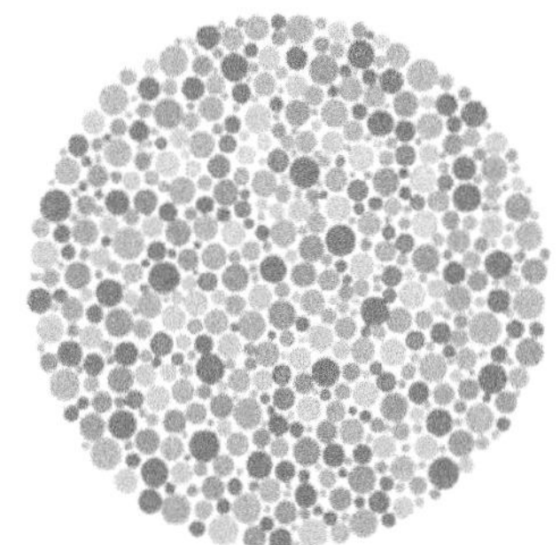

Source: Taken from https://onlinelibrary.wiley.com/doi/full/10.1111/aos.14219.

Figure 83.2 Colour range variations between different pathologies.

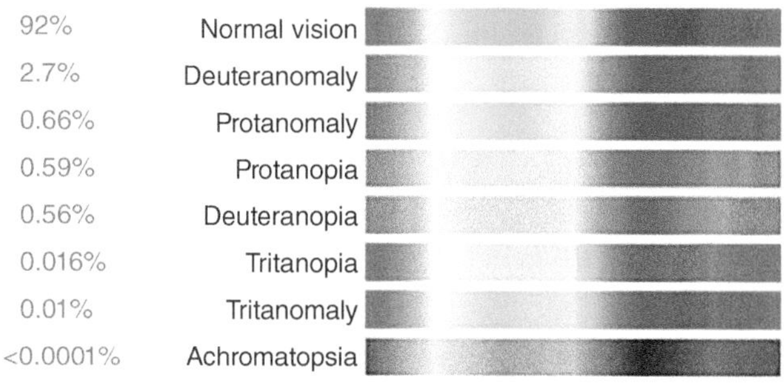

84 Retinitis pigmentosa

Background

Retinitis pigmentosa (RP) was first described by a Dutch ophthalmologist, Dr Franciscus Donders, in 1857. The term 'retinitis' is a misnomer, originating from the initial (incorrect) presumption that this was an inflammatory condition. The term 'pigmentosa' originates from the observation of retinal pigment around blood vessels. RP encompasses a diverse group of inherited diffuse retinal degenerative diseases, characterised by photoreceptor dysfunction and degeneration (initially rods, with cone involvement at later stages).

Aetiology

RP is the commonest inherited retinal dystrophy, affecting approximately 1 : 5000. RP can be broadly divided into non-syndromic and syndromic forms.

Genetics

Non-syndromic RP is considered genetically heterogeneous, as it can exhibit sporadic, AD, AR, X-linked, or digenic inheritance. There are over 165 known genes associations. Overall, sporadic cases account for the largest proportion of RP cases (40–50%), followed by AD RP (adRP) (15–25%), AR RP (arRP) (5–20%), and X-linked RP (xlRP) (5–15%). *RHO* alterations are the commonest cause of adRP; *EYS,* and *USH2A* alterations are the commonest cause of arRP, and *RPGR* alterations accounting for the majority of xlRP. A comprehensive list of all of the different genes associated with RP can be found at the RetNet website: https://sph.uth.edu/retnet/.

Syndromic forms of RP have the pigmentary retinopathy along with systemic features. These include Usher syndrome (AR), Kearns-Sayre syndrome (mitochondrial inheritance), Bardet-Biedl syndrome (genetically heterogeneous), abetalipoproteinemia (AR), and Refsum disease (AR).

Pathophysiology

The pathophysiology of RP is complex. The genes discussed are known to be involved in various pathways such as visual cascade and visual cycle, retinal catabolic pathways, and mitochondrial metabolism. They tend to be preferentially expressed in the retina. One of the genes studied in detail is *RHO* (encoding for the rhodopsin protein), which is the commonest gene associated with adRP. In *rho* knockout mice, rhodopsin filled vesicles accumulate at the inner and outer segment junction of the photoreceptor. This is hypothesised to arise due to abnormal transport of the mutant rhodopsin to the membranes of the outer segments, leading to photoreceptor loss through apoptosis.

Symptoms

Nyctalopia (night blindness) is the commonest presenting symptom in RP. Tunnel vision or reduced visual acuity may also be reported. However, reduced visual acuity tends to be a later feature. RP is a progressive disease thus can remain undiagnosed for a number of years. One of the complications of RP is development of cystoid macular oedema. This can occur at any age and would affect central vision. Earlier age of onset of disease is associated with a more severe disease course. In syndromic forms, systemic symptoms can be present in addition to nyctalopia.

Clinical features

The classic triad associated with RP includes bone-spicule retinal pigmentation, arteriolar attenuation, and waxy disc pallor (Figure 84.1). The bone-spicule pigmentary changes tend to occur in the mid-periphery of the retina and may increase in density and spread over time. The large choroidal vessels may remain unmasked over time resulting in a tessellated fundus appearance.

RP may be associated with other ocular pathologies such as myopia, optic disc drusen, keratoconus, and posterior subcapsular cataracts.

Syndromic forms of RP can have systemic manifestations such as sensorineural hearing loss (Usher syndrome), chronic progressive ophthalmoplegia with ptosis (Kearns-Sayre syndrome), ataxia, and endocrinological abnormalities. In Bardet-Biedl syndrome, systemic features can include truncal obesity, postaxial polydactyly, cognitive impairment, male hypogonadotropic hypogonadism, complex female genitourinary malformations, and renal abnormalities. In abetalipoproteinemia, there is failure to thrive in infancy and spinocerebellar ataxia. Refsum disease can present with ataxia, neuropathy, ichthyosis (scaly skin), cardiac arrhythmia, and hearing loss.

Diagnosis

Full field electroretinogram (ERG) is a sensitive diagnostic test which will show reduced scotopic response (rod function) which will be affected to a greater extent in relation to the photopic responses (cone function). As the disease progresses, photopic responses reduce and eventually the ERG becomes extinguished. Therefore, constant monitoring of VF is helpful for observing disease progression. Optical coherence tomography can help distinguish from other inherited cone disorders and monitor for intraretinal fluid (cystoid macular oedema).

Currently, the most effective genetic testing strategy is via the use of a multigene RP panel that includes all known RP-associated genes. Single gene testing has been replaced by multigene panels in most scenarios except if there is strong evidence of X-linked

Clinical Genetics and Genomics at a Glance, First Edition. Edited by Neeta Lakhani, Kunal Kulkarni, Julian Barwell, Pradeep Vasudevan, and Huw Dorkins.

non-syndromic RP. *RPGR* mutations account for 80% of X-linked RP therefore Sanger sequencing could be a cost-effective approach.

Management

There are no specific curative treatments for RP. Treatments are aimed at addressing manifestations of the disease and improving quality of life. Patients should be advised to avoid smoking. Short-wave-length light exposure may accelerate the retinal degeneration, therefore UV-A and UV-B blocking sunglasses are advised for outdoor use. For cystoid macular oedema there is evidence supporting the use of systemic and topical carbonic anhydrase inhibitor. Surgery should be offered for cataracts as this can improve vision. The use of Vitamin A palmitate is no longer recommended. There is limited evidence base on the use of nutritional supplements. Low vision aids and rehabilitation can improve quality of life.

The future

Gene therapy trials using adeno-associated virus (AAV) and stem cell therapies have shown promising results. Retinal prostheses are have been trialled with some success in severe sight loss. The Argus II epiretinal prosthesis system has been licensed in Europe and received FDA approval for advanced RP.

Figure 84.1 Appearance of a normal eye and an eye affected by RP.

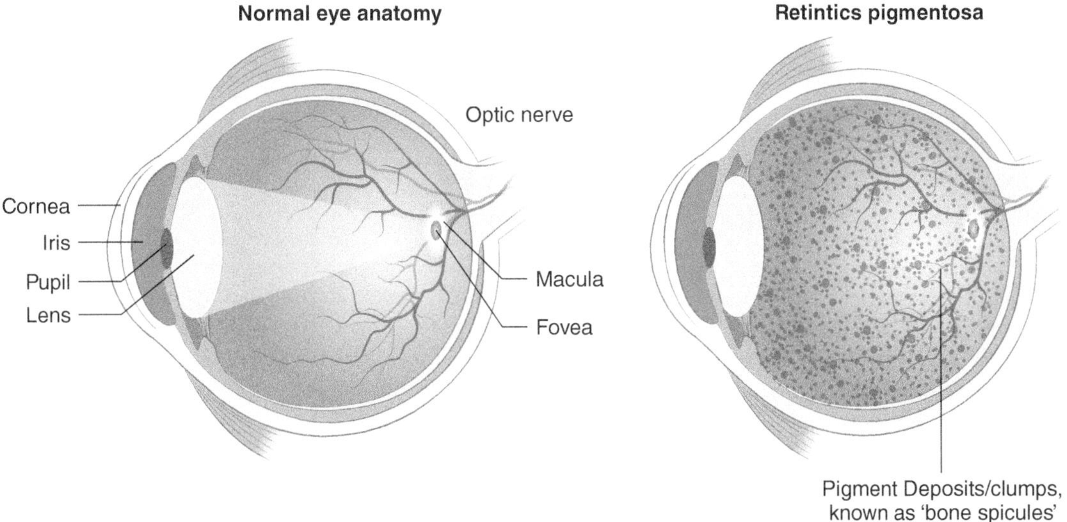

85 Primary congenital glaucoma

Background

Glaucoma is a heterogeneous disease characterised by progressive optic neuropathy, with associated visual field loss. It is the third leading cause of blindness worldwide. 'Glaucosis' was first mentioned in Hippocractic writings (400 BC), referring to a blinding disease in the elderly. The etymological origin for the word glaucoma is from the two Greek words 'glaukos' and 'glausso', meaning to glow or shine. It was considered to refer to the 'hot eye' seen in acute glaucoma. After the discovery of the ophthalmoscope in 1850, excavated optic nerves with neuroretinal rim loss associated with elevated intraocular pressure (IOP) were observed, providing evidence that raised IOP was damaging the optic nerves.

Aetiology

Primary congenital glaucoma (PCG) refers to glaucoma present at birth. PCG has varying prevalence in different countries. In western countries it varies between 1 : 5000–22 000 but is more prevalent in the Middle East (1 : 2500), Romani population of Slovakia (1 : 1250), and the Indian state of Andhra Pradesh (1 : 3300). In these high prevalence populations it is the most common cause of childhood blindness. This is attributed to the higher levels of consanguinity in these populations.

Genetics

Three main genes alterations are responsible for PCG: *CYP1B1*, *LTBP2*, and *TEK*. Mutations in *CYP1B1* result in the commonest cause of PCG. The prevalence of the alterations varies among different populations. For example, p.Glu387Lys accounts for all pathogenic variants in the Rom Slovakian population, whereas p.Gly61Glu accounts for over 70% of mutations in Saudi Arabia. *LTBP2* alterations account for <40% of PCG alterations. *TEK* alterations in PCG are rare and just over 10 families have been described in the literature. *CYP1B1* and *LTBP2* are inherited in an AR manner (AR), while *TEK* is inherited in as AD.

The exact mechanism by which protein abnormalities result in the development of glaucoma is unclear. In human and mouse models with *CYP1B1* alterations, different morphological abnormalities that affect aqueous outflow have been observed. These include small or absent Schlemm's canal, basal lamina extending from the cornea over the trabecular meshwork, fibres resembling smooth muscle at anterior positions in the trabecular meshwork, and attachments of the iris to the trabecular meshwork and peripheral cornea (synechiae). *LTBP2* has high levels of expression in the trabecular meshwork and ciliary processes. However, *LTBP2* knockout mice die before embryonic day 6.5. Based on the expression patterns, it is hypothesised that *LTBP2* alters the elasticity of ciliary body structures, thus influencing aqueous outflow. The TEK receptor is highly expressed in the Schlemm's canal endothelium and is required for Schlemm's canal development. Thus, *TEK* mutations are hypothesised to affect aqueous outflow.

In addition to PCG, there are several other associated genetic conditions that may present with secondary glaucoma in childhood. These include aniridia (*PAX6* alterations, AD inheritance), anterior segment dysgenesis syndromes (many genes), Axenfeld-Reiger anomaly (*FOXC1* or *PITX2* alterations, AD inheritance), congenital hereditary endothelial dystrophy (*SLC4A11* mutations, AR inheritance), Lowe syndrome (*OCRL* alterations, X-linked), and Sturge-Weber syndrome (*GNAQ* alterations, somatic alterations).

Pathophysiology

Aqueous humour production and outflow is central to the maintenance of IOP. Aqueous humour is produced by the ciliary body, with aqueous outflow occurring via two routes: trabecular (>70%) and uveoscleral. Inadequate drainage of aqueous humour is hypothesised to result from developmental defects of the trabecular meshwork and anterior chamber angle. This results in elevated IOP and stretching of the sclera that produces an enlarged globe (buphthalmos). Raised intraocular pressure is an important risk factor in not only developing glaucoma, but also in progression of the disease. Treatment is therefore aimed at reducing the progression of neuroretinal rim loss and associated visual field loss by controlling the IOP.

Symptoms

The classic symptoms experienced in the first year of life are tearing, photophobia, and irritability. The spectrum of symptoms and signs depends on the severity of the disease. In very severe cases, a cloudy cornea or corneal opacity is seen.

Clinical features

Interestingly, *CYP1BI* alterations have also been identified in patients with juvenile open-angle glaucoma. Thus, eliciting a family history of early onset glaucoma should trigger screening. On examination, the following features maybe seen: corneal oedema, breaks in Descemet's membrane (Haab's striae), enlargement of the globe (buphthalmos), increased corneal diameter, atrophy of iris, thinning of anterior sclera, and progressive optic atrophy. IOP will be typically elevated. There are an absence of signs of anterior segment dysgenesis.

Patients with *LTBP2* alterations can have additional clinical features not seen in individuals with *CYP1B1* or *TEK* mutations. These include ectopia lentis, high-arched palate, and mild-to-moderate osteopenia. In secondary glaucoma, additional ocular or systemic phenotypes are present. These can range from ophthalmic features such as anterior segment dysgenesis to systemic manifestations (Table 85.1).

Clinical Genetics and Genomics at a Glance, First Edition. Edited by Neeta Lakhani, Kunal Kulkarni, Julian Barwell, Pradeep Vasudevan, and Huw Dorkins.

Table 85.1 Clinical features of the conditions causing secondary glaucoma.

Aniridia
- Nystagmus
- Foveal hypoplasia
- Optic nerve abnormalities.

Axenfeld-Rieger syndrome
- Posterior embryotoxon
- Iris hypoplasia
- Ectropion uvea
- Tends to be bilateral

Lowe syndrome
- Affected boys tend to have dense congenital cataracts
- Congenital hypotonia
- Developmental delay
- Proximal renal tubular dysfunction

Sturge-Weber syndrome
- Facial cutaneous malformations (port-wine stains),
- Leptomeningeal angiomatosis
- Seizures may be present

Diagnosis

The following criteria are used for diagnosis:
- Elevated IOP (>21 mm Hg) on at least two separate occasions (measured using applanation tonometry, I-care tonometry, or pneumotonometry)
- Cloudy cornea and increased corneal diameter
- Breaks in Descemet's membrane
- Buphthalmos
- Anomalously deep anterior chamber

If the clinical features are inconclusive, molecular genetic testing can provide confirmation, utilising either a:
- Multigene panel approach: includes all the PCG genes (*CYP1B1*, *LTBP2* and *TEK*) and genes causative of secondary glaucoma, *or*
- Serial single-gene testing followed by deletion/duplication analysis: if no pathogenic variants are identified.

The genetic testing strategy is governed by ethnicity, family history, and parental consanguinity. For instance, for a patient with Romani Slovakian ancestry, the p.Glu387Lys testing could be performed first. Similarly, patients of Saudi Arabian ancestry, the p.Gly61Glu testing could be performed first.

Management

The main aim of treatment is to reduce IOP to reduce the risk complications such as corneal opacification and glaucomatous optic neuropathy. This can be achieved using surgical approaches and medical treatment.
- In primary congenital glaucoma, surgical treatment is the first line and mainstay treatment. Surgical approaches include goniotomy (create openings in the trabecular meshwork while visualising anterior chamber structures using a gonio lens) and trabeculectomy.
- Patients with *CYP1B1* mutations tend to have better operative success rates (measured by level of IOP control) compared to those without *CYP1B1* mutations.
- If surgical approaches fail, diode laser ablation (cyclodiode) or glaucoma drainage implants can be used. Pharmacological treatments (e.g. timolol) are typically used as a temporary measure to control IOP and establish a clear cornea for surgery.

The future

Hand-held optical coherence tomography has revolutionised the field of paediatric ophthalmology and imaging. This technology allows non-invasive visualisation of anterior chamber structures and the optic nerve head in infants and children. This has huge potential for diagnosis and monitoring progression of the disease.

86 Bardet–Biedl syndrome

Background

Bardet–Biedl syndrome (BBS) is a systemic disorder with a variety of clinical features. It was previously termed Laurence-Moon-Biedl-Bardet syndrome (with the first case reportedly described by Laurence and Moon in 1866, although BBS and Laurence-Moon syndrome (LMS) is now felt to be distinct conditions.

Epidemiology

This is a rare condition, with estimated average prevalence of around 1 in 100 000–250 000 in most areas globally. There are higher rates in some populations (e.g. Bedouin peoples of Kuwait - 1 in 13 500, or regions of Newfoundland - 1 in 1500). Equal male to female rates.

Genetics

Inheritance is AR. Over 20 different gene alterations have been described, including *BBS1, BBS2, ARL6 (BBS3), BBS4, BBS5, MKKS (BBS6), BBS7, TTC8 (BBS8), BBS9, BBS10, TRIM32 (BBS11), BBS12,MKS1 (BBS13), CEP290 (BBS14), WDPCP (BBS15),SDCCAG8 (BBS16), LZTFL1 (BBS17), BBIP1 (BBS18), IFT27 (BBS19), IFT72 (BBS20),* and *C8ORF37(BBS21)*; 20–30% of affected individuals do not have an identified alteration. There is no clear link between alteration and severity, although *BBS1* alterations have milder visual involvement, whereas *BBS2, BBS3,* and *BBS4* alterations have more severe visual problems.

Pathophysiology

The underlying cause is primary ciliary dysfunction (ciliopathy), hence the widespread clinical manifestations. The BBS proteins encoded by the various BBS genes are found in the cilia and basal body of cells, and are involved in intraflagellar transport, a process required for cilia development and maintenance. The individual proteins come together to form a complex, known as the 'BBSome', which plays a role in intracellular transport and cilia function. From an ophthalmological perspective, photoreceptor cells are provided nutrient via the IFT of retinal cilia; abnormal ciliary function in BBS may therefore cause retinal pathology.

Symptoms and clinical features

There are six classical features: retinal degeneration (visual loss), (truncal) obesity, learning difficulties, renal anomalies, polydactyly, and hypogenitalism. In addition, affected individuals may have distinctive facial features, dental abnormalities, and a partial or complete anosmia. Additionally, BBS can affect the cardiac (e.g. valvular stenosis), liver, and gut manifestations.

- Vision loss is one of the major features, with loss of vision caused by retinal abnormalities. Problems with night vision become apparent by mid-childhood, followed by blind spots that develop in the peripheral vision. Retinitis pigmentosa may start with progressive loss of colour discrimination. These abnormalities can progress, resulting in tunnel vision. Poor visual acuity is common, often resulting in blindness by adolescence or early adulthood. Additional features include strabismus, cataracts, and glaucoma.
- Truncal obesity is a characteristic feature. Abnormal weight gain typically begins in early childhood (in the first year of life in 90%) and remains an ongoing issue. The weight is disproportionately distributed on the abdomen and chest. Complications of obesity can include type 2 diabetes (up to 50%), hypertension, and hypercholesterolemia.
- Mild-to moderate developmental/intellectual difficulties include impaired speech, delayed development of motor skills such as standing and walking, behavioural problems such as emotional immaturity and inappropriate outbursts, and clumsiness or poor coordination.
- Renal abnormalities are variable, including hydronephrosis and infections (e.g. pyelonephritis). These can result in renal failure.
- Alongside, polydactyly (extra digits), affected individuals may have also have brachydactyly (short digits) or syndactly (fused digits).
- In addition to genital abnormalities (commonly hypoplasia), most affected males produce reduced amounts of sex hormones (testicular hypogonadism, cryptotchidism, delayed puberty). Affected females may have anatomical abnormalities of the genitourinary tract, including underdeveloped uterus, fallopian tubes, or ovaries. Menstrual cycles may also be irregular. Infertility may arise in both sexes (Figure 86.1).

Diagnosis

Diagnosis is through a combination of family history and clinical features, with relevant specialty examination (e.g. ophthalmological) when appropriate. Molecular genetic testing may confirm diagnosis in some patients. In parents with a family history of BBS, prenatal ultrasound may identify characteristic features early (e.g. renal hypertrophy, polydactyly). Several conditions have similar clinical features and must be differentiated from BBS (Table 86.1).

Management

- Multidisciplinary care is required, with diet and lifestyle advice an important consideration to deal with the associated obesity and sequelae (e.g. diabetes). This includes input from

Clinical Genetics and Genomics at a Glance, First Edition. Edited by Neeta Lakhani, Kunal Kulkarni, Julian Barwell, Pradeep Vasudevan, and Huw Dorkins.

Figure 86.1 Clinical features of Bardet-Biedl syndrome.

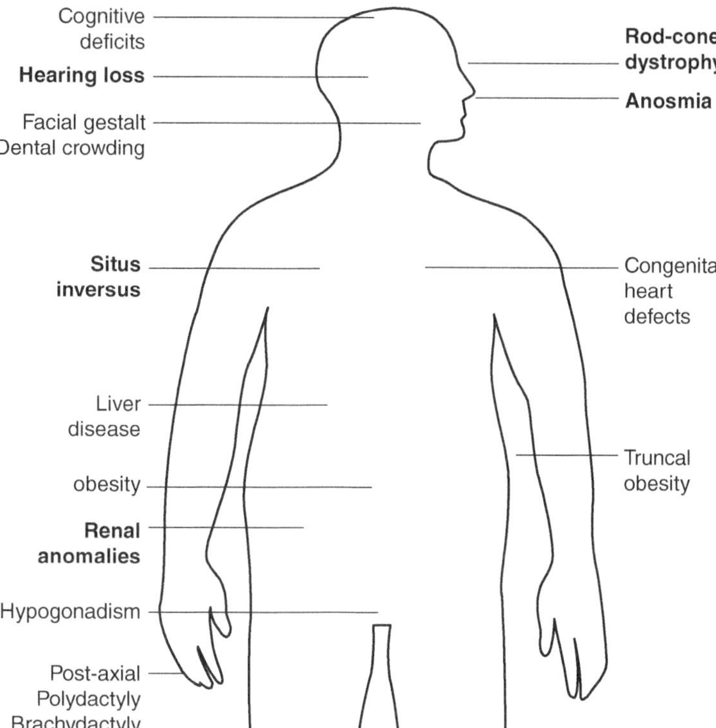

Table 86.1 Several conditions have similar clinical features and must be differentiated from BBS. Most of these follow AR inheritance, and include:

- *LMS:* Features include visual degeneration and pituitary dysfunction. Early (childhood) neurological problems (loss of movement) may develop due to peripheral nerve abnormality
- *Alstrom syndrome:* Features include visual and auditory problems, alongside obesity, diabetes, and renal dysfunction
- *Meckel syndrome:* Features include encephalocele, polydactyly, and renal cysts. Similarly to BBS, liver cirrhosis and genital abnormalities may develop, with similar genetic alterations (e.g. *BBS2, BBS4, BBS6*)
- *McKusick-Kaufman syndrome (MKKS):* Features include polydactyly, congenital cardiac defects, and (in females) hydrometrocolpos (maternal oestrogen-induced accumulation of secretions in the vagina and uterus secondary to an intact hymen). The *MKKS* gene is also known as BBS6, hence the association with BBS
- *Biemon II syndrome:* Features include iris coloboma, learning difficulty, obesity, genitourinary abnormalities, and polydactyly
- *Prader-Willi syndrome*: Features include hypotonia, feeding difficulties, and failure for infants to thrive. Individuals later develop short stature, excessive appetite, cognitive impairment/learning difficulties, behavioural difficulties, and genital abnormalities

dieticians and physiotherapists. Bariatric surgery has limited evidence.

- Ophthalmologists play an important role in screening and correcting abnormalities (e.g. refractive/acuity errors). This is of particular importance in children where visual impairment can affect development and education.
- Specific treatments depending upon the particular clinical features affecting an individual. For example, a hand surgeon specialising in congenital hand abnormalities may be consulted for removal of extra digits, or end-stage renal failure may require dialysis and transplantation. Other supportive specialists also play important roles, e.g. speech therapists.
- Genetic counselling can assist affected individuals with coordinating care and advising on risk in future pregnancies.

The future

Research is ongoing into stem cell treatments, suppressor therapies, and gene therapy, alongside ongoing advances in subspeciality management of each of the individual features of this condition.

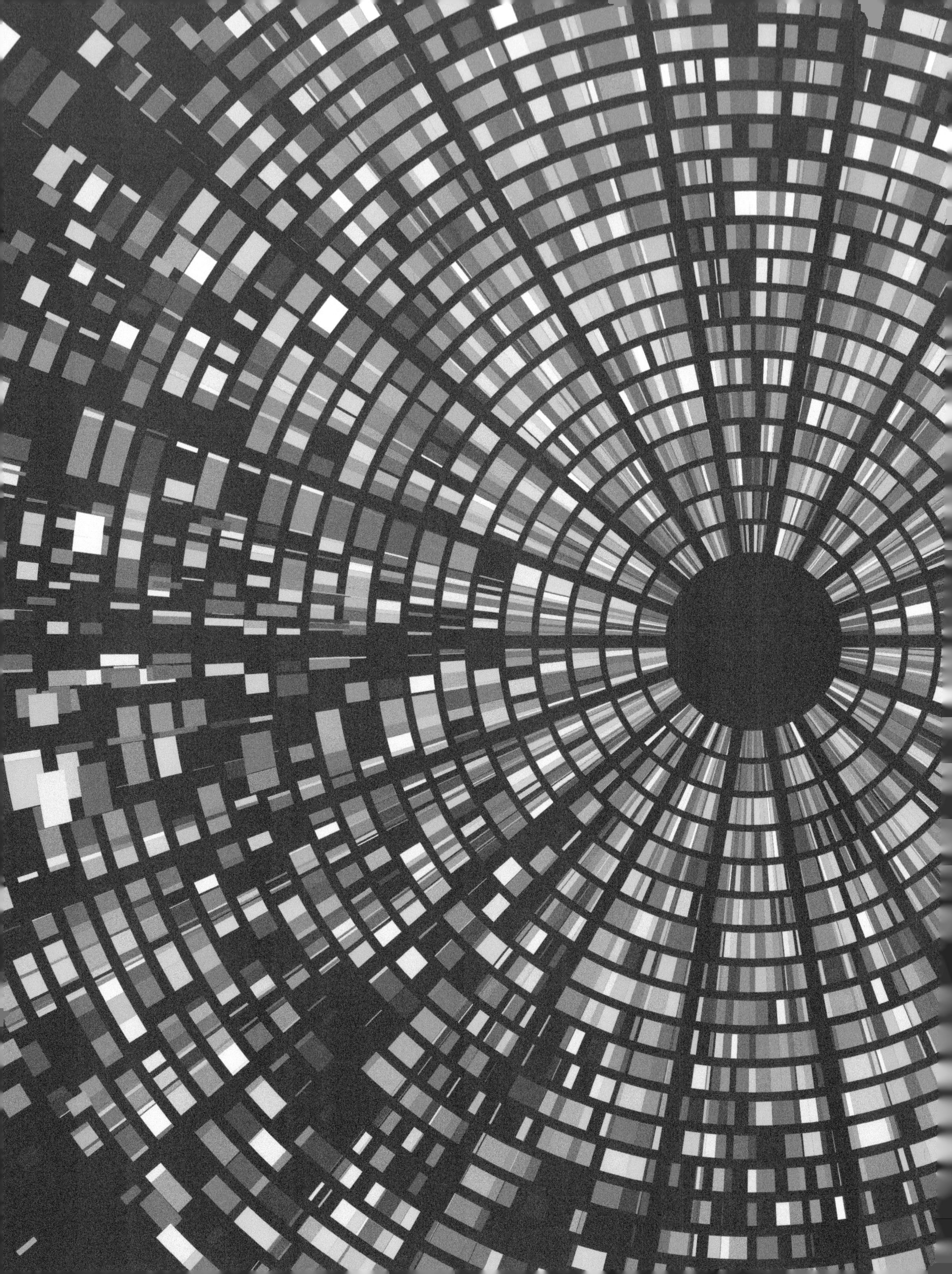

Renal

Chapters

87 Polycystic kidney disease

Background

Cystic kidney diseases comprise a group of inherited disorders. Renal cysts are a major component of the phenotype. Polycystic kidney disease (PKD) is the most common and refers to two specific conditions: autosomal recessive polycystic kidney disease (ARPKD) and autosomal dominant polycystic kidney disease (ADPKD). The molecular and cellular mechanisms of renal cyst formation is extremely complex. There are a number of interactions and shared phenotypic abnormalities in both diseases, often named the 'cystic phenotype'.

Aetiology

ADPKD affects 1 in 400–1000 live births and accounts for 5% of end-stage renal disease. ARPKD is much rarer than its dominant counterpart, with an incidence of 1 in 20 000 live births, corresponding to a carrier frequency of approximately 1 : 70. ADPKD tends to present later in life as a systemic disease characterised by bilateral, progressive enlargement of focal renal cysts, with variable extra-renal manifestations.

Genetics

PKD is mapped to chromosome 16 and chromosome 4 with 100% penetrance. These genes encode the proteins polycystin 1 (PC1) and polycystin 2 (PC2), respectively. The majority of ADPKD patients carry a germline alteration in the *PKD1* gene on chromosome 16p13 (ADPKD1), whereas about 15–20% harbour an alteration in the *PKD2* gene on chromosome 4q21 (ADPKD2).

ARPKD is rarer, and the clinical course is much more severe. ARPKD is primarily caused by alterations in polycystic kidney and hepatic disease 1 (*PKHD1*), which encodes fibrocystin (also known as polyductin), a protein that localizes to the primary cilium and basal body.

Pathophysiology

- **ARPKD:** The majority of patients present in infancy with ectasia and cystic dilatation of the renal collection tubules, which prevents the normal development of renal nephrons. They remain as primitive ducts lined by undifferentiated epithelium, and there is no distinction between the renal cortex and medulla. The rate of progression to renal failure is variable and the prompt diagnosis of a fetus during pregnancy is crucial in optimising long-term outcomes and prognosis.
- **ADPKD:** Cyst formation and progressive growth is a complex dynamic process with multiple interacting signalling components that contribute to disease. Normal renal epithelial cells transform from mature, differentiated, non-proliferative, absorptive cells, to a partially de-differentiated secretory cell.

Symptoms

- ARPKD typically manifests either perinatally or in childhood, with many patients dying in infancy. Affected fetuses display oligohydramnios, with enlarged kidneys, pulmonary hypoplasia, and contracted limbs with club feet.
- 30–50% of affected neonates die shortly after birth from respiratory insufficiency due to pulmonary hypoplasia and thoracic compression by the excessively enlarged kidney.
- Patients with ADPKD may present with abdominal, flank, or back pain due to cyst enlargement or bleeding. Urinary tract infection may also be a presenting feature, including acute pyelonephritis, infected cysts, or a perinephric abscess.

Clinical features

- **ARPKD:** The early appearance of ARPKD is dominated by its renal manifestations and associated sequelae, but liver involvement is also commonly present. Congenital hepatic fibrosis is characteristic of ARPKD and correlates with the severity of the renal cystic disease. This may lead to portal hypertension, oesophageal varices, and hepatosplenomegaly. Hypertension usually develops during the first months of life. Careful blood pressure monitoring is essential in preventing sequelae of hypertension (e.g. cardiac hypertrophy, congestive heart failure) and deterioration of renal function.
- **ADPKD:** About 2% of ADPKD patients present with early clinical manifestations before the age of 15 years. These cases are typically associated with significant perinatal morbidity and mortality and may be indistinguishable from ARPKD.
- Clinical symptoms usually arise in adulthood, and there can be considerable phenotypic variability. Chronic renal failure presents in about 50% of patients by the age of 60 years. Polycystic liver disease is the most common extra-renal manifestation. Cysts in other epithelial organs such as the pancreas and diverticulosis are also common. Among the cardiovascular co-morbidities, intracerebral aneurysms play a significant role and are present in about 8% of ADPKD patients, along with hypertension and valvular malformations. Rarely, symptoms related to renal failure may be present.

Diagnosis

- **ARPKD:** Diagnosis may be suspected on prenatal ultrasonography, with bilaterally enlarged and hyperechoic kidneys, with poor cortico-medullary differentiation and multiple cysts. Oligohydramnios may also be present. Amniocentesis and chorionic villus sampling may be used for prenatal diagnosis.
- **ADPKD:** Diagnosis is based on DNA analysis, ultrasonography, and CT. ADPKD is now increasingly diagnosed in the fetus based on antenatal scans (and subsequently in a parent and the extended family). Diagnostic criteria based on ultrasound imaging for ADPKD1 are (Figure 87.1):
  - ≥2 cysts in 1 kidney, or 1 cyst in each kidney in an at-risk patient ≤30 years

Clinical Genetics and Genomics at a Glance, First Edition. Edited by Neeta Lakhani, Kunal Kulkarni, Julian Barwell, Pradeep Vasudevan, and Huw Dorkins.

- ≥2 cysts in each kidney in an at-risk patient aged 30–59 years
- ≥4 cysts in each kidney for an at-risk patient aged ≥60 years

- Genetic testing may be performed. The major indication is for genetic screening in young adults with negative who are being considered as potential kidney donor.

Management

There is no cure for PKD. Approximately, half of the children with this disease die within the first month of life, usually due to pulmonary complications. Management involves reducing the sequelae of renal and extra-renal manifestations and optimising pre-existing renal function. Drug therapy may be required to maintain electrolyte levels and to control hypertension. Pain control may be needed due to enlarging cysts and nephrectomy can be offered. A proportion of patients will require renal replacement therapy in the form of dialysis or kidney transplant. Liver transplantation can also be performed in cases of portal hypertension due to polycystic liver or hepatomegaly.

The future

Much research has focussed on targeting the complex cellular signalling features of a cystic cell. Tolvaptan can slow the increase in total kidney volume and slowed the decline in loss of renal function; it is approved in Europe, but there are concerns about its therapeutic effectiveness and potential for hepatic injury.

Figure 87.1 Clinical features of (a) ARPKD and (b) ADPKD.

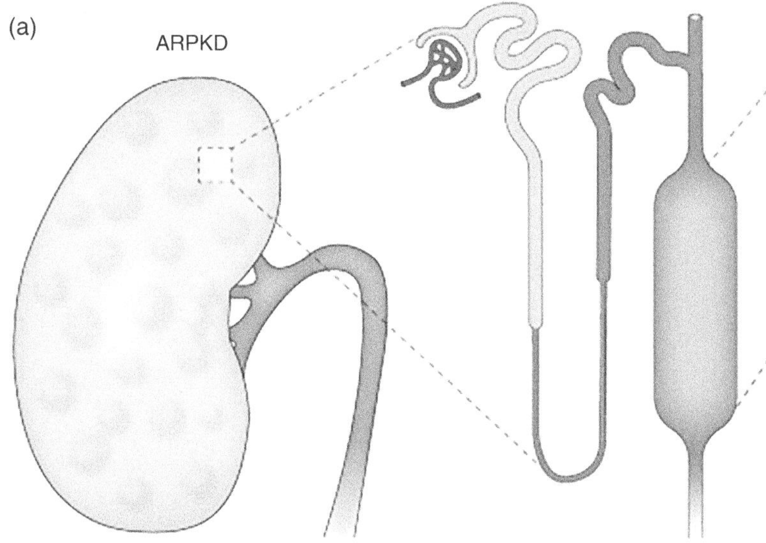

Source: Polycystic kidney disease.

- Typically paediatric onset
- Mutations in *PKHD*1 and *DZIP*1*L*
- Cystic kidneys (collecting ducts and distal tubules) and bile ducts
- Hepatic fibrosis
- Hypertension in up to 75% of children (often during the first few months of life)
- Intracranial aneurysms only described in case reports
- ESRD in 60% of patients by 20 years of age

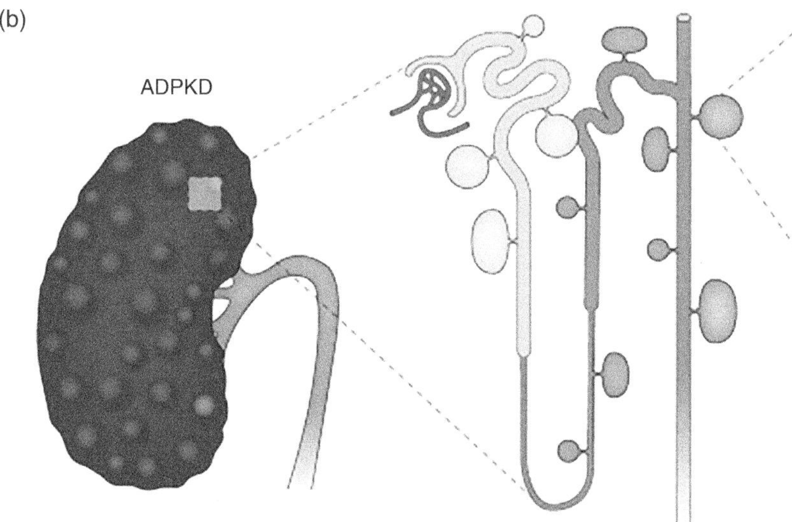

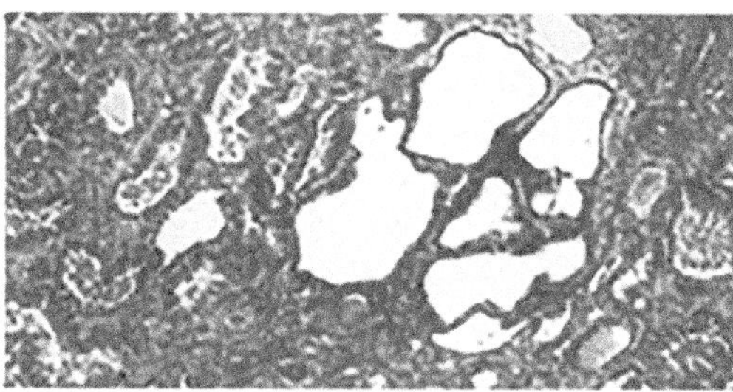

- Typically adult onset
- Mutations in *PKD*1 (~80%) or *PKD*2 (~15%)
- Cystic kidneys (all nephron levels but mainly distal regions), bile ducts and liver
- Hypertension in at least 20–40% of children and adolescents and in most adult patients (50–70% of patients before GFR decline)
- Intracranial aneurysms in ~8% of patients (increased three-fold in patients with a positive family history)
- ESRD in 50% of patients by 60 years of age

Source: https://www.nature.com/articles/s41572-018-0047-y

88 Nephronophthisis

Background

Nephronophthisis (NPHP), or 'wasting of the nephrons' is a chronic tubulointerstitial nephritis, overlapping with other ciliopathy syndromes. It is the most frequent genetic cause of end-stage renal disease (ESRD) in the first three decades of life.

Aetiology

Estimated incidence of NPHP is 1 in 5000.

Genetics

NPHP is an AR condition. Over 20 monogenic recessive genes have been identified, with *NPHP1* being the most common, accounting for 25% of cases. *NPHP1* encodes nephrocystin-1, a protein that interacts with components of cell to cell, and cell to matrix signalling. It also interacts with the products of other NPHP genes, including nephrocystin-2, nephrocystin-3, and nephrocystin-4.

Pathophysiology

The proteins mutated in cystic kidney diseases result in alterations to structures named cilia and the centrosomes of renal epithelial cells (Figure 88.1). Primary cilia are sensory organelles that connect a variety of stimuli to mechanisms of epithelial cell polarity and cell cycle control. Patients subsequently have multiple organ involvement, including retinal degeneration, cerebellar hypoplasia, liver fibrosis, and situs inversus.

Symptoms

- Initial symptoms are relatively mild, except in infantile NPHP type 2. The disease may become apparent in early childhood or adolescence and the clinical presentation is insidious.
- Patients can experience polyuria and polydipsia (due to the renal concentrating defect), but these can be overlooked in the presence of a normal urinalysis and blood pressure. Secondary enuresis may be present. Most patients are therefore not diagnosed until after the onset of renal failure and sequelae such as anaemia.

Clinical features

Three clinical forms of NPHP have been described, based on the onset of ESRD: infantile, juvenile, and adolescent NPHP, which manifest with ESRD at the median ages of 1, 13, and 19 years, respectively.

- **Infantile NPH:** Can present in utero with oligohydramnios sequence (limb contractures, pulmonary hypoplasia, and facial dysmorphisms) or with renal manifestations that progress to ESRD.
- **Juvenile NPH:** This is the most prevalent subtype. It typically presents with polydipsia and polyuria, growth failure, and anaemia, or other findings related to chronic kidney disease. Hypertension is typically absent due to salt wasting. ESRD develops at a median age of 13 years. Ultrasound findings show increased echogenicity, reduced corticomedullary differentiation, and renal cysts. Histologic findings include tubulointerstitial fibrosis, thickened, and disrupted tubular basement membrane and corticomedullary cysts.
- **Adolescent/adult NPH:** Clinically similar to juvenile NPH, but ESRD develops at a median age of 19 years.

The eyes are the most frequently affected extra-renal organ, with patients most commonly developing retinitis pigmentosa, which leads to progressive visual loss and night blindness.

Diagnosis

- Typically relies on the identification of characteristic clinical and imaging findings (Figure 88.2).
- Establishing the genetic cause of the NPH phenotype is possible in approximately 30–40% of individuals.
- A detailed family history and physical examination including blood pressure, growth parameters, and developmental assessment should be performed to evaluate for extra-renal manifestations. Laboratory tests of renal function, anaemia, and metabolic bone disease should be performed. Urinalysis for specific gravity can evaluate concentrating ability and proteinuria.
- Renal ultrasound typically demonstrates increased echogenicity of the kidneys and reduced corticomedullary differentiation.
- Renal biopsy is characterized by a diffuse chronic tubulointerstitial nephritis and by the presence of microcystic dilatation of proximal tubules and Bowman space. Pathologically, it differs from later-onset NPHP by the absence of medullary cysts and thickened tubular basement membranes and by the presence of cortical microcysts.

Management

- There is no treatment available for NPHP and management strategies are based on reducing progression to renal failure.
- Water/electrolyte imbalances and anaemia must be corrected if present, and hypertension should be managed. Children with significant growth retardation can have hormonal treatment. Where significant ESRD is present, renal dialysis or transplantation may be required. Disease recurrence has not been reported in kidneys that were transplanted to patients with NPHP.
- All patients should be under surveillance, with regular blood pressure monitoring, to identify the features that appear with time, such as retinal dystrophy. Patients must avoid nephrotoxic agents, including nonsteroidal anti-inflammatory drugs, aminoglycoside antibiotics, and radiocontrast.

The future

Research into a vasopressin V2 receptor antagonist, OPC31260, has demonstrated that the renal cystic phenotype of *pcy* mice, (the equivalent of human NPHP type 3) can be strongly mitigated or even reversed.

Clinical Genetics and Genomics at a Glance, First Edition. Edited by Neeta Lakhani, Kunal Kulkarni, Julian Barwell, Pradeep Vasudevan, and Huw Dorkins.

Figure 88.1 Pathophysiology of NPHP.

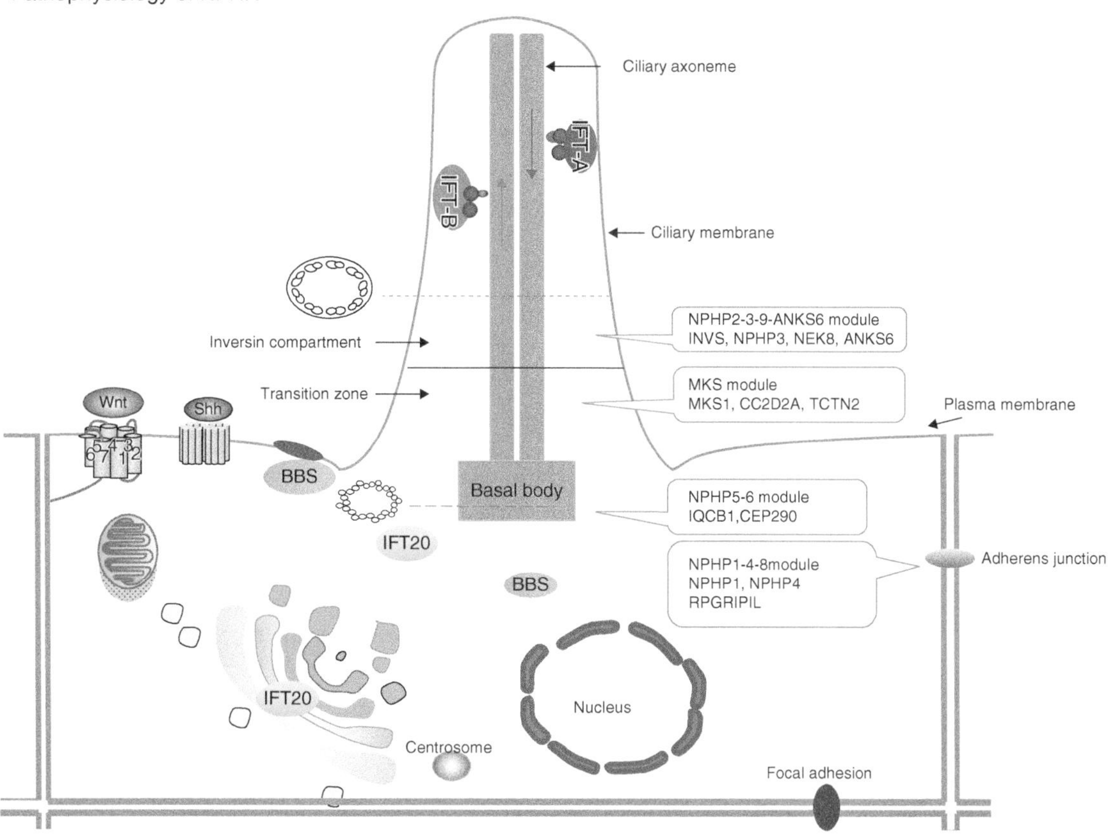

Figure 88.2 Features and investigation of the different forms of NPHP.

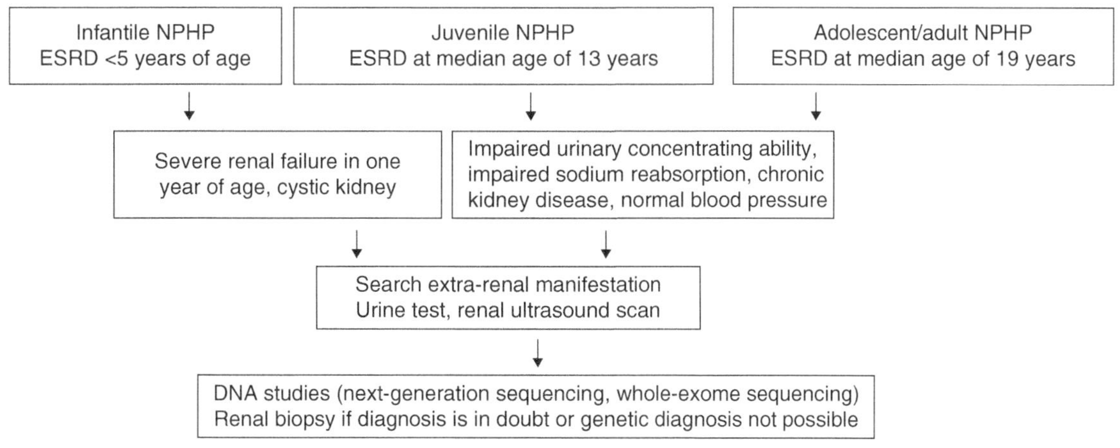

Source: Both taken from https://onlinelibrary.wiley.com/doi/full/10.1111/nep.13393

89 Medullary cystic kidney disease

Background

Medullary cystic kidney disease type 1 (MCKD1) leads to renal fibrosis and impaired kidney function, usually beginning in adulthood.

Aetiology

The incidence of end-stage renal disease (ESRD) caused by MCKD is 0.1%.

Genetics

MCKD1 is an AD inherited condition. It is caused by alterations in the *MUC1* and *UMOD* genes, which encodes the proteins mucin-1 and uromodulin, respectively. These proteins are essential in the production of the lubricating substance mucus, as well as the lining of renal tubules.

Two genetic loci have been identified for MCKD: MCKD1 on 1q21 and MCKD2 on 16p12. Mutations in uromodulin, the Tamm-Horsfall protein, have been shown to cause MCKD type2 (MCKD2), familial juvenile hyperuricaemic nephropathy, and glomerulocystic kidney disease. Uromodulin is expressed in the thick-ascending limb of the nephron; it is the matrix protein for casts and is the most abundant protein in the urine.

Pathophysiology

Mucin-1 and uromodulin are expressed in the thick ascending limb and distal convoluted tubule of the kidney. Alterations lead to the production of deposits within cells of the renal tubules, leading to cell death, which causes a progressive loss of kidney function.

Symptoms and clinical features

- Due to a urinary concentrating defect, patients experience polyuria, polydipsia, and secondary enuresis.
- Kidney function may remain stable or demonstrate a slow decline, and usually results in ESRD in the 4th–6th decades of life. Renal replacement therapy may be required and disease recurrences have not been observed following kidney transplant.
- The key significant extra-renal manifestation associated with MCKD is hyperuricaemia with gouty arthritis. No other distinctive findings on physical examination are associated with MCKD.
- There are no distinctive findings on physical examination with MCKD.

Diagnosis

- Laboratory evaluation includes urinalysis, where a low specific gravity is found, reflecting a significant urinary concentration defect. Urinalysis is otherwise unremarkable, without significant proteinuria or haematuria.
- Serum biochemistry evaluation for electrolytes, creatinine, phosphate, parathyroid hormone level, and uric acid should be performed.
- Renal ultrasound may demonstrate a normal or reduced kidney size, with increased echogenicity, loss of corticomedullary differentiation, and medullary cysts. Cysts range in size from 1 to 15 mm and usually arise from the distal convoluted tubule or medullary collecting duct. They may not be seen on imaging early in the course of disease.

Management

- No disease-specific therapy is currently available. Management involves treatments to reduce the progression of kidney failure and specific manifestations such as anaemia, acidosis, hyperparathyroidism, urinary tract infection, and hypertension if present.
- Xanthine oxidase inhibitors and uricosurics can be used to treat hyperuricaemia and prevent episodes of gout.
- Patients should receive genetic counselling regarding family risk and planning.

The future

It has been observed that if the angiotensin-converting enzyme gene (ACE) is knocked out in mice, they develop a renal syndrome that resembles MCKD. Increased levels of cyclic adenosine monophosphate (cAMP) have been seen in the renal tubular epithelial cells of a mouse model of MCKD, suggesting that cAMP is functioning as a second messenger in the abnormal proliferation of renal epithelial cells, although the mechanism is unclear. These pathways may yield potential future therapeutic targets.

Clinical Genetics and Genomics at a Glance, First Edition. Edited by Neeta Lakhani, Kunal Kulkarni, Julian Barwell, Pradeep Vasudevan, and Huw Dorkins.

Urine culture

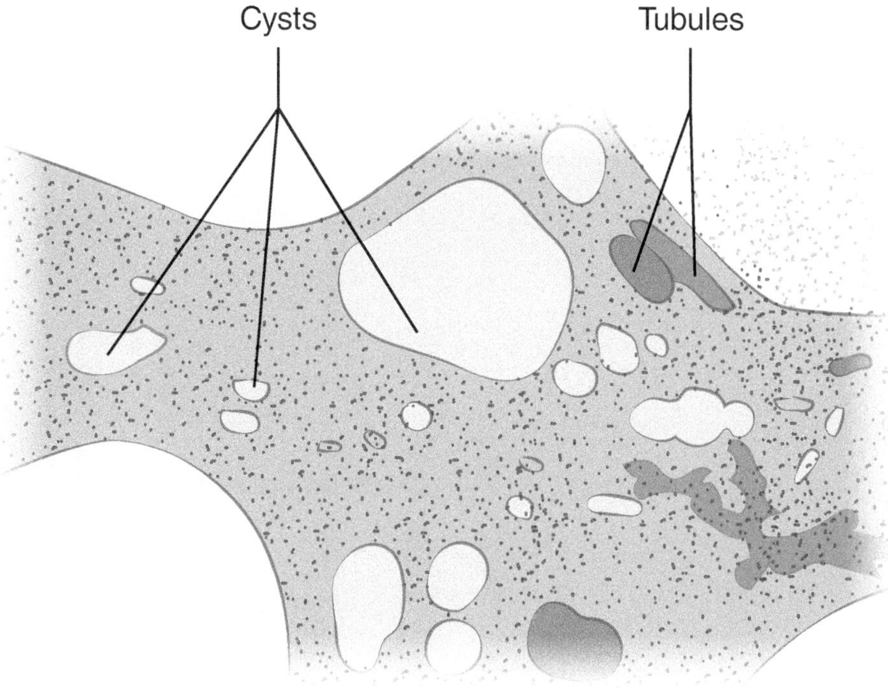

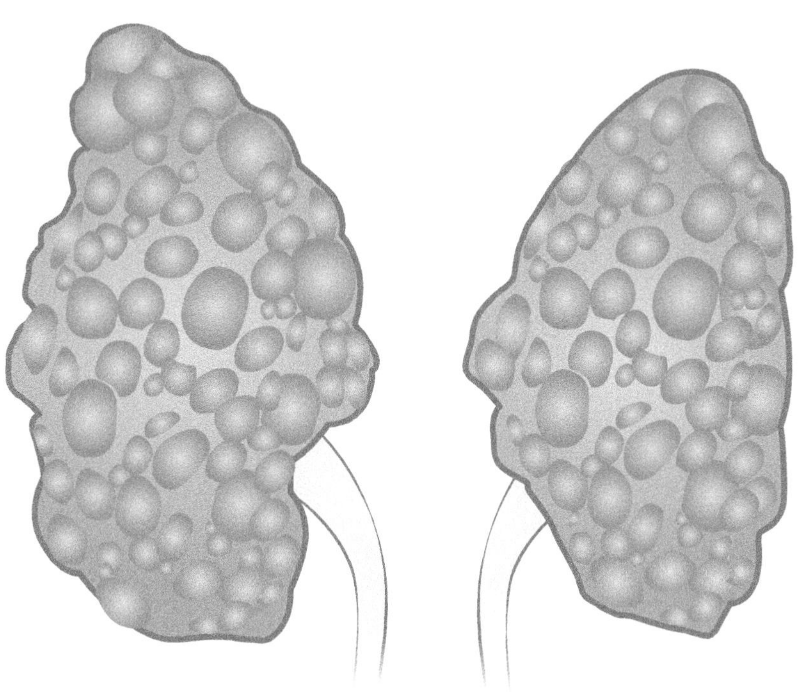

90 Alport syndrome

Background

Alport syndrome (also known as hereditary nephritis) is an inherited syndrome caused by defects in synthesis of type IV collagen, a major component of tissue basement membranes.

Aetiology

Alport syndrome is rare, with an incidence of 1 in 5000 live births.

Genetics

Alport syndrome is inherited in either an X-linked form (*COL4A5* gene on Xq22) by males or an AR form by either gender (*COL4A3* and *COL4A4* genes on 2q). Genes are located on chromosomes 2, 13, and X. These encode chains of collagen type IV, a component of the glomerular basement membrane (GBM) in the kidney. Affected patients can present with a wide spectrum of phenotypes, depending on the nature of the alteration they carry. Thin basement membrane nephropathy (TBMN) is usually caused by heterozygous alterations in the *COL4A3* and *COL4A4* genes and may represent a carrier state of AR Alport syndrome. They often present with isolated haematuria.

Aetiology

Genetic alterations lead to an abnormality in type IV collagen, which results in splitting of the GBM, podocyte effacement, glomerulosclerosis with extracellular matrix deposition, renal fibrosis. Ultimately, this results in ESRD, early in life.

Pathophysiology

Collagen type IV is composed of six different α chains, which assemble into three different heterotrimers in a tissue-specific distribution. These heterotrimers are essential for basement membrane structure and function. As the GBM is a key component of the filtration barrier, patients with Alport syndrome develop proteinuria. Over time, these changes may result in the accumulation of extracellular matrix and glomerulosclerosis, kidney fibrosis due to fibroblast formation (Figure 90.1).

Figure 90.1 Pathophysiology of Alport syndrome.

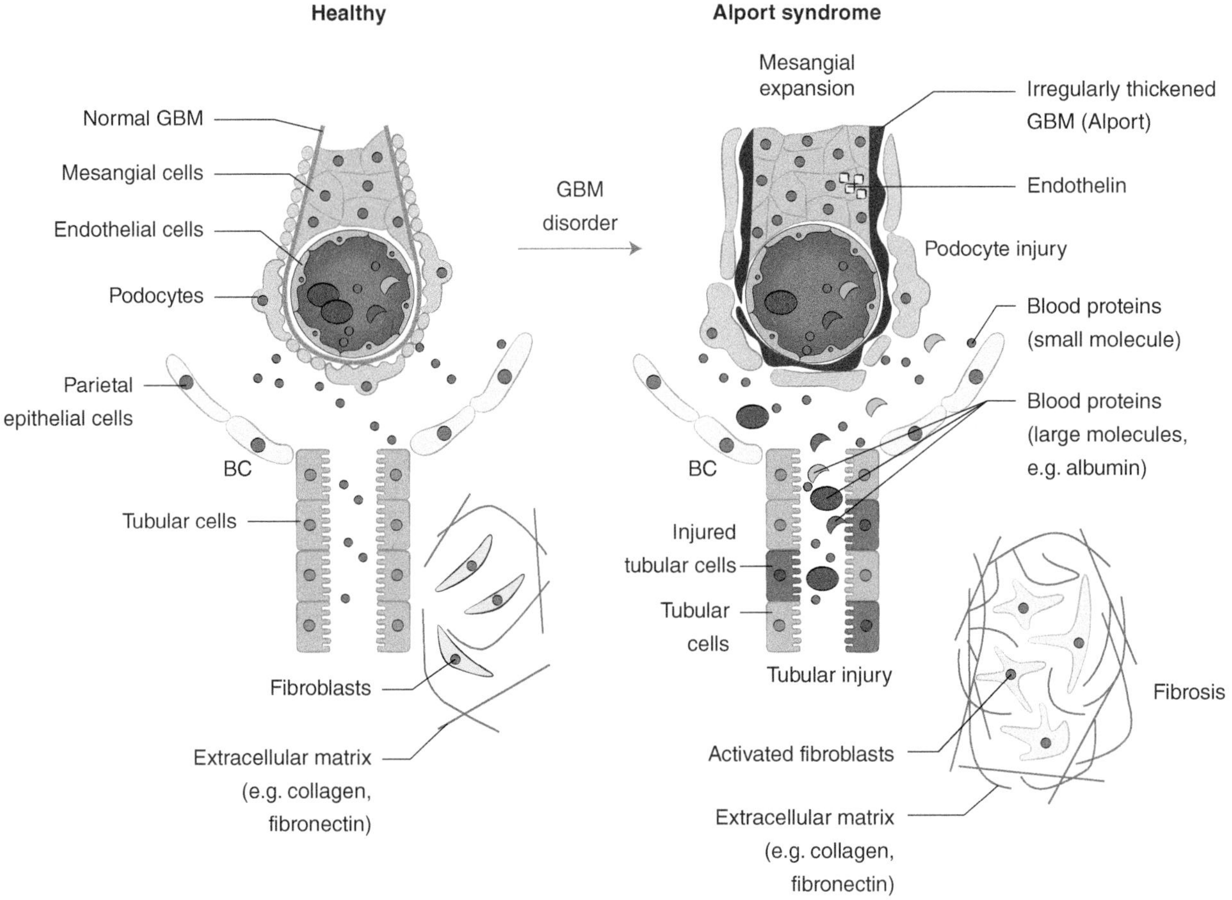

Clinical Genetics and Genomics at a Glance, First Edition. Edited by Neeta Lakhani, Kunal Kulkarni, Julian Barwell, Pradeep Vasudevan, and Huw Dorkins.

Symptoms and clinical features

- Presentation is typically with upper respiratory tract infections with visible or non-visible haematuria. Renal failure occurs in the second to third decade of life.
- Patients with AR Alport syndrome and males with X-linked Alport syndrome develop proteinuria in early adulthood, with subsequent nephrotic syndrome. Hypertension is also common.
- Progressive hearing loss is usually clinically significant by the second decade.
- Anterior lenticonus is associated with established progression to ESRD and occurs in 15% of males with X-linked disease.

Diagnosis

- Diagnosis is confirmed by renal biopsy, which demonstrates a thickened GMB that is split and replaced with small, dense granulations. Renal function may initially be unaffected, and imaging is typically normal, but is important to exclude alternative diagnoses.
- Genetic screening by linkage analysis or gene sequencing is possible, although challenging due to the large number of disease-causing alterations.

Management

- Patients are advised to follow low-phosphate, low-protein, and low-salt diets.
- Treatment with the calcineurin inhibitor ciclosporin is described, offering some preservation of renal function, but the evidence is limited to small studies.
- Treatment of hypertension can reduce proteinuria and delay the progression of renal failure. Renal transplantation is an effective treatment after ESRD develops. Following transplantation, exposure to these previously absent type IV collagen subunits in the renal allograft may trigger a significant immune response. Post-transplantation anti-GBM disease has been in patients with Alport syndrome.
- Ophthalmology and audiology review should also be performed early to identify problems.
- All patients should be offered genetic counselling.

The future

Bone marrow transplantation has been shown to ameliorate renal disease in a murine model of Alport syndrome, although clinical trials in humans have not yet been conducted. Increased use of angiotensin-converting enzyme inhibitors and angiotensin II receptor blockers may slow progression of excretory dysfunction and delay the onset of ESRD, although the evidence for this also remains very limited.

91 Cystinosis

Background

Cystinosis is an inherited metabolic disorder of systemic cystine accumulation, resulting from defective lysosomal transport of the amino acid cystine. The commonest organ manifestations are renal (non-glomerular) and ophthalmic.

Aetiology

This is an extremely rare condition, with approximately only 180 patients in the United Kingdom. Cystinosis occurs in all ethnic groups and has a higher prevalence in communities with a higher rate of consanguinity.

Genetics

Cystinosis, like many other metabolic disorders, is inherited in an AR manner. Alterations in *CTNS* (encoding the protein cystinosin) on chromosome 17p13 lead to either a lack of production of cystinosin or its defective action, causing lysosomal cystine accumulation. The commonest alteration is a 57 kb deletion.

Pathophysiology

Lysosomes are intracellular organelles that accumulate breakdown products from the intracellular degradation of macromolecules. Lysosome cell membranes contain a variety of distinct transporters, one of which is cystinosin. Cystinosin acts as the lysosomal cystine/H^+ symporter, mediating cystine transport out of the lysosome. Defects in the transporter result in lysosomal accumulation of cystine and cystinosis. There is high lysosomal density in the cornea and proximal renal tubule, making the eyes and kidneys most susceptible to the disease.

Symptoms and clinical features

- Symptoms typically develop in the first year of life, with many non-specific symptoms, including poor feeding, failure to gain weight, vomiting, and slow gross motor development (Figure 91.1).
- While kidney dysfunction predominates in the first decade, systemic cystine accumulation causes multiple organ dysfunction.
- Poor growth, hypothyroidism, and hypergonadotrophic hypogonadism with delayed puberty is common. Impaired glucose tolerance results in the development of diabetes mellitus.
- Several neurological features may be present including swallowing difficulties, myopathy, visuospatial, and motor problems. Progressive corneal crystal deposition and clouding is also common.

Diagnosis

- Genetic testing via a PCR-based test can identify the most common alteration (*CTNS* deletion).
- Cystine crystals can also be demonstrated via slit-lamp examination of the eye or via tissue biopsy.
- Patients may have hyperchloraemic metabolic acidosis, hypokalaemia, and hypophosphataemia. On biopsy, histological sections show variation in size and shape of proximal tubules and irregularity of the brush border. There is also variation in the appearances of podocytes, sometimes forming a multinucleate giant cell.

Management

- The goal is to treat volume depletion, replace solute losses, and correct acidosis.
- Untreated children risk life-threatening dehydration and electrolyte imbalance. They can progress to ESRD by 10 years. Renal transplantation is then an option, and the disorder does not recur within the kidney.
- Large amounts of fluids and electrolytes are required, often exceeding conventionally defined limits. Urinary losses must be carefully monitored and replaced. The rehydration fluid should contain glucose, sodium, potassium, and bicarbonate, ensuring adequate ongoing fluid intake and nutrition is required with some children requiring enteral feeding support. Acidosis must be slowly corrected with sodium bicarbonate supplements (IV or oral) or combined sodium and potassium citrate solutions.
- Recombinant growth hormone may be necessary in children with sustained poor growth.
- Delayed-release cysteamine bitartrate is available for the management of nephropathic cystinosis for patients older than two years. This reacts with intralysosomal cystine to form mixed-disulphide cysteamine–cysteine, which can then leave the lysosome using the lysine transporter.
- Adults with cystinosis usually require standard management of their renal replacement therapy and more specialist assessment of the treatment and multi-system problems of cystinosis every 3–4 months.

The future

Effective cysteamine treatment has changed the outlook for cystinosis, from inevitable renal replacement therapy within the first decade to a disorder requiring intense medication but with prospects of reasonable growth and kidney survival through childhood. There is also encouraging evidence that cysteamine ameliorates the longer-term complications. A better understanding of the underlying pathogenetic mechanism by which cystine accumulates within the lysosome and affects cell dysfunction should open new avenues of therapy.

Clinical Genetics and Genomics at a Glance, First Edition. Edited by Neeta Lakhani, Kunal Kulkarni, Julian Barwell, Pradeep Vasudevan, and Huw Dorkins.

Figure 91.1 Clinical features of cystinosis.

Eyes
- Corneal cystine crystals (photophobia,blepharospasm)
- Filamentary keratopathy
- Iris thickening
- Corneal erosions
- Band keratopathy
- Retinopathy (impaired colour vision, visual field constriction, retinal blindness)
- Cataract

Endocrinology + Reproduction
- Hypothyroidism
- Growth retardation
- Delayed puberty
- Insulin-dependent diabetes mellitus
- Azoospermia
- Primary hypogonadism

Kidney
- Renal Fanconi syndrome (polydipsia, polyuria, dehydratation, proximal renal tubular acidosis, urinary loss of electrolytes, glucosuria, aminoaciduria)
- Glomerular proteinuria
- Deterioration of renal function

Skin
- Hypohydrosis
- Heat intolerance
- Hypopigmentation of skin and hair

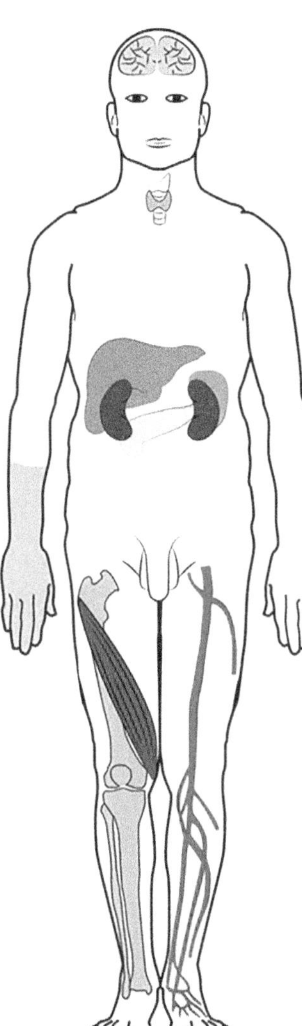

Neurology
- Neurocognitive impairment
- Non-verbal learning difficulties
- Impairment in visual-motor function
- Cystine encephalopathy (cerebellar and pyramidal signs, mental deterioration, pseudo-bulbar palsy, distal myopathy, weakness of the extremities, dysphagia, pulmonary insufficiency)
- Behavioural problems

Gastrointestinal
- Hepatomegaly
- Splenomegaly
- Exocrine pancreas insufficiency

Haematology
- Cystine crystal accumulation in bone marrow (Pancytopenia)

Bone and Muscle
- Hypophosphatemic rickets (genua vara, frontal bossing, rachitic rosary, metaphyseal widening)

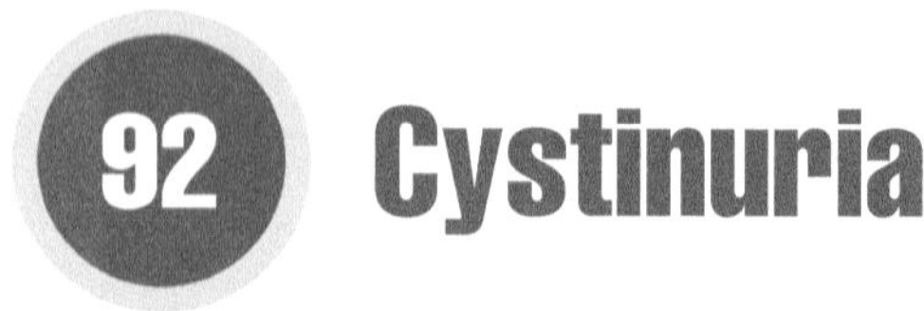

92 Cystinuria

Background

Cystinuria is a rare recessive condition characterised by the accumulation of the amino acid cysteine in the kidneys and bladder.

Aetiology

Incidence varies widely, for example, from 1 in 2500 (in Jewish Israelis of Libyan origin) to 1 in 100 000 (in Sweden).

Genetics

Cystinuria is caused by a defective dibasic amino acid transporter of cystine, lysine, arginine, and ornithine in the renal proximal tubules and small bowel. Alterations in the *SLC3A1* or *SLC7A9* gene lead to this defect. *SLC3A1* alterations are inherited in a true AR mechanism, whereas in *SLC7A9*, inheritance is AD, with incomplete penetrance. Individuals with a single copy of the altered gene can present with disease, but the presence of two altered genes leads to a more severe presentation.

Pathophysiology

The genes encode a protein complex in the kidneys that enables the reabsorption of certain amino acids, including cysteine, into the blood from the filtered fluid that becomes urine. As a result, the amino acids become concentrated in the urine. Cystine is relatively insoluble compared with the other dibasic amino acids and accumulates, leading to crystal formation (Figure 92.1).

Symptoms

The most common symptom of urinary tract stones is ureteric colic – a severe waxing and waning pain felt anywhere from the loin to the groin. Haematuria may also be present, as can symptoms of a urinary tract infection.

Clinical features

There are no specific features on clinical examination, but in patients with severe urinary tract infection (pyelonephritis), fever, tachycardia, and hypotension could be present.

Diagnosis

- As a rare condition, the diagnosis is often missed or delayed. Screening should be considered in patients with recurrent or bilateral stones, patients who first present at a young age (<30 years old), or those with siblings with stone disease.
- Microscopic evaluation of urine to identify cystine crystals is performed. Sodium cyanide-nitroprusside is used as a screening test and only requires a urine sample. Cyanide reduces cystine to cysteine, which then binds to nitroprusside, resulting in a red to purple colour change. The sensitivity of this test is 72% with a specificity of 95%. In patients who form renal calculi, stone analysis can be undertaken, which demonstrates cystine composition or raised levels of urinary dibasic amino acids.
- Genetic testing can be performed to identify the known alterations.

Management

- A multimodal approach is required from diagnosis, to treatment, and the prevention of sequelae, the most important being the formation of renal stones and deteriorating renal function.
- The primary objective of treatment is to reduce the cystine concentration in the urine. The ratio of soluble to insoluble cystine is affected by its urinary concentration, urinary pH, and urine volume.
- Adequate hydration is the most important (and most simple) method to prevent stone formation in cystinuria. Consumption of large amounts of fluid both day and night helps maintain a high volume of urine and reduces cystine concentration in the urine. For practical reasons, 3–4 l/day are recommended. Caffeinated drinks should be avoided.
- Alkalinisation of the urine is important. Patients with consistently low urinary pH despite adequate fluid intake can take an alkalinising agent, such as potassium citrate or sodium bicarbonate, which can increase urinary pH and the solubility of cysteine. This treatment is accompanied by dietary salt and animal protein restriction.
- Thiol-binding drugs such as D-penicillamine and mercaptopropionylglycine (also known as tiopronin) can be very effective. A soluble drug-product 50 times more soluble than cystine is formed, which can then be excreted in urine. Adverse effects include nonspecific allergy, nausea, leucopenia, thrombocytopenia, proteinuria, and systemic-lupus-erythematosus-like syndromes, so patients should be regularly monitored.
- The management of cystine stones is identical to that of all other stone types – conservatively or with surgery. The choice of intervention will depend on numerous factors, such as stone size, location, previous intervention, availability of equipment, and surgeon/patient preference. Patients with cystinuria often have multiple procedures and high recurrence rates; a balance between the safety of the procedure and stone clearance must be achieved.
- Genetic counselling is recommended for patients and their families. Other treatment is symptomatic and supportive.

The future

Future research into cystinuria should aim to focus on collaboration, both at national and international levels, owing to the small number of affected patients. Current research is predominantly focussed on the basic science, involving α-lipoic acid (α-LA) (a nutritional supplement) and tolvaptan (an arginine vasopressin receptor antagonist), which decrease urinary supersaturation in kidney stone formers by considerably increasing diuresis.

Clinical Genetics and Genomics at a Glance, First Edition. Edited by Neeta Lakhani, Kunal Kulkarni, Julian Barwell, Pradeep Vasudevan, and Huw Dorkins.

Figure 92.1 Pathophysiology of cystinuria.

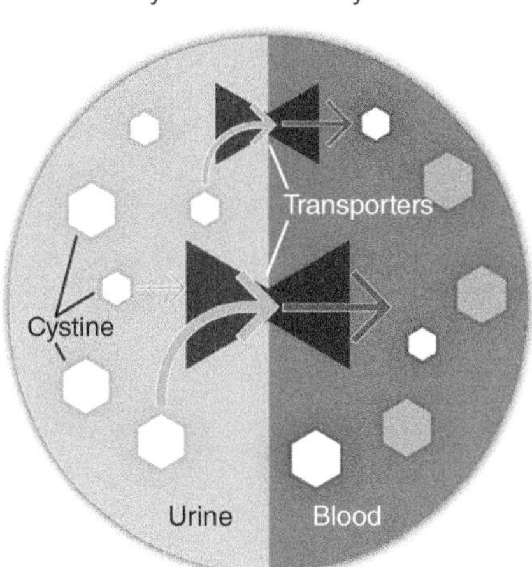

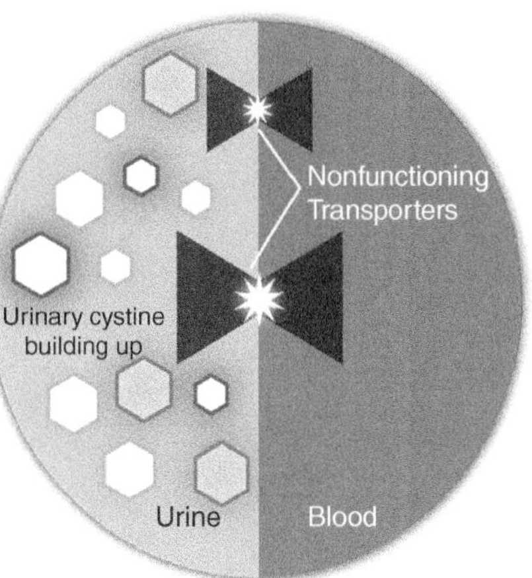

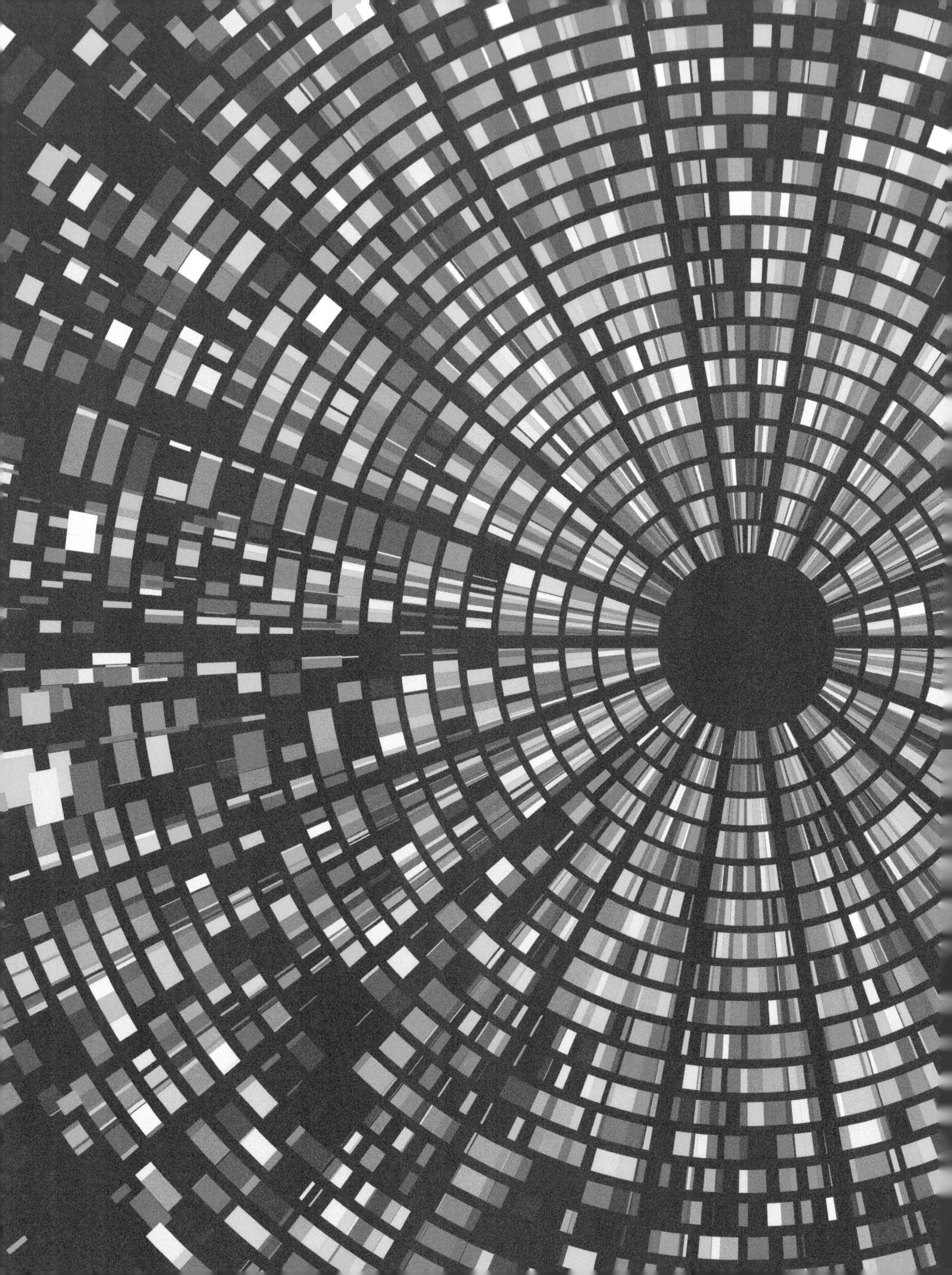

Musculoskeletal

Chapters

93 Marfan syndrome

Background

Marfan syndrome (MFS) is a systemic connective tissue disorder. As a result, manifestations are wide ranging, with abnormal tissue growth in multiple sites, classically including the heart, vessels, bones, joints, and eyes. Clinical phenotype, severity and presentation age are variable, including among affected members of the same family. A multidisciplinary approach to management is therefore required.

Aetiology

Global incidence is 1 in 5000–10000, equal in both sexes, and with no ethnic predilection.

Genetics

MFS is caused by an alteration in the fibrillin-1 (*FBN1*) gene on the long arm of chromosome 15. Around 75% of cases are inherited, with the remainder *de novo* alterations, with both somatic and germline mosaicism possible. Inheritance is in a AD manner, resulting in a 50% risk to all offspring. In cases of *de novo* alteration (with unaffected parents), recurrence risk is low. Penetrance is age-dependant and variable, even within families, leading to variable expression. Approximately 75% of individuals with MFS have a positive family history of MFS. Neonatal forms or more severe forms of MFS are usually caused by *de novo* alterations.

Pathophysiology

Fibrillin-1 is a component of the microfibrils of the extracellular matrix; it is a glycoprotein associated with elastin, commonly found in the cardiac valvular tissues, suspensory ligament of the eye, and in skin, tendons, cartilage, and periosteum. Abnormal *FBN1* results in reduced normal microfibril formation, resulting in excess growth factors (such as transforming growth factor beta, TGF-β). Their increased availability causes tissue overgrowth and generalised joint laxity.

Symptoms and clinical features

New patients may present in differing ways, with any of the general, cardiac, skeletal, or ocular manifestations (Figure 93.1). Tall stature and arachnodactyly are commonly presenting features. MFS can present at different ages, with a continuum of phenotypes of differing severity. As a result, diagnosis may not be made until later in life.

Neonates and infants presenting with the rapidly progressive, early-onset phenotype are often floppy and long. They may develop severe and rapidly progressive scoliosis, joint contractures, arachnodactyly and aortic disease. This form is often more severe and may be fatal. 'Classic' MFS may be milder overall.

Other associated syndromes/variants also exist, such as Shprintzen-Goldberg syndrome (heterozygous *SKI* alteration, AD), a rare condition presenting in infants with features that

Figure 93.1 Clinical signs associated with Marfan syndrome.

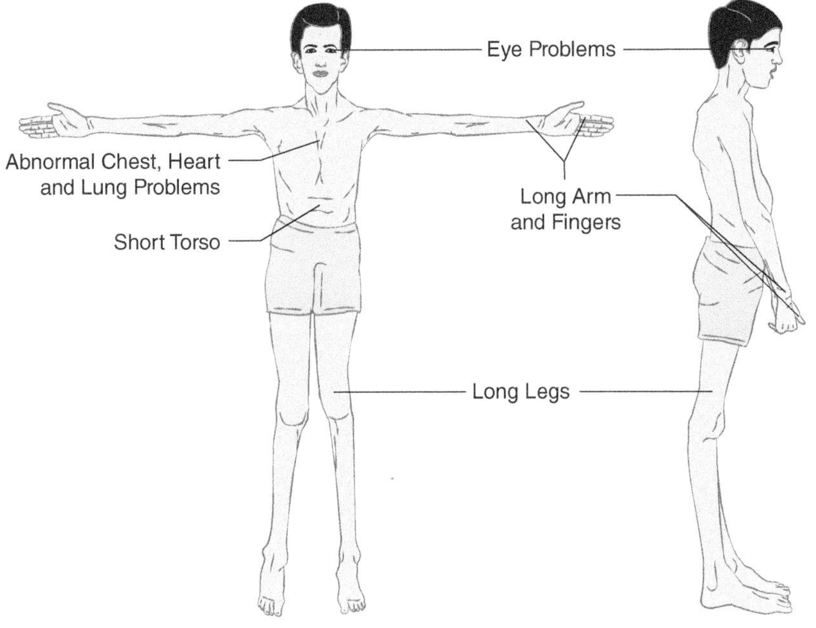

Signs and Symptoms of Marfan Syndrome
- Disproportionately long legs, arms, toes and fingers
- Extremely tall and slender build
- Long, narrow face
- High arched neck and crowded teeth
- Indented or protruding sternum
- Dislocated lenses of the eyes
- High pressure in the eye
- Cystic changes in the lungs
- Flexible joints
- Flat feet
- Curved spine
- Abnormal heart sounds

Clinical Genetics and Genomics at a Glance, First Edition. Edited by Neeta Lakhani, Kunal Kulkarni, Julian Barwell, Pradeep Vasudevan, and Huw Dorkins.

overlap MFS and Crouzon syndrome. Other differential conditions may have similar presentations, including homocysteinuria (learning difficulty, high urinary homocysteine levels); Stickler syndrome (distinctive facial features, ocular problems, hearing loss, joint problems); Loeys-Dietz syndrome; X-linked thoracic aortic aneurysm and dissection; Ehlers-Danlos syndrome.

The features of MFS can be divided into systems:

- **Skeletal system:** Bone overgrowth; excessive growth of the long bones leads to increased height (taller than predicted for their family) and arachnodactyly. Patients have disproportionately long arms in comparison to the trunk size, leading to an increase in the ratio of the arm span to height and decreased ratio of the upper segment to lower segment. Scoliosis can be caused by bone overgrowth and ligament laxity. Overgrowth of the ribs cause the sternum to be pushed inwards (pectus excavatum) or outwards (pectus carinatum). Joint laxity or conversely, reduced joint mobility, particularly in the elbow and digits. Protrusio acetabuli (deformity of the medial wall of the acetabulum).
- **Cardiovascular system:** Cardiovascular manifestations are the major cause of morbidity and mortality and can include aortic dilatation/dissection, and mitral and tricuspid valve prolapse or regurgitation.
- **Ocular system:** Myopia is one of the most common ocular manifestations. Ectopia lentis (upward dislocation of the lens of the eye) is present in around 60% of individuals with MFS. Other ocular manifestations may include retinal detachment, glaucoma, and early cataract formation.
- **Respiratory system:** Bullae can develop in the lungs causing predisposition for a spontaneous pneumothorax.
- **Skin:** Striae can be caused by rapid growth, typically on the back.
- **Facial features:** Long, narrow face, with dysmorphic features. Downward slanting palpebral fissures. Enophthalmos (deep set eyes). Micrognathia and retrognathia. Malar hypoplasia. Narrow and high-arched palate. Dental overcrowding.

Diagnosis

The diagnosis of MFS is usually based on clinical examination along with family history, echocardiogram results and ophthalmology findings and supported by the results of genetic testing. The physical features are reviewed in a systemic score that helps make a clinical diagnosis of MFS. This is based on a set of defined clinical criteria, the Revised Ghent Criteria (Loeys et al. 2010) to help facilitate diagnosis (Table 93.1).

In cases of known *FBN1* mutation in first-degree relatives, prenatal testing (CVS, amniocentesis) is possible. Pregnant women require additional assessment, particularly of cardiac valvular abnormalities. Parents (and/or siblings) of affected children should receive clinical assessment, ophthalmic slit-lamp examination, and cardiac echosonography. Children of affected parents should have periodic assessment.

Management

Regular surveillance off affected individuals and those at higher risk is essential. With appropriate management, the life expectancy of individuals with MFS is roughly that of the general population. Treatment depends upon the clinical manifestation:

Table 93.1 Revised Ghent Criteria (2010) and Loeys et al. (2010).

Index case & no family history

- Aortic Root Dilatation Z score ≥ 2 AND Ectopia Lentis
- Aortic Root Dilatation Z score ≥ 2 AND *FBN1*
- Aortic Root Dilatation Z score ≥ 2 AND Systemic Score ≥ 7 pts
- Ectopia lentis AND *FBN1* with known Aortic Root Dilatation

Family history present

- Ectopia lentis AND Family History of Marfan syndrome (as defined above)
- A systemic score ≥ 7 points AND Family History of Marfan syndrome (as defined above)
- Aortic Root Dilatation Z score ≥ 2 above 20 yr old, ≥ 3 below 20 yr old) + Family History of Marfan syndrome (as defined above)

Note: Without discriminating features of Shprintzen-Goldberg syndrome, Loeys-Dietz syndrome, or vascular Ehlers-Danlos syndrome ***and*** after *TGFBR1/2*, collagen biochemistry, *COL3A1* testing if indicated. Other conditions/genes will emerge with time.

- **General:** Growth should be monitored regularly in children, although growth-slowing medical/surgical intervention is rare. Dental overcrowding may need orthodontic input.
- **Ophthalmic:** Highly myopic/raised axial globe length patients should avoid contact sports or high-velocity activities with sudden acceleration/deceleration. Periodic surveillance, including for glaucoma, is needed, especially in children and teenagers, with early intervention to correct acuity disturbances. Acute retinal detachment should be suspected in sudden visual field loss.
- **Cardiovascular:** Beta and angiotensin receptor blockers may help reduce progression of valvular root dilatation. Annual cardiac surveillance (including echo/cardiac MRI) is recommended for most, with more frequent review for those with significant valvular disease (aortic root dilatation >4.5 cm) that is rapidly increasing (>3 mm/year). Pregnant women should have an echo in each trimester. Surgery may be needed for aortic root dilatation >5 cm. Acute dissection requires emergency intervention. Mortality is most commonly (>80%) due to cardiovascular complications.
- **Orthopaedic:** Scoliosis, when severe or progressive, may require bracing or surgery. Non-operative management is preferred for patello-femoral joint instability as recurrence is common after surgery. Orthotic insoles can be given for symptomatic pes planus.
- **Respiratory:** Pleurodesis if recurrent pneumothorax. Avoid risky activities (e.g. scuba diving).

The future

Future gene therapy for AD-inherited disorders such as MFS present a therapeutic challenge as this would necessitate suppression of the disease-causing allele without affecting expression of the wild-type allele. Trials using gene editing technology such as CRISPR (Clustered Regularly Interspaced Short Palindromic Repeats) are ongoing.

Reference

1. Loeys, B.L., Dietz, H.C., Braverman, A.C., et al., (2010). The revised Ghent nosology for the Marfan syndrome. *Journal of Medical Genetics*, 47 (7): 476–485.

Ehlers-Danlos syndrome (EDS)

Background

These are a group of disorders affecting the connective tissues. With connective tissues playing important structural roles in multiple systems, including the skin, bones, vasculature, and viscera, abnormalities yield a broad range of phenotypes, from joint laxity to vascular dissection.

Aetiology

Combined prevalence (all types) is around 1 in 5000. Hypermobile (1 in 5–20 000) and classical types (1 in 20–40 000) are commonest.

Genetics

Eleven subtypes of EDS were originally described (I to XI), although the Villefranch nomenclature (1997) simplified this to a more descriptive classification. This has since been revised (2017) to include recently identified and rarer subtypes; 13 subtypes are currently included (Table 94.1).

Over 19 gene alterations have been associated with EDS, with most affecting collagen production. Inheritance is variable, with *de novo* alterations in a proportion.

Pathophysiology

Most gene alterations result in impaired collagen production, processing, or assembly. Some gene alterations associated with rarer subtypes have functions unrelated to collagen synthesis yet still result in similar clinical features.

Symptoms

Skin and joint laxity is a common presenting feature, present in most subtypes of EDS. Table 94.1 outlines some of the features of the rarer subtypes that patients may also present with, including life-threatening vascular rupture and haemodynamic compromise.

Table 94.1 Subtypes of Ehlers-Danlos syndrome.

Type	Inheritance, alteration, protein	Main features
Classical	AD. *COL5A1/2* (usually; type 5 collagen); *COL1A1* (rarely; type 1 collagen)	Second commonest. Joint hypermobility and dislocations, skin laxity and fragility. Cigarette-paper scars. Occasional scoliosis and cardiac valvular prolapse
Classical-like	AR. *TNXB* (tenascin XB)	Joint hypermobility, elastic and fragile skin. No scar atrophy (as with other types)
Hypermobile	AD. Unknown (usually); *TNXB* (rarely)	Majority of cases. Joint hypermobility and dislocations. Associated with chronic fatigue, anxiety, depression, headaches, limb/joint pain
Cardiac-valvular	AR. *COL1A2*. Type 1 collagen	Cardiac abnormalities (e.g. mitral/aortic valvular insufficiency), lax and fragile skin that is easily bruised, atrophic scarring, joint laxity
Arthrochalasia	AD (usually); AR (rare) *COL1A1/2* (some). Type 1 collagen	Very rare (few cases only). Short stature, skin and joint laxity, dislocations (hip dislocation at birth). Skin biopsy useful in diagnosis
Vascular	AD (usually); AR (rare). *COL3A1* (most); *COL1A1* (rare). Type 1 collagen	Spontaneous life-threatening vascular or visceral (e.g. bowel, uterus) rupture. Skin bruising. Clubfoot. Variable skin laxity
Dermatosparaxis	AR. *ADAMTS2*. ADAMTS-2	Very rare (few cases only). Very fragile skin with excess sagging, wrinkles, folds (skin biopsy useful in diagnosis)
Kyphoscoliotic	AR. *PLOD1, FKB14*. LH1, FKB22, ZNF469	Severe scoliosis, retinal detachment, skin, and joint laxity
Periodontal	AD. *C1R*. C1r	Early dental disease, joint laxity and dislocations, pretibial skin discolouration, early osteoarthritis, scoliosis
Spondylodysplastic	AR. *B4GALT7, B3GALT6, SLC39A13*. *B4GalT7, B3GalT6, ZIP13*	Short stature, skeletal abnormalities (e.g. bowing of long bones)
Musculocontractural	AR. *CHST14, DSE*. D4ST1, *DSE*.	Muscle hypotonia, joint contractures
Myopathic	AD or AR. *COL12A1*. Type 12 collagen	Muscle hypotonia, joint contractures
Brittle cornea syndrome	*ZNF469, PRDM5*. Proteins of same names	Blue sclerae, corneal rupture post-minor trauma, keratoconus/keratoglobus, skin and joint laxity

Clinical Genetics and Genomics at a Glance, First Edition. Edited by Neeta Lakhani, Kunal Kulkarni, Julian Barwell, Pradeep Vasudevan, and Huw Dorkins.

Clinical features

Table 94.1 summarises the clinical features of the various subtypes of EDS. The key features include:

- **Joint hypermobility:** Occurs in most types, particularly the hypermobile-type. High Beighton score (Figure 94.1).
- **Hypotonia:** Associated with hypermobility, particularly in neonates and young children. Particularly seen with the musculocontractural and myopathic forms.
- **Developmental delay:** Motor skills, in particular those involving truncal tone (e.g. sitting, standing, walking) may be delayed due to hypermobility and hypotonia.
- **Joint instability/dislocation:** This is associated with a loss of function and pain. With some types (e.g. arthrochalasia), there may be hip dysplasia, with dislocations at birth.
- **Excess skin elasticity:** The skin is often described as softer and more fragile than normal, resulting in bruising with minimal trauma and impaired wound healing ('cigarette paper scars'). Some types (e.g. dermatosparaxis) have particularly saggy excess skin folds.
- **Vascular abnormalities:** Life-threatening vascular dissection and visceral rupture are associated with the vascular-type (and also the classical, classical-like and kyphoscoliotic types to an extent). Cardiac valvular function is impaired in the cardiac-valvular type. Visceral rupture may occur with lesser trauma (gut) or pregnancy (uterus).
- **Ophthalmic abnormalities:** Brittle cornea syndrome features thinning of the cornea.
- **Musculoskeletal abnormalities:** Short stature/limb deformity are seen with the spondylodysplastic-type, with features including bowing of the long bones. Progressive scoliosis is seen with the kyphoscoliotic-type and can restrict respiratory function. Joint contractures are found in the musculocontractural and myopathic types
- **Dental abnormalities:** Abnormal teeth and gums in the periodontal-type

Diagnosis

In most cases, diagnosis is clinical. The hypermobility-type is commonest (80%), for which there is no known laboratory or imaging diagnostic test. Adjuncts to clinical diagnosis for the rarer types include molecular genetic testing, skin biopsy, and cardiac echosonography.

Management

Usually supportive, for example with splinting and physiotherapy to address the joint laxity, alongside avoidance of excess pressure. Activity modification may be required if certain features are present (e.g. recurrent dislocation).

The future

As a rare disease, diagnosis of EDS is often made late, or never at all, given the differing and overlapping presentations with other conditions. Improved understanding of the underlying molecular genetic basis of the rarer types alongside other measures (e.g. uptake of patient registries led by the Ehlers-Danlos Society) will help gather more data on this condition and guide future management.

Figure 94.1 Beighton score (out of 9).

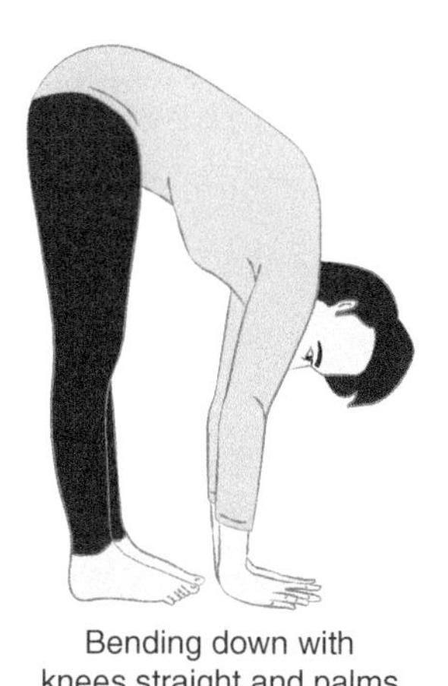
Bending down with knees straight and palms flat on the ground = max. 1 point

Flexing thumb to touch volar forearm = max. 2 points (1x each side)

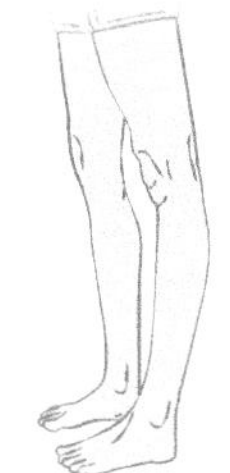
Hyperextension of knees = max. 2 points (1x each side)

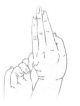

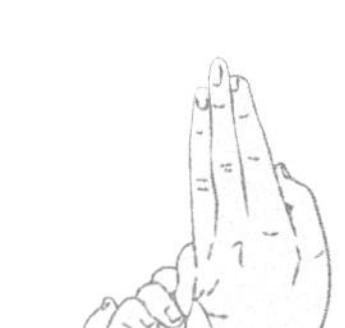
Hyperextending little finger >90 degrees (towards dorsal forearm) = max. 2 points (1x each side)

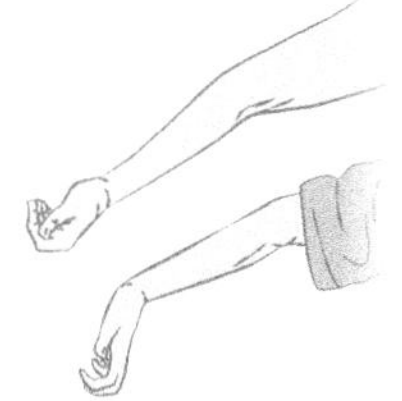
Hyperextension of elbows = max. 2 points (1x each side)

95 Congenital limb deficiencies

Background

Congenital limb deficiencies encompass a vast spectrum of limb defects that may either exist in isolation or as the MSK manifestation of a broader underlying syndrome. They range from hypoplasias (i.e. smaller digits/limbs) to complete absence. This chapter is not exhaustive, and it is important to be aware of other conditions related to a failure of normal MSK development, such as hypoplasias/microdactyly (smaller size) and hyperplasias/macrodactyly (larger size) - e.g. of the thumb, or a whole limb), failure of normal differentiation of structures (e.g. tarsal coalition, clavicle pseudoarthrosis, radio-ulnar synostosis), and accessory structures. These conditions can involve the joints (e.g. arthrogryphosis, congenital knee dislocation, radial head dislocation), pelvis (e.g. developmental dysplasia of the hip), spine (e.g. congenital scoliosis), or trunk (e.g. Sprengel's) (Figure 95.1).

Aetiology

Overall prevalence of limb deficiencies is approximately 5–6/10 000 live births, although there is a wide range. Causes include underlying genetic disorders (e.g. Fanconi anaemia), extrinsic growth restriction (e.g. amniotic band constriction), vascular insufficiency, drugs (e.g. thalidomide), and iatrogenic injury (e.g. chorionic villus sampling). They are commoner in multiple pregnancies.

Genetics

While some abnormalities (e.g. pure syndactyly, clinodactyly, small finger polydactyly, occasionally camptodactyly, tibial hemimelia, Madelung's) may have a Mendelian (AD) inheritance in some/all cases, there is often variable penetrance/expression (Tables 95.1–95.3). Others may be sporadic (e.g. proximal femoral focal deficiency, PFFD). Most abnormalities have a multifactorial, complex, or unclear genetic basis due to both, the complex interplay between soft tissues, bone, joints, and neurovascular structures in their 3D development, alongside the influence of underlying syndromes. The Sonic Hedgehog (*SHH*) gene plays an important role in embryological limb development via its influence at the zone of polarising activity (ZPA) and is implicated in a number of deficiencies, including congenital radial longitudinal deficiency (radial clubhand), PFFD, and fibular deficiency.

Pathophysiology

When limb abnormalities occur with visceral abnormalities, this may be due to a common timing of intrauterine insult, as the embryological development of limbs and viscera both take place between weeks 4 and 12. Limb growth is a complex process involving three main axis: (i) apical ectodermal ridge (AER, proximo-distal growth), (ii) zone of polarising activity (ZPA, radio-ulnar growth), and (iii) dorsal ectoderm (volar-dorsal).

Table 95.1 Features of common underlying syndromes associated with limb abnormalities.

Syndrome	Incidence	Inheritance	Alteration	Features and associations
Fanconi anaemia	1 : 160 000	AR (usually). XLR (rare)	>15 genes implicated (majority involve *FANCA, FANCC, FANCG*)	Marrow failure (aplastic anaemia), myelodysplasia, malignancy (AML), genito-urinary tract abnormalities, short stature, hearing loss, ear malformation, microcephaly
Holt-Oram	1 : 100 000	AD	*TBX5* alterations	Absent or long thumb, cardiac abnormalities
Poland syndrome	1 : 20 000	Sporadic (usually). AD (rare)	Unknown	Underdeveloped muscles on one half of body (often pectoralis major), brachydactyly, syndactyly, radial/ulnar longitudinal deficiency
TAR (thrombocytopaenia absent radius)	<1 : 100 000	AR	*RBM8A* gene, chromosome 1 deletion	Syndactyly, clinodactyly, other skeletal abnormalities, cardiac and renal malformations
VACTERL association (vertebral defects, anal atresia, cardiac defects, trachea-oesophageal fistula, renal abnormalities, limb abnormalities)	1 : 10 000–1 : 40 000	Sporadic	Multifactorial	Limb abnormalities in up to 50%: missing thumbs, hypoplastic forearms and hands

Clinical Genetics and Genomics at a Glance, First Edition. Edited by Neeta Lakhani, Kunal Kulkarni, Julian Barwell, Pradeep Vasudevan, and Huw Dorkins.

Table 95.2 Features of upper limb abnormalities.

	Incidence	Pathophysiology	Presentation	Associated conditions
Syndactyly	1 : 1000–2000. Commoner in Caucasians. 50% bilateral. 2 : 1 (M:F)	Failure of apoptosis in digit separation. Simple (soft tissue) vs complex (bony) vs complicated (abnormal bones); complete (full length) vs incomplete (partial length)	Digits appear fused. Long/ring commonest	Poland, Holt-Oram, Down's, Carpenter syndromes Arachnosyndactyly. (Apert syndrome)
Polydactyly	1 : 1000–10 000. Thumb commoner in Caucasians; Little finger commoner in Afro-Caribbean (1 : 150)	Duplication	Extra part/full digits. Pre-axial (thumb) vs central vs post-axial (small finger)	Pre-axial: Triphlangism (Wassel VII) associated with Holt-Oram, Fanconi's anaemic, cleft palate, tibial defects Post-axial in Caucasians may be syndromic
Clinodactyly	1–20 : 100	Unclear. Initial soft tissue imbalance leading to bony/joint abnormality	Radio-ulnar plane curvature. Middle phalanx commonest	Down's, Poland, Kleinfelter syndromes
Camptodactyly	<1 : 100. Unilateral 1/3, bilateral 2/3	Soft tissue imbalance across the proximal interphalangeal joint (PIPJ) later joint abnormality	Flexion deformity, usually at PIPJ	Rare
Congenital radial longitudinal deficiency (radial clubhand)	1 : 150–100 000 (bilateral in 50–70%)	Sporadic, unclear cause. Longitudinal deficiency of radius (Bayne & Klug classification, ranges from absent radial epiphysis to total radial aplasia)	Hand abnormality (appears radially deviated at wrist). Thumb often absent (although often present with TAR)	Fanconi, Holt-Oram, TAR, VACTERL, VATER. Remember FBC and chromosomal breakage analysis (Fanconi), renal ultrasound, and cardiac echo
Congenital ulnar longitudinal deficiency (ulnar clubhand)	Less common than radial	Sporadic, unclear cause. Ranges from hand deficiency and small ulna to absent ulna and radio-humeral synostosis	Short, bowed forearm. Ulnar digits absent. Painless usually. Reduced elbow function	Rare
Madelung deformity	Rare. 1 : 4 (M:F)	Asymmetric growth arrest of volar and ulnar distal radial physis due to abnormal band between radius and lunate (Vickers ligament)	Volar and ulnar title of hand on wrist. Prominent ulnar head. Ulna longer than radius	Cf. Leri-Weill dyschondrosteosis

Disturbances in the developmental pathway result in characteristic patterns of deformity. Anatomically, limb abnormalities can be pre-axial (radial/tibial sided), central, or post-axial (ulnar/fibular side). Many detailed classification systems exist (e.g. Swanson, Eurocat) to stratify the pattern of the abnormality.

Symptoms and clinical features

Most congenital limb deficiencies exist as a spectrum, ranging from minor growth deficiencies to complete absence of all or part of a limb (Figure 95.1). Congenital amputations are rare (trans-radial is commonest) and occur due to a failure of formation, for example due to amniotic band constriction; their genetic basis is unclear and they are not usually associated with underlying syndromes.

Examination should be holistic. Remember to look for features of any underlying syndrome (e.g. visceral malformations, developmental delay, dysmorphism, neurological deficit), functional impact (e.g. range of motion, strength), and other associated limb abnormalities. Minor upper limb deficiencies may be functionally compensated, whereas more complete deficiencies may result in marked difficulties in activities of daily living. Lower limb long bone deficiencies often result in leg length discrepancies (LLD) and abnormalities of gait.

Diagnosis

Initial investigations should involve radiographs of the affected limb (including joints above and below), other investigations for underlying causes and their severity (e.g. ECG, cardiac echo, renal ultrasound), followed by focused genetic testing (genomic array, gene panel, WES/WGS, karyotype, DNA) as appropriate.

Management

In many cases, the management strategy of the MSK component of these pathologies is initial observation, with non-operative measures (physiotherapy, orthotics and prosthetics) for functional support. Surgery may be required to improve function. Examples of management include:

- **Digits:** Splinting/stretching may help minor angular deformities. Surgery in early childhood can improve function (e.g. with duplication or absence of digits).

Table 95.3 Features of lower limb abnormalities.

	Incidence	Pathophysiology	Presentation	Associated conditions
Proximal femoral focal deficiency (PFFD)	1 : 50 000–200 000. Bilateral 15%	Primary ossification centre defect	LLD. Short thigh. Spectrum ranging from short femur, absent femur, pseudoarthrosis of femoral neck, to absent hip. (AD). Feet usually normal	Fibular hemimelia (50%). ACL deficiency. Coxa vara. Knee contractures. Dysmorphic facies
Fibular deficiency (hemimelia)	1–10 : 100 000. Commonest congenital long bone deficiency	Unclear. Vascular, infection, traumatic and environmental aetiologies all hypothesised	Short limb: spectrum from short (partial) to completely absent fibula. Dimpling of anterior tibial skin. Equino-valgus foot. Antero-medial tibial bowing. Missing lateral toes and valgus knees. Small tibial spine, shallow intercondylar notch	Ball and socket ankle joint (ankle instability). Tarsal coalition. CTEV. Femoral abnormalities (PFFD, coxa vara). Developmental dysplasia of hip. Cruciate ligaments deficient. Valgus knees. Leg length discrepancy (short femur/tibia)
Tibial deficiency (hemimelia)	Less common than fibular	Unclear	Short limb, ranging from short to absent tibia). Antero-lateral tibial bowing. Flexion contracture of knee. Hand and foot deformities	Ulnar aplasia, pre-axial polydactyly
Tibial bowing	Antero-lateral (AL) and antero-medial (AM) rarer than postero-medial (PM)	AL (tibial pseudoarthrosis association); AM (fibular deficiency); PM (physiological, intrauterine malposition). Amniotic band or other compression implicated	Bowing and shortening of limb. Foot deformities. Features of underlying syndrome (e.g. café au lait spots of NF). Pathological fractures	AL (50% have NF1; pseudoarthrosis) AM (fibular hemimelia); PM (calcaneovalgus foot)
Congenital talipes equinovarus (CTEV) – clubfoot	1 : 1000 (2 : 1, M:F)	Multifactorial, involving bone, soft tissues and neurovascular structures (abnormalities of multiple tissue types)	'CAVE' (midfoot Cavus & Adductus, hindfoot Varus & Equinus). Small foot and calf (hypotrophy of limb). Pirani score helps to objectively determine response to treatment. Usually diagnosed on antenatal ultrasound.	80% isolated limb abnormality. Arthrogryphosis. Tibial hemimelia. Myelodysplasia. Diastrophic dysplasia. Pierre Robin. Larsen.

- **Upper limb deficiencies:** Passive stretching of tight structures. Surgical options for radial longitudinal deficiency include centralisation of carpus on wrist provided there is good elbow/biceps function, alongside tendon transfers. Madelung's rarely requires surgery.
- **Lower limb deficiencies:** Heel raises for LLD, braces to prevent progression of angular deformity, passive terminal prosthesis (fitted when the child is old enough, usually >6 months). Surgical options include limb lengthening (e.g. with a circular frame), osteotomy (correct malalignment), fixation of (pathological) fractures, epiphysiodesis of longer limb (to slow growth allowing deficient side to catch up), amputation.
- **CTEV:** Ponsetti regime (serial manipulation and casting) is common in the United Kingdom, with excellent results. Denis Brown boots and bars are then worn to around four years. Minor surgical interventions include Tendo-Achilles tenotomy before the final cast, and occasional tendon transfers. Extensive releases are rare.

The future

These abnormalities are rare their causes are often multifactorial. A better understanding of the underlying molecular genetic and extrinsic basis of these complex developmental pathologies may help both, their prevention (e.g. avoidance of implicated drugs during pregnancy), and their early (intrauterine) detection.

Figure 95.1 Examples of congenital abnormalities.

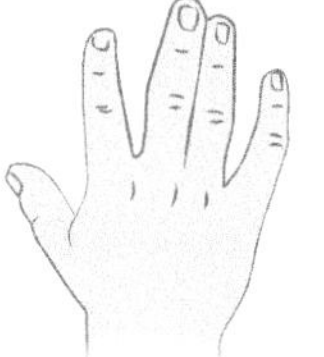

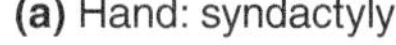

(a) Hand: syndactyly

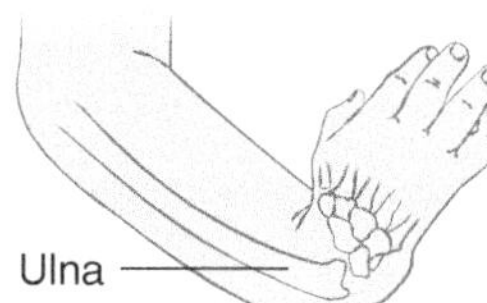

(b) Upper limb: Radial longitudinal deficiency

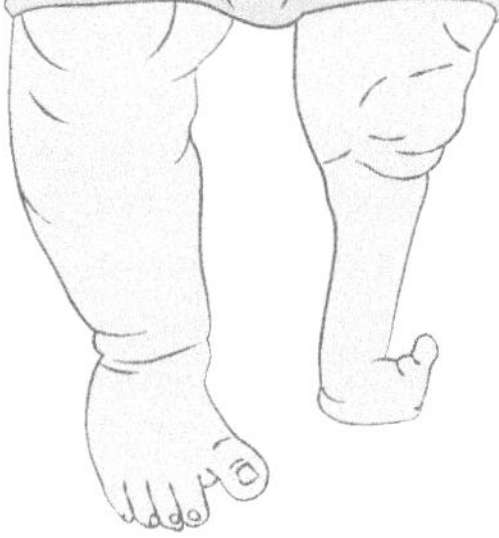

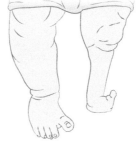

(c) Lower limb: Fibular hemimelia

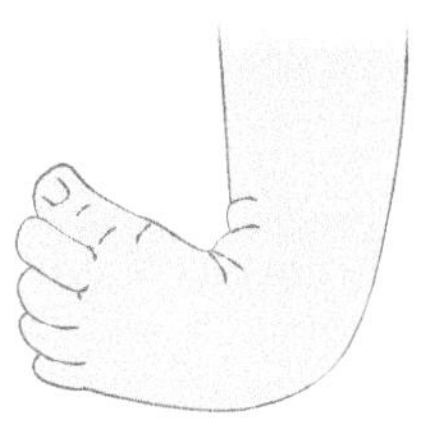

(d) Lower limb: CTEV

96 Duchenne muscular dystrophy

Background

Described for the first time in 1834 by Giovanni Semmola and again by Gaetano Conte in 1836, Duchenne muscular dystrophy (DMD) was eventually named after a French neurologist called Guillaume-Benjamin-Amand Duchenne in 1861. Duchenne was given the privilege as he detailed the case of a young boy who had the condition and was the first to carry out a biopsy to obtain tissue from a living patient for microscopic examination.

Genetics

DMD has X-linked recessive inheritance (Figure 96.1) and is caused by alterations in the dystrophin gene at cytogenetic location Xp21.1—p21.2 (short arm of the X chromosome, loci 21) (Figure 96.2). These alterations can be germline or *de novo* and out of frame alterations result in a truncation of the protein product of the Dystrophin gene. Females are usually carriers for DMD, while males are affected. The *child* of a carrier mother has a 50% chance of inheriting the defective gene. The *daughter* of a carrier mother has a 50% chance of being a carrier. If the receiving child is male, then he will develop DMD as his father will pass him his Y chromosome and the altered X chromosome from the mother will prevail. Female offspring inherit a normal X from their father and thus are carriers. Female carriers of an X-linked recessive condition, such as DMD, can show symptoms depending on their pattern of X-inactivation.

Penetrance is complete in males therefore inheritance of the gene will lead to development of the condition.

Normal skeletal muscle tissue contains only small amounts of dystrophin (about 0.002% of total muscle protein). It is located primarily in muscles used for movement (skeletal) and in the heart (cardiac). Small amounts of dystrophin are also present in nerve cells in the brain.

In skeletal and cardiac muscles, dystrophin (Figure 96.3) is part of a group of proteins (a protein complex) that work together to strengthen muscle fibres and protect them from injury as muscles contract and relax. The dystrophin complex acts as an anchor, connecting each muscle cell's structural framework (cytoskeleton) with the lattice of proteins and other molecules outside the cell (extracellular matrix). The dystrophin complex may also play a role in cell signalling by interacting with proteins that send and receive chemical signals.

Figure 96.1 Inheritance pattern of DMD.

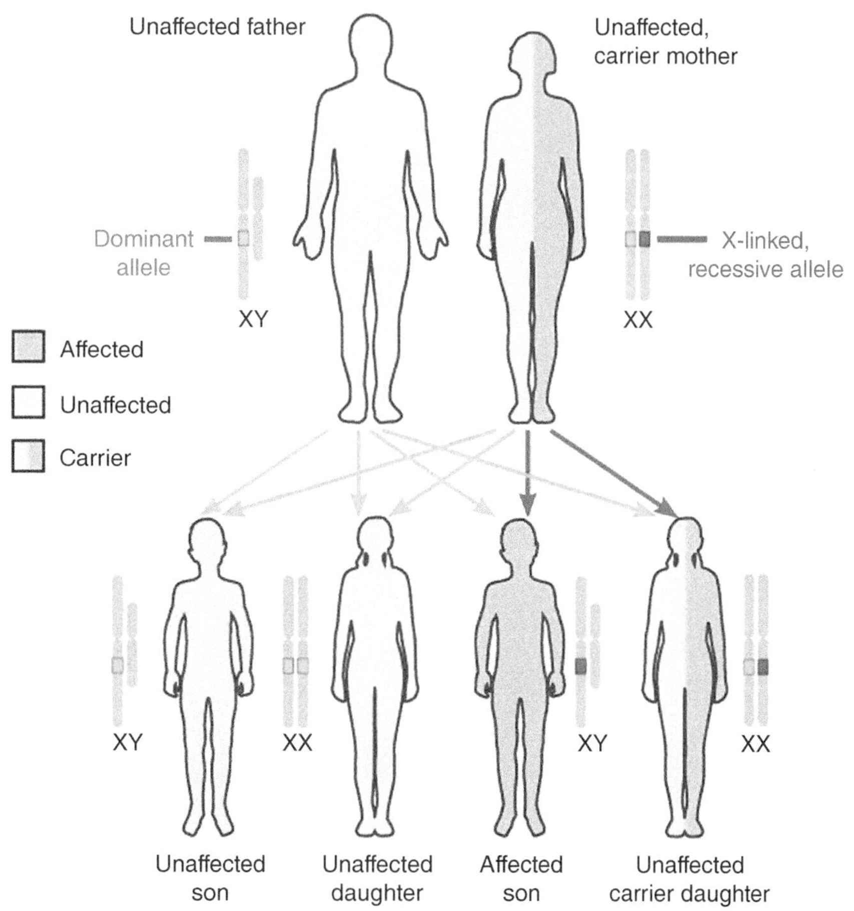

Clinical Genetics and Genomics at a Glance, First Edition. Edited by Neeta Lakhani, Kunal Kulkarni, Julian Barwell, Pradeep Vasudevan, and Huw Dorkins.

Figure 96.2 X-chromosome and location of affected genes.

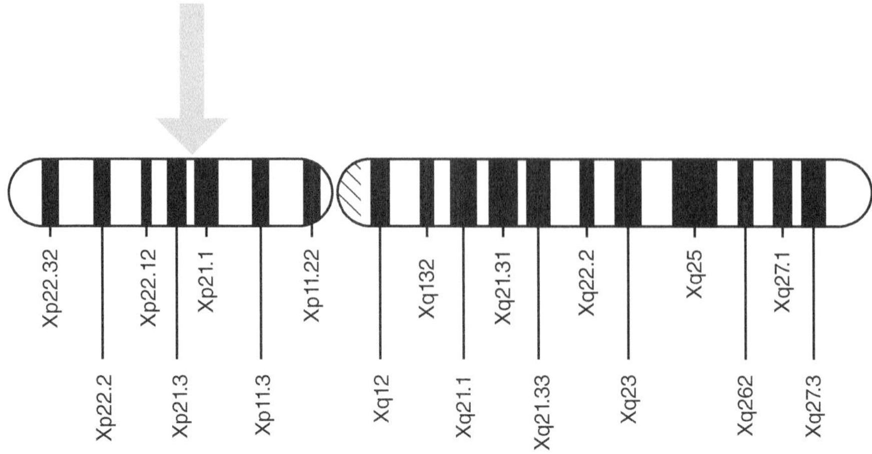

Figure 96.3 Function of dystrophin.

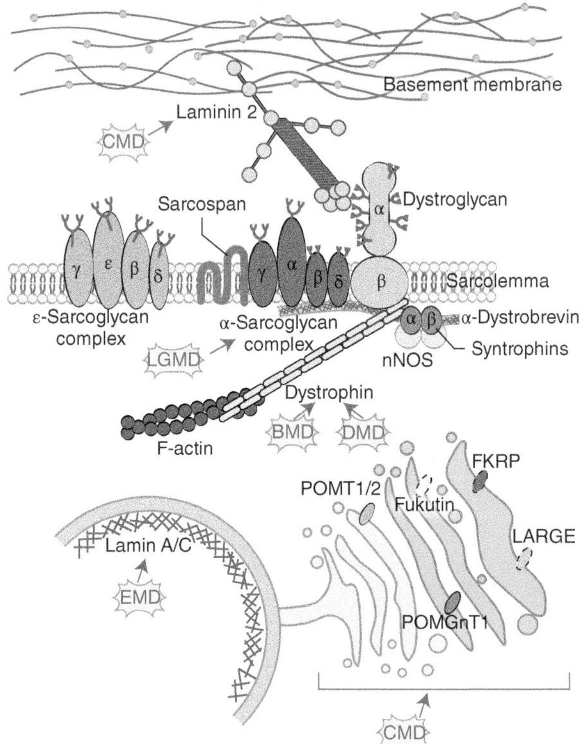

Little is known about the function of dystrophin in nerve cells. Research suggests that the protein is important for the normal structure and function of synapses, which are specialised connections between nerve cells where cell-to-cell communication occurs.

Aetiology

This severe, progressive condition affects between 3600 and 6000 live male births. There is an equal distribution across all ethnicities.

Symptoms

The main symptom of Duchenne muscular dystrophy is progressive muscle weakness. Symptoms usually appear before the age of 6 years when the weakness differentiates affected individuals from their peers. This is often manifested by an abnormal gait when walking or running. Toe walking is a compensatory adaptation to knee extensor weakness. There will be frequent falls and eventual loss of the ability to walk, usually by the age of 12 years. Skeletal deformities including scoliosis and increased lumbar lordosis, leading to shortening of the hip-flexor muscles. In addition, contractures, especially of the Achilles tendon and hamstring muscles restricts function.

Figure 96.4 Gowers sign.

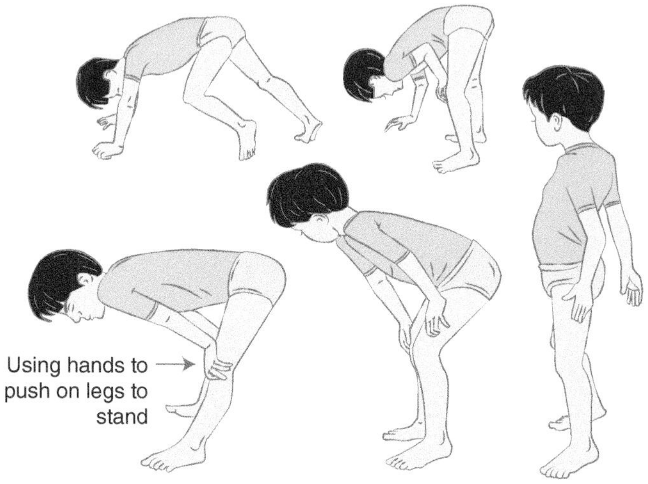

Pseudohypertrophy (enlarging) of tongue and calf muscles can occur, as the muscle tissue is eventually replaced by fat and connective tissue, hence termed 'pseudohypertrophy'. There is a higher risk of development of neurobehavioral disorders (e.g., ADHD), learning disorders (dyslexia), and non-progressive weaknesses in specific cognitive skills (in particular, short-term verbal memory), which are believed to be the result of absent or dysfunctional dystrophin in the brain.

Clinical features

Muscle wasting begins in the legs and pelvis, then progresses to the muscles of the shoulders and neck, followed by loss of arm and respiratory muscles. Calf muscle enlargement (pseudohypertrophy) is apparent. Cardiomyopathy (DCM) is common, but the development of congestive heart failure or arrhythmias (irregular heartbeats) is much rarer.

A positive Gowers' sign (Figure 96.4) is a compensatory manifestation of impairment of the lower extremities muscles; the child helps themselves stand using their upper limbs first by rising to stand on their arms and knees, and then 'walking' their hands up the legs to stand upright.

Diagnosis

Not walking by the age of 16–18 months, a positive family history, Gowers sign, and abnormal muscle function are all indicative of DMD. Genetic testing can reveal alterations in the Xp21 gene and is the mainstay of diagnosis. Creatine kinase (CPK-MM) levels in the bloodstream are usually extremely elevated and are characteristic of the condition. Electromyography (EMG) shows that weakness is caused by destruction of muscle tissue rather than damage to nerves. A muscle biopsy (immunohistochemistry or immunoblotting) or blood test can confirm the absence of dystrophin, although improvements in genetic testing often make this unnecessary.

Clinical features

Management is generally aimed at controlling the onset of symptoms to maximise the quality of life. Corticosteroids early in disease progression have been shown to increase energy and strength, and defer symptom progression for a small period. Randomised control trials have shown that beta2-agonists increase muscle strength but do not modify disease progression. Physical therapy is helpful to maintain muscle strength, flexibility, and function. Mild physical activity such as swimming is encouraged. Inactivity can worsen function. Orthotics (such as braces and wheelchairs) may improve mobility and the ability for self-care. Form-fitting removable leg braces that hold the ankle in place during sleep can defer the onset of contractures.

Appropriate respiratory support as the disease progresses is important. Non-invasive oxygen therapy through to continuous positive pressure ventilation is often needed. Children are monitored regularly and treatment is stepped up where appropriate. Recurrent chest infections secondary to difficulty in clearing secretions or difficulty swallowing lead to repeated hospital admissions.

Nutritional assessment, psychosocial management, and cardiac management are all critical components of the MDT approach to the management of DMD.

Comprehensive multi-disciplinary care standards/guidelines for DMD have been developed by the Centers for Disease Control and Prevention (CDC) and were published in two parts in The Lancet Neurology in 2010 and updated in 2018.

Ataluren (Translarna) is used to treat some children with DMD that can still walk. It's only effective for children with MD with a specific gene nonsense gene alteration.

Ataluren can help slow down the progress of muscle weakness. It's prescribed as a sachet of granules which can be mixed into liquids or food like yoghurt and eaten.

The future

The future of DMD treatment and management is changing to incorporate current developments in research. Exon-skipping, stem cell replacement therapy with IV administration of pericytes, analog up-regulation, and gene replacement all show potential.

Charcot–Marie–Tooth (CMT)

Background

Also known as hereditary motor and sensory neuropathy (HSMN) or peroneal muscular atrophy, these are a heterogeneous group of disorders affecting the motor and sensory peripheral nerves, resulting in muscle weakness/atrophy and sensory loss. CMT was first reported in 1886 by Jean Martin Charcot and Pierre Marie, with Howard Henry Tooth also reporting similar cases of distal lower limb muscle weakness.

Aetiology

Prevalence is around 1 in 2500-3000, making this one of the commonest neuromuscular disorders.

Genetics

A careful family history is important, as this may suggest a pattern of inheritance, which can be AD, AR or XLR. Over 60 associated genes are potentially affected, which play roles in myelin formation, gene transcription, mitochondrial function, and intracellular membrane transport. The commonest defect (70–80%) is a 1.5Mb duplication at 17p11.2, which encodes for *PMP22* (peripheral myelin protein), and results in overproduction and demyelination (CMT1A). Note that in sporadic cases, a *de novo* alteration may be the explanation, but there are also many other non-genetic causes of peripheral neuropathy to consider.

Pathophysiology

Impaired peripheral nerve conduction due to either (predominantly) axonal abnormalities, demyelination, or a combination. Classically, CMT has been divided into demyelinating and axonal forms although as demyelination makes axons more susceptible to degeneration, there is overlap. Given the heterogeneity in presentation and underlying genetics, CMT may not be diagnosed until later in life, or may even remain either undiagnosed or misdiagnosed.

Figure 97.1 Classic clinical features: inverted champagne bottle legs (a, b), cavus foot (c–e), clawed hands (f).

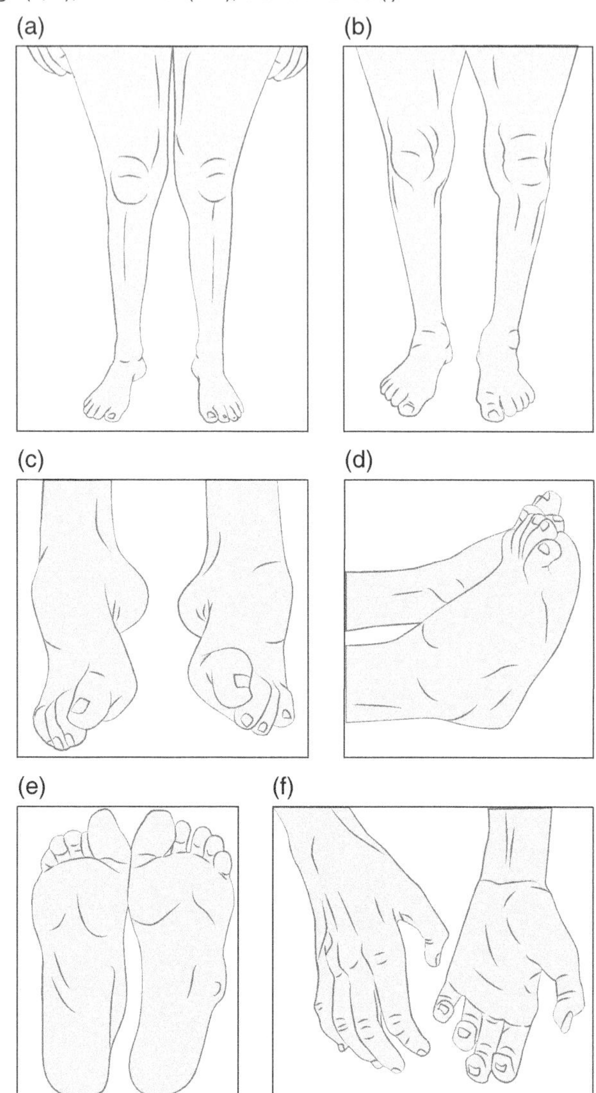

Symptoms

Patients classically present in adolescence (or earlier) with progressive deformity, weakness, or sensory disturbance, initially in the legs, then later in the hands. Difficulty walking due to foot drop is the commonest mode of presentation, alongside loss of peripheral (hand/feet) sensation (resulting in clumsiness or falls), and a high-arched appearance to the feet. In milder cases, presentation may be later in adult life, or related to difficulty with sports or fitting footwear.

Clinical features

Severity is variable; while some individuals (10%) with the genetic alterations may be asymptomatic, others may be severely affected and wheelchair bound in early adulthood. Prenatal diagnosis is possible.

- **General appearance:** 'Inverted champagne bottle' appearance of lower limbs due to wasting of calf muscle bulk (Figure 97.1).
- **Pes cavus (cavo-varus) foot deformity:** Tibialis posterior and peroneus longus tendons are strong (strong hindfoot inversion and first metatarsal depression), while tibialis anterior and peroneus brevis tendons are weak (weak ankle dorsiflexion and foot eversion). This results in a high-arched foot. The Coleman block test can help determine whether the hindfoot is fixed or flexible, thereby helping guide surgery. The long toe extensors compensate for tibialis anterior weakness, leading to lesser toe clawing.
- **High stepping/slapping gait:** Occurs due to weakness of dorsiflexion and eversion (foot drop). Heel walking is impaired.

Clinical Genetics and Genomics at a Glance, First Edition. Edited by Neeta Lakhani, Kunal Kulkarni, Julian Barwell, Pradeep Vasudevan, and Huw Dorkins.

- **Hand weakness:** Finger abduction weakness secondary to wasting of interossei. Disproportionate wasting of thumb abduction over first dorsal interosseous function is suggestive of CMT1X
- **Reduced peripheral sensation:** Impaired vibration sense in feet and hands.
- **Reduced deep tendon reflexes:** Loss of ankle reflex may be present, followed by loss of others.
- **Prominent peripheral nerves:** Enlarged peripheral nerves may be felt (e.g. greater auricular nerve enlargement behind the ear is suggestive of CMT1A).
- **Tremor:** Roussy-Levy syndrome (a form of CMT11).

Several similarly presenting differential diagnoses exist. Learning difficulties are not a feature and may suggest an alternative differential (e.g. Smith Magenis syndrome). *PMP22* deletion (rather than duplication) causes HNPP (hereditary neuropathy with liability to pressure palsies). Features may also be similar to other conditions such as spinal muscular atrophy (HSP22/27), Friedreich's ataxia frataxin, familial brachial plexus neuropathy, or transthyretin-related familial amyloid neuropathy (TTR-FAP).

Diagnosis

- **Neurophysiology (nerve conduction studies):** Slowed median nerve conduction nerve velocity (usually 10-38 m/s compared to normal >40 m/s) in certain types (e.g. CMT1A).
- **Molecular genetic (DNA) testing:** Performed particularly if there is a positive family history. May require gene panel, WES or WGS due to genetic heterogeneity.
- **Alterations:**
  - **HSMN1/CMT1A (70-80%):** *PMP22* duplication in majority. AD inheritance. Distal muscle weakness/atrophy, mild sensory glove and stocking loss, depressed reflexes, pes cavus, occasional tremor. Abnormal myelin, slow NCS.
  - **HSMN1X/CMTX (10-20%):** Connexin 32 (*GJB1*) alteration. XL semi-dominant inheritance (no male-to-male inheritance but note symptomatic females may present after males so appearance my initially mimic AD). Clinically like HSMN1. Demyelination, although some have a more axonal form (overlap with HSMN2).
  - **HSMN2/CMT2 (10%):** *KIF1B-MFN2* (commonest alteration), also *RAB-7, 6ARS*, or neurofilament triplet L protein mutations. AD inheritance. Clinically like a less-severe HSMN1. Axonopathy, with slightly reduced/normal neurophysiology.
  - **HSMN3/CMT3 (congenital):** Dejerine-Sottas syndrome. Often reclassified into one of the other types based on the alteration. *De novo* AD usually with *PMP22* (CMT1A), although may be *MPZ* (CMT1B, reclassified as HSMN1) or *EGR2* (CMT1D and 4). AD inheritance for CMT1A/B/D. AR inheritance for CMT4. Severe demyelinating neuropathy in childhood with marked weakness. Myelin abnormal with markedly slow neurophysiology.
  - **HSMN4/CMT4 (rare):** One of a number of genes, including *EGR2* (CMT4E), *PRX* (CMT4F). AR inheritance. Early childhood presentation. Abnormal myelin or axonopathy.
  - **Complex (rare):** Variable genetics. Neuropathy alongside visual/auditory/phonation disturbance.
- **Sural nerve biopsy:** If genetic testing unhelpful.
- **Ophthalmology assessment:** Pigmentary retinopathy or optic atrophy.
- **Phytanic acid:** Differential is Refsum disease, which may resemble HSMN 2/3 with associated night blindness and pigmentary retinopathy.
- **MRI:** If developmental regression.

Management

In the absence of a cure, treatment is primarily supportive, aiming to deal with the symptoms and complications:

- **Foot drop:** Physiotherapy (stretching). Splinting (with an ankle foot orthosis, AFO).
- **Foot deformity:** Stretching to prevent Achilles tendon shortening. Supportive footwear with ankle support. Surgery to restore alignment if severe deformity.
- **Sensory loss:** Protective measures to prevent ulceration and injury, including supportive footwear and regular nail care to prevent infection.
- **Spine:** Serial assessment to screen for scoliosis (secondary neuromuscular), although this is rarely severe. Commoner if early onset.
- **Strength/function:** Physiotherapy (exercises) to improve core strength and stability. Mobility/walking aids as required.
- **Medication:** Medication may help cramps. Avoid neurotoxic drugs (e.g. vincristine, nitrofurantoin).
- **Lifestyle:** Care with activities due to weakness and sensory impairment. May require driving regulatory body to be informed (e.g. in the UK, the DVLA must be notified).

The future

Prognosis is variable, with the condition only slowly progressive in some affected individuals resulting in near-normal life expectancy, whereas in the most severe cases, complications (e.g. respiratory) may result in premature death. Despite the perception that feet involvement is usually first, evidence suggests that hand dysfunction is also present early on in the disease process, highlighting the importance of screening and early physiotherapy. Novel drug treatments, including gene therapy, are the subject of ongoing research.

98 Ankylosing spondylitis

Background

Ankylosing spondylitis (AS) is a chronic seronegative spondyloarthritis. The name is derived from the Greek: 'ankylosis' (joint stiffening) and 'spondylos' (vertebra). While the axial skeleton is primarily affected, resulting in progressive spinal fusion, sacroiliitis, hypokyphosis, and extra-articular manifestations are also present. While the skeletons of Egyptian mummies have demonstrated the condition, it was formally first described in the 1600s by Irish physician Bernard Connor.

Aetiology

Global prevalence ranges from 0.7 to 49 per 10 000, with significant variation between ethnic groups; the disease is more prevalent in Caucasian populations. Male-to-female ratio is approximately 3 : 1.

Genetics

Individuals with human leucocyte antigen (HLA)-B gene variants (particularly *HLA-B27*) are at higher risk of developing AS. This relationship, first recognized 40 years ago, is one of the strongest associations of a single gene variant in a complex genetic disease. While the majority (over 90%) of individuals diagnosed with AS are *HLA-B27* positive, not everyone with a HLA-B variant will necessarily develop AS. Furthermore, there is ethnic variation; for example approximately 50% of Afro-Americans with AS have the *HLA-B27* variant, compared to around 90% of Caucasian Europeans. For relatives of an affected individual, risks of developing AS are 63% in monozygotic twins; 8.2% in first-degree relatives; 1% in second-degree relatives; 7.9% parent-child. Between siblings, AS occurs almost exclusively in those that are *HLA-B27*-positive. Variations in over 40 other genes/genetic regions, including *ERAP1, CARD9, STAT3, IL1A, and IL23R*, have also since been associated with ankylosing spondylitis, although their link is not clearly established. Signalling in the IL-23/IL-17 axis has been implicated in a common susceptibility factor in several types of seronegative spondyloarthritis, including AS.

Table 98.1 Diagnostic criteria for AS: Modified New York classification.

Any one of the following clinical criteria:
- Low back pain >3 months improved by exercise and not relieved by rest;
- Limitation of lumbar spine in sagittal/frontal planes;
- Limitation of chest expansion (relative to age/sex).

+ any one of the following radiological criteria:
- Bilateral grade 2–4 sacroiliitis;
- Unilateral grade 3–4 sacroiliitis.

Pathophysiology

AS is a systemic disease that is part of the spondyloarthritis family. CD4/8 T cells have been suggested to play a role, given their interaction with *HLA-B27* (Figure 98.1). The HLA complex is involved in distinguishing the immune response to self versus foreign pathogens. Bony fusion in the spine occurs due to ossification of the intervertebral discs, resulting in syndesmophyte formation and a bamboo-spine appearance.

Symptoms

The primary symptom is chronic (inflammatory) back pain, which characteristically affects individuals <40 years of age (peak onset between 20 and 30 years), develops insidiously, improves with exercise, is not relieved by rest, with night pain/stiffness often present that is relieved upon waking and mobilising. This results in progressive stiffness of spinal movements, resulting in reduced chest expansion and pain in other joints (e.g. hips and knees). Other joints (e.g. thoracic, peripheral) may also be affected in up to 50% patients, alongside enthesitis (inflammation of tendon/ligament insertions).

Clinical features

Clinical examination can reveal stiffness and pain of movements (e.g. using Schober's test to assess lumbar spine flexion), as well as demonstrating the various extra-articular manifestations (Figure 98.2). In the later stages, osteoporosis and osteopaenia are not uncommon, secondary to both inflammation and disuse. Spinal complications can occur, including fractures, atlanto-axial subluxation, and neurological compromise (e.g. cauda equina syndrome and cord injury). Extra-articular manifestations can have a complex relationship, and include the 'A's: heart (aortic regurgitation, aV node block), lungs (apical fibrosis), eyes (anterior uveitis), and amyloidosis, as well as affecting skin (psoriasis), bowel (inflammatory bowel disease, IBD), kidneys, and psychological well-being. Disease severity correlates with prognosis.

Diagnosis

This is primarily clinical. Inflammatory back pain is present in approximately 80% individuals with AS. Neck pain can also be a prominent component, alongside progressive postural deformity (stooped posture secondary to flexion deformity of the cervical spine, thoracic kyphosis, and loss of lumbar lordosis). Laboratory blood markers include HLA-B27, which is not diagnostic, but can help confirm the diagnosis. Presence of this marker also correlates with presence of extra-articular features, such as anterior uveitis. Elevated blood inflammatory markers (e.g. CRP/ESR) and ALP may suggest active disease. Plain radiographs of the spine and pelvis can demonstrate spondylitis (eventually resulting in the classic 'bamboo spine') and sacroiliitis, although there can be a lag of up to 10 years before radiographic changes are evident. Sacroiliac joint

Clinical Genetics and Genomics at a Glance, First Edition. Edited by Neeta Lakhani, Kunal Kulkarni, Julian Barwell, Pradeep Vasudevan, and Huw Dorkins.

Figure 98.1 Possible contributions to spondyloarthritis (SpA) pathogenesis.

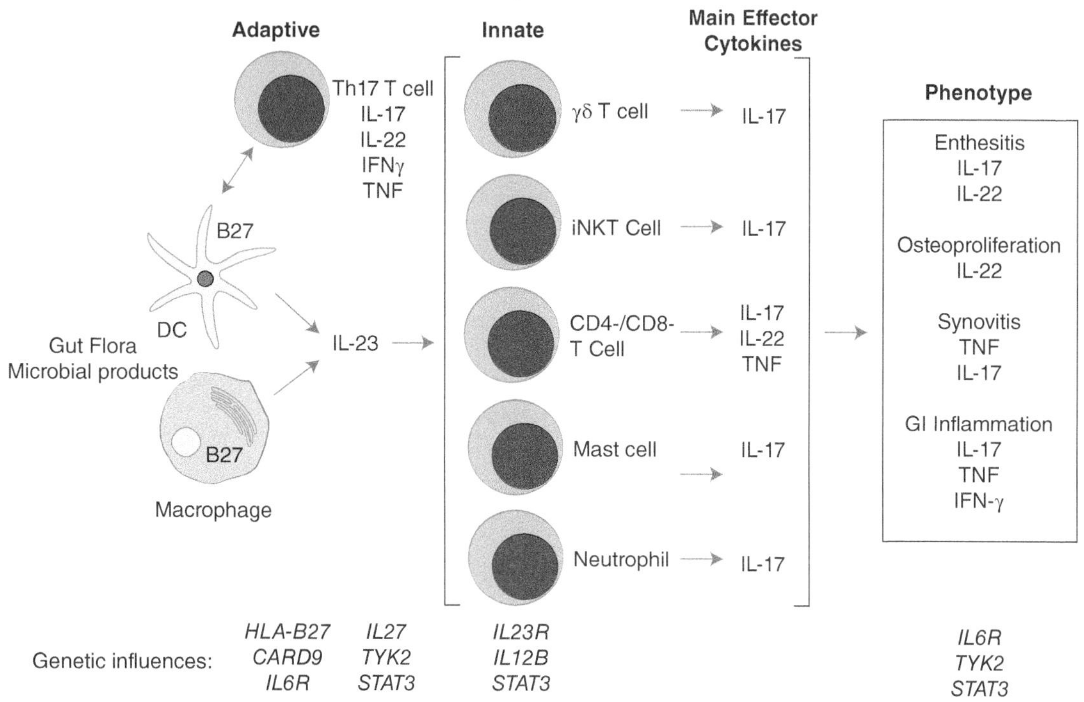

From: Arthritis Rheumatol. 2014 Feb; 66(2): 231–241. doi: 10.1002/art.38291 (https://www.ncbi.nlm.nih.gov/pmc/articles/PMC4058712/figure/F1/).

Figure 98.2 Clinical posture and spinal features of AS.

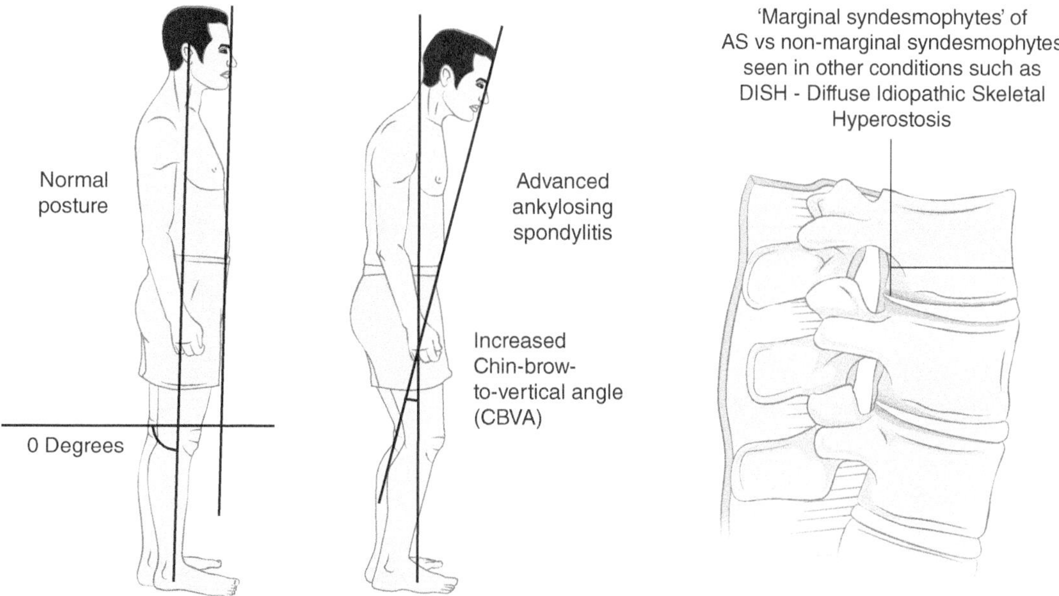

changes characteristically progress from normal (grade 0-1), to sclerosis and erosive changes (grade 2), to joint space narrowing (grade 3), to eventual complete ankylosis (grade 4). MRI can be more sensitive in early disease, demonstrating oedema. Ultrasound can help diagnose enthesitis. Various scoring systems exist, such as the 1984 modified New York classification, which can help establish a diagnosis (Table 98.1). Factors that correlate with faster disease progression include male gender, pre-existing radiographic damage, presence of HLA-B27, and history of smoking.

Management

Management is primarily symptomatic. Analgesics, particularly anti-inflammatories, therefore play an important role. Progression can be slowed with the help of disease-modifying anti-rheumatic drugs (DMARDs), such as sulfasalazine. Biological agents, including TNF-α antagonists (e.g. infliximab), can be used acute flares. Physiotherapy plays an important role in symptom in control. Functional scoring systems (e.g. Bath Ankylosing Disease Activity Index, BASDAI) can help monitor disease activity. Surgery is an option for deformity correction, although this is not without considerable peri-operative risk.

The future

Better diagnostic tools and disease-modifying treatment modalities are key to earlier diagnosis and delaying progression of this chronic condition. In particular, therapies involving the IL-23/IL-17 axis are of greater potential as several genes in these pathways have been demonstrated to act as determinants of AS risk.

99 Skeletal dysplasias

Background

These are a range of over 450 congenital structural bone and cartilage abnormalities that result in the disturbance of normal growth and development of the trunk or limbs. Also known as osteochondrodysplasias, these disorders can also have effects on muscle, ligaments, and tendons. Most are rare; while this topic will provide an overview, only a selection of the more common dysplasias will be considered in detail.

Aetiology

Incidence ranges widely; see Table 99.3 for specific conditions.

Genetics

The molecular basis for over 300 of these disorders has been identified. Inheritance is generally Mendelian and can be AD, AR, XLD, XLR, or Y linked. Some dysplasias may exhibit less common features such as somatic mosaicism (one parent mildly affected, children more severely affected) or gonadal mosaicism (unaffected heterozygous parent for a dominant disorder with alteration in one progenitor germ cell lineage, and familial recurrence). In some disorders, the type and location of the alteration within the disease-producing gene may guide severity/prognostic information (e.g. in OI, *COL1A1* nonsense/stop alterations yield milder phenotype, missense alterations yield more severe forms).

Pathophysiology

Skeletal dysplasias may broadly be categorised based upon their common genetic or phenotypic features. Table 99.1, while far from exhaustive, highlights those that are either more common or better known, to demonstrate the way in which these disorders can be stratified.

Other classifications may also be helpful, such as Fairbank's or Rubin's (Table 99.2).

Symptoms

Patients may present with either a growth problem (e.g. abnormal stature, deformity, or malalignment of limbs), abnormal facies (specific to the condition, e.g. frontal bossing), functional limitation (e.g. joint contractures), or a complication (e.g. delayed development, seizure, fracture). Presentation is usually in infancy or childhood. There may be a family history of early arthritis (e.g. hip osteoarthritis secondary to an epiphyseal/articular pathology).

Clinical features

Clinical findings are broad ranging and depend on the specific dysplasia (although there is considerable overlap):

- **Facies:** Characteristic facial appearances (frontal bossing, triangular/trefoil, midface hypoplasia).
- **Dentition:** Abnormalities may be due to a collagen disorder.
- **Hair:** Thinning.

Table 99.1 Grouping of common skeletal dysplasias by genetic basis.

Disorder group	Disorder	Inheritance	Gene
FGFR3	Achondroplasia	AD	*FGFR3*
	Hypochondroplasia		
	Thanatophoric dysplasia		
COMP	Pseudochondroplasia	AD (usually)	*COMP*
	Multiple epiphyseal dysplasia (MED)	xxxx	
Sulphate	Diastrophic dysplasia	AR	*SLC26A2*
	Achondrogenesis IB, Atelosteogenesis II		
Osteogenesis imperfecta (OI) and reduced bone density	Osteogenesis imperfecta (moderate, severe, lethal)	AD	*COL1A1, COL1A2*
	Osteogenesis imperfecta (moderate, severe, lethal)	AR	*CRTAP, P3H1, PPBI, FKBP10, HSP47, SP7, WNT1*
Type II collagen	Spondyloepiphyseal dysplasia congenita (SEDC)	AD	*COL2A1*
	Kniest dysplasia		
	Achondrogenesis		
Type XI collagen	Fibrochondrogenesis	AD	*COL11A1/2*
	Fibrochondrogenesis	AR	*COL11A1*

Adapted from: 'Krakow, D. Skeletal Dysplasias. Clin Perinatol. 2015 Jun; 42(2): 301–319'.

Clinical Genetics and Genomics at a Glance, First Edition. Edited by Neeta Lakhani, Kunal Kulkarni, Julian Barwell, Pradeep Vasudevan, and Huw Dorkins.

Table 99.2 Rubin's classification (based upon anatomical site of abnormality).

- I. Epiphyseal dysplasias
  - A. Epiphyseal hypoplasias
    - 1. Failure of articular cartilage: spondyloepiphyseal dysplasia, congenita and tarda
    - 2. Failure of ossification of center: multiple epiphyseal dysplasia, congenita and tarda
  - B. Epiphyseal hyperplasia
    - 1. Excess of articular cartilage: dysplasia epiphysealis hemimelica
- II. Physeal dysplasias
  - A. Cartilage hypoplasias
    - 1. Failure of proliferating cartilage: achondroplasia, congenita and tarda
    - 2. Failure of hypertrophic cartilage: metaphyseal dysotosis, congenita and tarda
  - B. Cartilage hyperplasias
    - 1. Excess of proliferating cartilage: hyperchondroplasia
    - 2. Excess of hypertrophic cartilage: enchondromatosis
- III. Metaphyseal dysplasias
  - A. Metaphyseal hypoplasias
    - 1. Failure to form primary spongiosa: hypophosphatasia, congenita and tarda
    - 2. Failure to absorb primary spongiosa: osteopetrosis, congenita and tarda
    - 3. Failure to absorb secondary spongiosa: cranio-metaphyseal dysplasia, congenita and tarda
  - B. Metaphyseal hyperplasia
    - 1. Excessive spongiosa: familial exostosis
- IV. Diaphyseal dysplasias
  - A. Diaphyseal hypoplasias
    - 1. Failure of periosteal bone formation: osteogenesis imperfecta, congenita and tarda
    - 2. Failure of endosteal bone formation: idiopathic osteoporosis
  - B. Diaphyseal hyperplasias
    - 1. Excessive periosteal bone formation: Engelmann's disease
    - 2. Excessive periosteal bone formation: hyperphosphatasemia

Adapted from: Rubin, P. Dynamic classification of bone dysplasias. Chicago. Year Book Medical Publishers. 1964, p. 82.

- **Height:** Most result in short stature (i.e. standing height less than third percentile for chronologic age). Standing and sitting height should both be compared with limb length to determine whether the loss is proportionate (both short trunk and limbs) or disproportionate (either short limbs or trunk).
  - **Short trunk:** Kniest syndrome, Morquio syndrome, metatrophic dysplasia, spondyloepiphyseal dysplasia (SED), spondyloepimetaphyseal dysplasia (SEMD).
- **Limb length and alignment:** Upper and (standing) lower limb alignment should be compared for any varus/valgus deformity or bowing. Limb span to determine which segment is shortened (aids diagnosis):
  - **Rhizomelic or proximal (i.e. humerus/femur):** Achondroplasia, hypochondroplasia, Jansen's metaphyseal dysplasia. SED congenita, diastrophic dysplasia, thanatophoric dysplasia. Commonest.
  - **Mesomelic or middle (forearm, lower leg):** Robinow and Reinhardt syndromes, Langer/Nievergelt mesomelic dysplasia.
  - **Acromelic or distal (hand):** Periphasal dysostosis, acrodysostosis.
  - **Micromelic or entire limb:** Robert's syndrome, Kniest dysplasia, achondrogenesis, fibrochondrogenesis.
- **Finger abnormalities:** Including polydactyly, brachydactyly and trident hand (equal finger length with excess gap between third and fourth fingers).
- **Limb/joint function:** Both fixed flexion deformity (e.g. elbow, hip, knee) and hypermobility may occur. Altered (waddling) gait due to hip or spinal pathology. Fractures with low energy trauma (abnormal bone mineral density/mineralisation). Clubfoot (talipes) may occur.
- **Neurological:** Developmental delay, including secondary to hydrocephalus and brain dysgenesis. Seizures. Spinal deformity (scoliosis), instability (cervical spine), cord compression, or foramen magnum stenosis.
- **Cardio-respiratory:** Functional compromise may occur (restrictive lung disease) in conjunction with a spinal or chest wall deformity. Sleep apnoeas due to soft tissue hypertrophy (e.g. adenoids). Cardiac pathology may occur.
- **Nutrition:** Poor feeding. Gastro-oesophageal reflux.

Table 99.3 summarises key features of the more commonly seen disorders.

Diagnosis

- **Before birth:** Diagnosis may occur in the pre/antenatal period with CVS/NIPT/imaging if there is a known family history. Screening modalities such as ultrasound can be used in early pregnancy to identify the more severe or fatal conditions, and in later pregnancy for a more precise diagnosis (although this may not be apparent until after birth) and for planning prior to delivery. DNA storage from deceased neonates is helpful where a diagnosis is required for future risk assessment.
- **After birth:** Once stable, clinical assessment will guide diagnosis. Features include:
  - **Clinical:** Birth weight/length and head circumference, dysmorphic features (characteristic facies, chest wall/trunk abnormalities, limb proportions/alignment), and other abnormalities (e.g. abdominal viscera/genitalia).
  - **Imaging:** Plain radiographs of the skull, chest, spine (including flexion/extension views), pelvis and limb (long bones, hands, feet) can then help stratify the disorder depending on anatomical involvement, with other imaging (e.g. cardiac echo) helpful. MRI brain/spine if required (e.g. stenosis).
  - **Blood tests:** Permit molecular genetic diagnosis (genomic array, WES/WGS) and identification of any metabolic/immunological abnormality (may also need urinalysis).
- **Differential diagnosis:** Include other causes of short stature, metabolic bone disease, glycogen storage disorders, endocrine disorders.

Management

- **Diagnosis and antenatal screening:** Knowing the mode of inheritance is important in both, surveillance of complications and prenatal counselling to prevent recurrence. Non-assortive mating (i.e. both parents with a dysplasia) is not uncommon, and must be considered.
- **Initial management:** For neonates with suspected dysplasias, management depends on whether the suspected genotype and phenotype (if known) yield a lethal condition (palliative care) or one that is survivable albeit with imminent potential complications (e.g. urgent medical care for cardio-respiratory or neurological issues).

Table 99.3 Features of more common/well-known dysplasias.

Disorder	Incidence & diagnosis	Features	Imaging	Complications
Achondroplasia *(FGFR3 on 4p, AD inheritance, incomplete penetrance, 90% sporadic de novo linked to increased paternal age)*	1 in 10 000–100 000 live births (commonest non-lethal skeletal dysplasia). Diagnosis in pregnancy (short femur on ultrasound scan), or at birth/in early infancy	Macrocephaly, frontal bossing, (usually) rhizomelic limb shortening, trident hand, spared soft tissues (appear excessive), ligamentous laxity, elbow contractures (+/– radial head dislocation), tibia vara, genu varum, ankle varus Hypochondroplasia is a less common and severe variant, with variable phenotype	X-ray: Large skull, short/flat vertebrae with premature fusion and broad pedicles, short/thick tubular bones, wide/flared metaphysis (V or U shape), spared epiphysis, champagne glass pelvis (inlet width > depth), flat acetabular roof, apparent femoral neck varus (GT overgrowth), thoraco-lumbar kyphosis (resolves)	Neurological (foramen magnum stenosis), apnoeas and hypotonias, resulting in sudden infant death. Spinal stenosis
Pseudochondroplasia *(COMP, AD inheritance usually)*	4 in 1 000 000. Diagnosis usually apparent within first 3 years.	Variable phenotype. Affects ephiphysis and metaphysis. Rhizomelic shortening, ligamentous laxity, genu varum or valgum (can be different on each side – 'windswept'). Skull and face unaffected	X-ray: Irregular/ fragmented epiphysis, dysplastic hip resulting in premature osteoarthritis, lower limb malalignment on long-leg views, odontoid hypertrophy (need C1-2 instability assessment pre-operatively), platyspondyly, anterior vertebral beaking	Premature arthritis (impaired articular cartilage). Atlanto-occipital instability (pain, fatigue, myelopathy)
Multiple epiphyseal dysplasia, MED *(COMP, 19, AD inheritance usually)*	1 in 10 000. Diagnosis usually in adolescence	Delayed walking (often with limp or waddling), joint pain and stiffness with flexion contractures, short stature in some, genu varum/valgum, short fingers/toes with clinodactyly, cleft palate, clubfoot, scoliosis	X-ray: Delayed, irregular ossification centres, reduced epiphyseal/carpal height, double layered patella, short metacarpals and phalanges, vertebral endplate changes. Changes in acetabulae and proximal femur with coxa vara (may mimic bilateral Perthes). MRI may show avascular necrosis of femoral epiphysis.	Premature osteoarthritis
Spondyloepiphyseal dysplasia, SED *(SEDC = COL2A1, AD inheritance with most spontaneous de novo alterations; SEDT = SEDKL, XLR or AR inheritance)*	SEDT XLR 1 in 150–200 000. SEDC rare (>175 cases reported). Diagnosis of SEDC (congenital) at birth, tarda (SEDT) later childhood.	Part of a heterogeneous group of type II collagenopathies. Short trunk, rhizo/mesomelic limb shortening (hands/feel/skull normal), micrognathia and flat midface (Pierre Robin sequence), cleft palate, wide set eyes, cervical spine instability and lumbar lordosis, barrel chest, hip flexion contractures and waddling gait (coxa vara), clubfoot, genu valgum (usually)	X-ray: Flattened and irregular epiphysis (appear late), platyspondyly, short thorax and ribs, pear/oval-shaped vertebrae, kyphoscoliosis, odontoid hypoplasia, absent pubic ossification, short long bones, unossified talus/calcaneus, coxa vara)	Respiratory problems (small thoracic cage), feeding difficulties (micrognathia). Recurrent ear infections. Neurological (spinal instability, myelopathy). Premature osteoarthritis (epiphysis abnormal, SEDT may mimic a bilateral Perthes). Ophthalmic (myopia, retinal detachment, cataracts). Renal (nephrotic syndrome). Variants (e.g. achondrogenesis II) are lethal.
Diastrophic dysplasia *(SLC26A2, AR inheritance)*	1 in 33 000 (Finland) to 500 000 (USA)	Short stature, joint contractures, hitchhiker thumbs, cauliflower ears, clubfoot, progressive scoliosis, cleft palate		Premature osteoarthritis
Osteogenesis imperfecta (OI) *(COL1A1/2, most = AD or sporadic de novo, severe = AR inheritance, rarely = XLR inheritance)*	1 in 10–20 000. Severe forms present in neonatal period	Macrocephaly, flat midface, short limbs, narrow trunk/thorax, blue sclerae, poor dentition. Normal hands/feet	X-ray: Multiple (healing) fractures (e.g. ribs), reduced skull ossification, osteopaenia, flat acetabulae	Fractures (reduced bone mineral density). Hearing loss. Respiratory difficulty. AR forms severe and maybe lethal
Osteopetrosis *(malignant AR inheritance = 50% TCIRG1, 15% CLCN7; benign AD inheritance = 75% CLCN7; rarely XL inheritance = IKBKG; 30% unknown)*	1 in 20 000 (AD) to 250 000 (AR). AR presents at birth/neonatal period. Benign presents later (maybe asymptomatic)	Scoliosis. AR may also have delayed growth with short stature, developmental delay, seizures, hepatosplenomegaly, dental abnormalities. XL may have lymphoedema and anhidrotic ectodermal dysplasia	X-ray: Rugger jersey spine, increased opacification of bones (lose distinction between cortices and medullary canal), endobones (mini bones in cortex)	'Marble bone' is brittle and susceptible to fracture (abnormal osteoclasts, fewer collagen fibrils). Premature osteoarthritis. Malignant form can yield pancytopaenia, blindness, deafness

- **Ongoing management:**
  - **Symptomatic/supportive care:** Remains the focus in the absence of a cure. Includes neonatal handling advice (bony fragility, spinal instability), physiotherapy (improve strength and joint movement), functional bracing (joints, spine), mobility aids, nutritional support (prevent obesity), dental (prevent crowding).
  - **Medical:** Drugs include growth hormone (if deficiency, for short term growth, minimal long term benefit), and other specific treatments (e.g. bisphosphonates for bone protection).
  - **Surgery:** Reserved for specific indications. Options include grommets for chronic otitis media, adenoidectomy/tonsillectomy for apnoeas, cleft palate repair, spinal decompression for stenosis, spinal fusion for instability, shunts for hydrocephalus drainage, joint preservation and deformity correction (e.g. osteotomy to restore alignment, complex clubfoot correction, limb lengthening), early joint replacement (premature osteoarthritis). Limb lengthening remains controversial due to surgical complexity/morbidity and limited potential height gain.

The future

Advances in molecular genetics have resulted in identification of the genetic basis of over two thirds of the skeletal dysplasias. This facilitates prenatal counselling and management of affected individuals and their families.

Glossary

Allele One of multiple alternative versions of a gene occuring at a particular locus (site) on a chromosome

Allele frequency Frequency within a population of each allele at a locus

Alteration Pathogenic variant of a gene, also known as 'mutation', this is a change in genetic material that can then be passed on to future generations; pathogenic alterations affect gene function

Amino acids Organic compounds containining both amino and carboxylic acid functional groups; these molecules combine to form proteins

Anticipation Progressively more severe disease phenotype in successive generations

Autosome Chromosome other than X or Y; there are 22 pairs of autosomes in human chromosomes

Autosomal dominant A type of Mendelian inheritance requiring only one copy of the altered allele to be inherited to cause disease; if there is one affected parent, then there is a 50% chance (i.e. 1 in 2) of the child inheriting the alteration

Autosomal recessive A type of Mendelian inheritance whereby two altered alleles must be inherited to manifest disease; a child usually inherits one altered copy of a gene from each unaffected carrier parent (i.e. each carry one copy of the altered gene)

Benign variant A genetic alteration that is not disease-causing

Chromosome Thread-like structure primarily composed of chromatin (DNA helix wrapped around core histones) that carries an ordered sequence of linked genes; the human nuclear genome is stored across 23 pairs of chromosomes

Consanguinity Related parents share a proportion of their genetic makeup

De novo When a gene alteration occurs for the first time

Dizygotic twins Two individuals born with genetic material from two separate eggs that have been fertilised by two different sperm

DNA Deoxyribonucleic acid; a polymer composed of two polynucleotide chains (sugar and phosphate backbone linked to nitrogen bases) that coil around each other to form a double helix that carries genetic instructions.

Epigenetics Heritable influence in either cell lines or individuals on chromosome/gene function that is not directly caused by a change in DNA sequence

Evolution DNA changes that influence the ability/likelihood of an organism to survive and reproduce successfully over future generations

Exome Protein cording portion of the genome

Exon Portion of the gene that codes the final protein product

Gene These form the baseline unit of inheritance and are sequences of DNA that code for formation of a polypeptide chain. Genes are comprised of exons (coding), introns (non-coding), and regulatory elements.

Genome Entire genetic complement of an organism, i.e. the entire complement of DNA instructions; in humans, the genome consists of 23 pairs of chromosomes in the cell nucleus and further small amounts of DNA in the mitochondria

Genotype The genetic constitution of an individual organism

Germline alteration Any detectable alteration within germ cells (i.e. those that ultimately form sperm and ova)

Germline mosaicism Presence of mosaicisim (i.e. a populaton of genetically distinct cells) in the gonad (testis/ovary); can therefore be inheritable

Heterozygous Presence of two different alleles at a particular locus

Homozygous Presence of two identical alleles at a particular locus

Imprinting Genetic mechanism for selective expression of genes, i.e. only one copy of a gene in an individual (from either the mother or father) is expressed with the other copy suppressed. Unlike alterations that can affect the ability of inherited genes to be expressed, genomic imprinting does not affect the DNA sequence itself - rather, gene expression is silenced by the epigenetic addition of tags to the DNA during egg or sperm formation, which usually remain throughout the individual's life

Inheritance How genetic material (and ultimately traits or conditions) are passed on in subsequent generations

Intron Transcribed but non-coding portion of the gene

Karyotype Chromosome complement of a cell/organism; in humans, the usual karyotype is 46XY (male) or 46XX (female)

Locus Unique site/region on a chromosome that corresponds to a specific DNA sequence/gene

Mainstreaming The process through which genetic testing to determine the cause inherited diseases and targeted molecular tests in tumours to identify drivers or therapeutic targets are carried out by specialists other than clinical genetics

Microarray A genetic test that identifies copy number variants

Monosomy Presence of only one copy of a chromosome (usually there are two)

Monozygotic twins Two individuals born with genetic material shared from the same sperm and egg

Mosaicism Presence of two or more cell populations from the same conception, with one having acquired a genetic difference

Mutation *See 'alteration'*

Nucleosome Basic subunit of a chromatin

Nucleotide Purine or pyramidine base to which sugar and phosphate groups are attached

Pathogenic variant A disease-causing alteration

Pedigree Diagram that demonstrates the inheritance of a trait/condition through successive generations of a family

Penetrance Probability of the carrier of an alteration showing features of the disease/condition (i.e. penetrance may be 'variable')

Phenotype Presence of features of a disease/condition

Polymerase chain reaction (PCR) Technique involving multiple cycles used to amplify the copies of a target DNA sequence

Clinical Genetics and Genomics at a Glance, First Edition. Edited by Neeta Lakhani, Kunal Kulkarni, Julian Barwell, Pradeep Vasudevan, and Huw Dorkins.

Polygenic Disease caused by the presence of alterations of multiple (>3) genetic loci

Polymorphism Presence of two or more non-pathogenic variants

Pre-implantation genetic diagnosis (PGD) In utero testing of fertilised uteros to identify a genetic disorder

Proband First person in a pedigree to be identified as affected by a genetic disorder

Somatic tissue Non-gamete tissue; altertions in these cells are not passed on, but may be pathological (e.g. cancers)

Trait A characteristic that may be seen/observed/measured (e.g. hair colour, behaviour, presence of a disease/condition)

Transcription Expression of a gene

Variant of uncertain significance Alteration with an uncertain link to a disease/condition

Variant Genetic alteration; may be classified as pathogenic, likely pathogenic, variant of uncertain clinical significance, likely benign, or benign. See ACMG guidance for details (Richards S et al. Genet Med. 2015 May;17(5):405-24. doi: 10.1038/gim.2015.30)

X-linked A type of Mendelian inheritance passed on through the X chromosome; may be dominant or recessive

Index

Clinical Genetics and Genomics at a Glance, First Edition. Edited by Neeta Lakhani, Kunal Kulkarni, Julian Barwell, Pradeep Vasudevan, and Huw Dorkins.